RECENT ADVANCES IN AEROSPACE MEDICINE

RECENT ADVANCES IN AEROSPACE MEDICINE

PROCEEDINGS XVIII INTERNATIONAL CONGRESS
OF AVIATION AND SPACE MEDICINE
AMSTERDAM 1969

Edited by

DOUGLAS E. BUSBY
Continental Airlines, Los Angeles,
California, U.S.A.

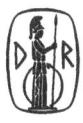

D. REIDEL PUBLISHING COMPANY

DORDRECHT-HOLLAND

Library of Congress Catalog Card Number 74–131264

ISB-13: 978-94-010-3319-0   e-ISB-13: 978-94-010-3317-6

DOI: 10.1007/978-94-010-3317-6

PREFACE

This book is a collection of scientific papers presented at the XVIII International Congress of Aviation and Space Medicine held in Amsterdam, The Netherlands, from 15–18 September 1969. It is dedicated to General E. de Vries and Dr. K. Vaandrager, President and Vice-President of the Congress, who wished that this unsurpassed exchange of scientific information by distinguished authorities of the international aerospace medical community be made readily available to all as a valuable source of information. I am deeply grateful to the Congress Committee for honoring me with this editorship, to the authors for submitting generally excellent manuscripts and to the publisher for compiling a book of such high quality.

This book contains both Main Theme papers, given by invited lecturers, and selected Free Communications at the Congress. Main Themes were 'physiology of atmospheric pressure' (papers by Ernsting, Meijne, Sluijter, Behnke), 'vestibular problems in aviation medicine' (papers by Melvill Jones, Benson, Oosterveld, Groen, Guedry and Benson, Brandt, Henriksson and Nilsson), 'aviation and cardiology' (papers by Blackburn, Wood) and 'space medicine' (paper by Berry). The Free Communications herein focus on many areas of continuing and timely interest to clinicians and investigators in aerospace medicine. Selection and health maintenance of pilots, medical problems in airline passengers, use of the centrifuge as a therapeutic device, and circadian rhythm effects on man's psychophysiological state receive particular attention.

Although the diversity of collected papers in aerospace medicine presents problems in arrangement for both broad and reference reading, the papers in this book fit well into sections dealing with man in the exploration of space, clinical aviation medicine, and man's responses to the various stresses imposed by the aerospace environment.

D. E. BUSBY

TABLE OF CONTENTS

SECTION III / MAN IN HIS GASEOUS ENVIRONMENT

SECTION IV / MAN IN HIS KINETIC ENVIRONMENT

SECTION V / MAN IN HIS THERMAL ENVIRONMENT

SECTION VI / MAN IN HIS TEMPORAL ENVIRONMENT

SECTION I

MAN IN THE EXPLORATION OF SPACE

SUMMARY OF MEDICAL EXPERIENCE IN THE APOLLO 7
THROUGH 11 MANNED SPACEFLIGHTS

C. A. BERRY

National Aeronautics and Space Administration, Manned Spacecraft Center, Houston, Tex., U.S.A.

1. Introduction

The goal of the Apollo Program was to land men on the Moon and return them safely to Earth. This goal was achieved in the Apollo 11 mission, with two astronauts stepping onto the lunar soil on July 20, 1969. A number of similar missions for further exploration of the Moon are planned.

The Apollo Program was a series of unmanned and manned spaceflights in both earth and lunar orbits, first to check out the operational safety of spacecraft components, and then to land on the Moon. Apollo manned spaceflights, summarized in Table I, gave a spaceflight experience of 3105 man-hours, including extravehicular lunar surface times of 2 hr, 14 min for astronaut Armstrong and 1 hr, 42 min for astronaut Aldrin. The total American spaceflight experience, including 54 man-hours in the Mercury Program and 1939 man-hours in the Gemini Program, is now 5098 man-hours.

Medical information gained especially in the Gemini Program (Gooch and Berry, 1969) was utilized extensively in planning the medical support and investigations (Graybiel *et al.*, 1967) conducted during the Apollo manned spaceflights (Berry and Catterson, 1967). Such significant biomedical observations in the Gemini Program as high energy cost of extravehicular activity, cardiovascular deconditioning, diminished exercise capacity and loss of red cell mass (Anon, 1966; Berry *et al.*, 1966; Fischer *et al.*, 1967; Kelly and Coons, 1967) had to receive thorough consideration, particularly with respect to their possible effect on astronaut performance during proposed lunar surface activity (Berry, 1968). Although the contribution of confinement *per se* to the deteriorative physiologic changes observed after flights of long duration in the small Mercury and Gemini spacecraft cabins could not be determined, it was thought that the freedom of movement and exercising allowed in the Apollo spacecraft would maintain the astronauts in optimum physical condition for the duration of the Apollo 11 mission.

2. Medical Objectives for Apollo Program

The following medical objectives were established for the Apollo Program:
(1) Assurance of crew safety.
(2) Assurance of mission completion and those activities contributing to mission management.
(3) Prevention of back contamination of the earth's biosphere.

TABLE I

Apollo manned spaceflights

Flights	Astronauts	Launch dates	Descriptions	Flight durations (hr:min:sec)
Apollo 7	Schirra Eisele Cunningham	Oct. 11, 1968	Earth orbital checkout of the command and service modules (CSM)	260:09:45
Apollo 8	Borman Lovell Anders	Dec. 21, 1968	First lunar orbit (10 orbits) flight for checkout of the CSM at lunar distance	147:00:11
Apollo 9	McDivitt Scott Schweikart	Mar. 3, 1969	First manned earth-orbital checkout of the lunar module (LM), CSM/LM rendezvous, and extravehicular activity (EVA)	241:00:54
Apollo 10	Stafford Young Cernan	May 18, 1969	First lunar orbit rendezvous and low pass over lunar surface	192:03:23
Apollo 11	Armstrong Collins Aldrin	July 16, 1969	First lunar landing and EVA on the lunar surface	195:18:35

(4) Continuance of the understanding of the biomedical changes incident to manned spaceflight.

To meet these objectives it was necessary to prepare a medical requirements document detailing a pre- and postflight medical evaluation program which would provide information to assure capability for the proper support of lunar landing. This program (Berry, 1967) was particularly important for the reason that all inflight medical and other experiments in the Apollo program were deleted after the fatal spacecraft fire in order to concentrate on the operational complexity of the Apollo missions. Areas of concern in planning the lunar mission have been summarized (Berry, 1969a).

Comparison of biomedical data obtained in the Gemini Program with that from Apollo missions prior to the lunar mission was vital to predicting the physiologic state of the astronauts at the time of lunar surface activity (Berry, 1969; Berry and Catterson, 1967). The provision of a microbial baseline for lunar quarantine operations and the further documentation of spaceflight effects on man were also valuable objectives.

The medical procedures conducted were developed by a multidisciplinary team in the Medical Research and Operations Directorate of the National Aeronautics and Space Administration Manned Spacecraft Center at Houston, Texas (Berry, 1969b). In addition to detailed physical examinations, exhaustive studies were performed in the areas of hematology, immunology, biochemistry, bone densitometry, cardio-vascular functions, exercise capacity and microbiology. These evaluations were supplemented by observations made during flight from continual monitoring of voice, electrocardiogram and respiration during Command Module (CM) operations, and monitoring of voice and electrocardiogram during Lunar Module (LM) operations. While only one crewman could be monitored at a time during Apollo 7 and 8 CM operations, all three CM crewmen could be monitored continuously for later missions. Only one crewman could be monitored at a time while in the LM except during lunar surface activity, when both could be monitored continuously.

3. Spacecraft Environment Characteristics

A. CABIN ATMOSPHERE

After the fire in the Apollo CM two years ago, it was decided that the CM cabin atmosphere should not be 100% oxygen. Calculations and studies demonstrated that if this atmosphere contained 60% oxygen and 40% nitrogen at launch, and the crew denitrogenated for 3 hr prior to launch, hypoxia and dysbarism could be avoided when the nominal cabin pressure of 5.0 psia was attained. The Apollo spacecraft have actually been launched with cabin atmospheres containing 64% oxygen and 36% nitrogen. The valve for dumping urine into space was left open at launch and for several hours thereafter to allow purging of the nitrogen from the atmosphere at a specified rate. An oxygen analysis on the Apollo 7 mission recorded the oxygen enrichment profile shown in Figure 1. The partial pressure of oxygen was never less than that at sea level.

Apollo astronauts removed space suit helmets and gloves usually within the first half-hour, always within the first hour after launch. Space suit doffing was completed

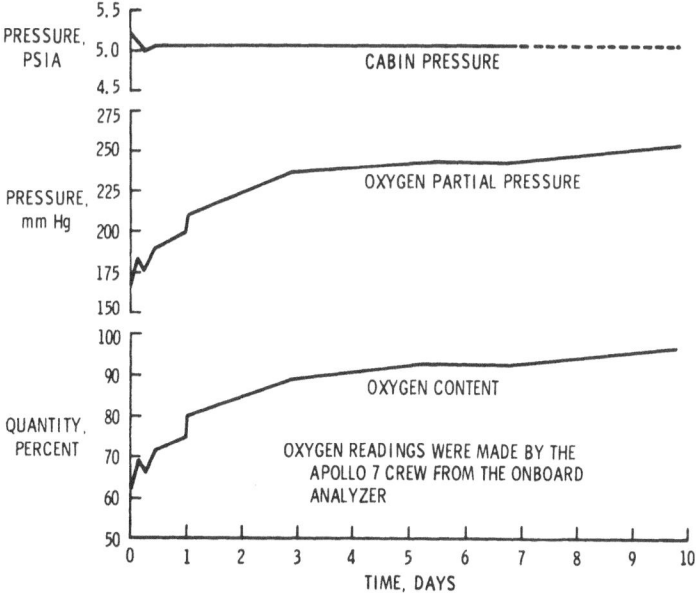

Fig. 1.   Cabin oxygen enrichment sequence during Apollo 7 10-day flight.

when convenient, and flight coveralls donned for the major portions of the missions. In the Apollo 7 mission, the crew donned their space suits in flight to check their capability to do so and their reentry configuration. They also donned their suits, without helmets and gloves, to use the foot restraints built for the suits during reentry. Since this mission, space suits have not been worn for reentry, but have been donned for critical mission phases such as separation and docking and, of course, lunar surface activity.

B. CM AND LM CABIN ATMOSPHERIC TEMPERATURES

The CM cabin temperature has been maintained about 70°F (range 62°F to 80°F), usually without the use of the cabin fans (Figure 2). Crews occasionally felt cool during translunar coast, but adjustment of the environmental control system returned the temperature rapidly to the comfort level.

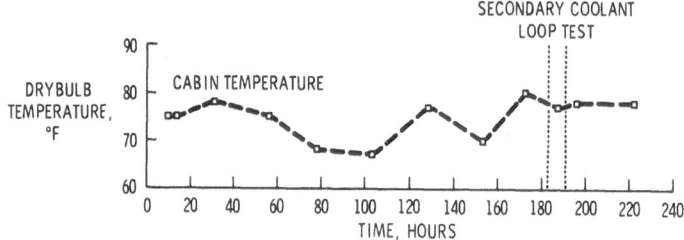

Fig. 2.   Representative Apollo CM cabin temperatures (Apollo 7 data).

The LM cabin temperature was kept between 65°F and 70°F, except during and immediately following depressurizations (Figures 3 and 4). The Apollo 11 astronauts did complain of sleep interference from chilling and shivering during their rest period on the lunar surface. Since their space suits, including helmets, were donned during this period, their discomfort was attributed primarily to operation of the liquid-cooled garment, the temperature of which is not reflected by the cabin gas temperatures (Figure 4).

C. NOISE AND VIBRATION

The cabin fans and glycol pump created a noise problem during preflight checkouts of the Apollo spacecraft. Glycol pump noise was attenuated with padding, and the cabin fans have generally not been used during flight. The cabin noise level during lift-off has been high, but an acceptable level has been reported during all missions, neither being distractive nor interfering with sleep.

The noise levels in the LM cabin were also reported to be high during the three LM flights, due primarily to the cabin fans. This noise was annoying to the astronauts when their space suit helmets were removed.

'Pogo' vibrations were reported during all spacecraft launches. However, any transmission of these vibrations to the crews was considered physiologically insignificant.

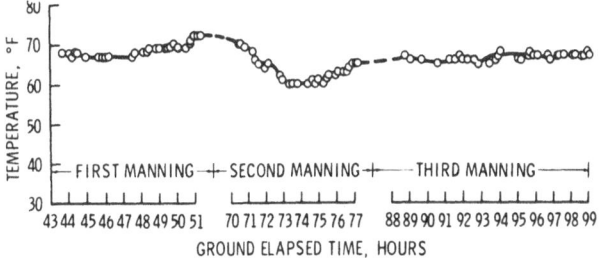

Fig. 3. Representative LM cabin temperatures (Apollo 9 earth-orbital data).

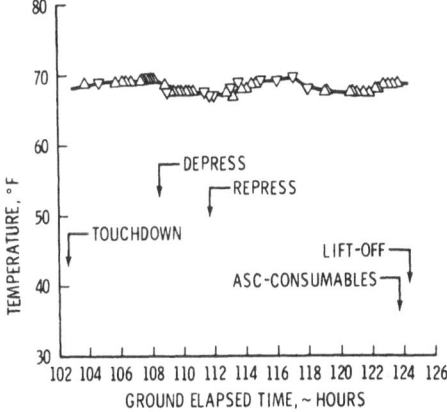

Fig. 4. Representative LM cabin temperatures (Apollo 11 lunar stay).

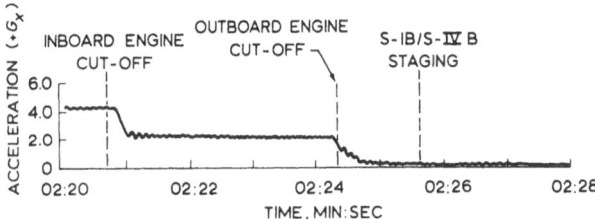

Fig. 5. Launch accelerations (Apollo 7 mission).

4. Accelerations and Impact

As anticipated and shown in Figure 5 accelerations $(+G_x)$ during launch have not been much greater than 4 g. Reentry from earth orbit has produced levels near 3.4 g and, as illustrated in Figure 6, reentry from lunar missions has produced levels near 6.7 g. Accelerations from S-IVB booster reignition for translunar injection, and all ignitions of the Service Module engine have been below 1 g. All these acceleration levels, which had been previously experienced by the crews suring centrifuge training, were well tolerated. Landing impacts, estimated from 6 to 8 g, were also well tolerated by the astronauts.

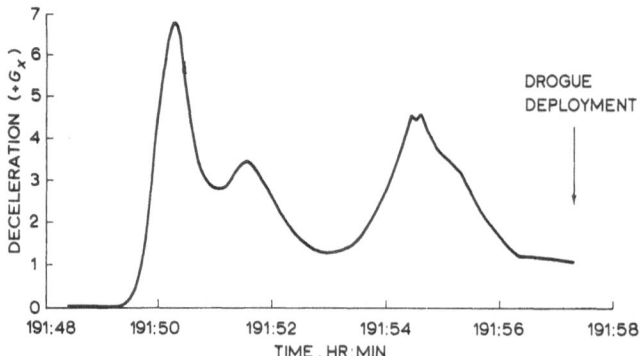

Fig. 6.   Re-entry decelerations from lunar mission (Apollo 10 mission).

5. Radiobiology

Only two of the five manned Apollo missions (Apollo 7 and 8) have occurred under the Van Allen, or natural radiation belt, which consists principally of protons and electrons trapped in the geomagnetic field. This belt, the boundaries of which are about 38° geomagnetic latitude, shields all the Earth but the polar regions from externally-generated radiations, such as solar flare protons. Earth orbital missions of 100 to 200 miles altitude stay well below the belt, except where the belt dips in the south Atlantic Ocean. Although orbiting Apollo and other flights have passed through this region once every seven orbits, it has not presented a radiobiological hazard. The polar regions, where spacecraft are exposed to untrapped space radiations, have been avoided in manned space missions.

Lunar missions passed through the Van Allen belt enroute to, and on return from the Moon. The skin radiation dosage received by the astronauts during belt passage has actually been of low magnitude, measured as approximately 10 millirad, due primarily the short transit times through the belt. It is important to point out that in the Apollo missions, beyond the Earth's protective 'magnetic umbrella', man is subjecting himself for the first time direct galactic radiations and particles from solar flares, should this event occur. However, measurements have shown that under normal circumstances galactic radiations are an insignificant hazard, giving only about a 10 millirad skin dose daily.

Since solar flares are random, occur infrequently, and are of short duration, the risk of exposure to a solar flare during a lunar mission is considered quite low, probably less than once in 5000 missions. Even if a solar flare should occur, radiation doses received by CM crewmen should be medically insignificant due to absorption of incident radiations by the thick CM wall and surrounding equipment. For example, it has been estimated that the solar flare of greatest magnitude in the last solar cycle would have given a CM crew a skin dose (0.7 mm depth) of 237 rad. Such doses would have a minimal effect on the average man. Although several flares can occur over several days duration, the probability of this event during the time required for an Apollo mission is quite low.

On the other hand, occurrence of a solar flare of large magnitude while astronauts occupy the LM and explore the lunar surface could present a significant medical hazard. Under the worst unprotected length-of-exposure conditions conceivable, it is estimated that skin doses could reach 691 rad (0.7 mm depth) and the depth dose (5.0 cm) 25 rad. Although this depth dose would not be expected to have a significant pathological effect, this skin dose could conceivably produce sufficient skin irritation and blepharitis to affect crew performance. Also, a skin dose of this magnitude is approaching the threshold for producing more serious latent radiation sequelae, such as dry and moist desquamation, ulceration, subcutaneous edema and fibrosis. Fortunately, there are certain operational constraints which can be used.

Radiations encountered during Apollo missions were measured by a variety of sophisticated devices, listed in Table II. Table III points out the average skin doses

TABLE II

Radiation instrumentation on Apollo missions

Instrument	Measurement	Location
Nuclear particle detection sytem	Telemetry (protons, 15–150 MeV; alpha particles, 40–300 MeV)	Service module
Van Allen belt dosimeter	Telemetry (skin depth dose rates)	Command module
Radiation survey meter (portable)	Direct visual (4 linear ranges, 0–0.1 to 0–100 rad/hr)	Command module
Personal radiation dosimeter	Direct visual (range 0.01–1000 rad)	Space suit
Passive radiation dosimeter	Postflight analysis (thermoluminescent dose)	Constant wear garment

TABLE III

Average radiation doses to skin during Apollo missions, measured by thermoluminescent dosimeter

	Average dose (rad)
Apollo 7	0.16
Apollo 8	0.16
Apollo 9	0.20
Apollo 10	0.47
Apollo 11	0.18

received by the astronauts during the five Apollo missions, as measured by the thermoluminescent dosimeter. It should be noted that these doses are much less than doses to various organs of the body during routine X-ray diagnostic procedures.

6. Toxicology

Three approaches were used to assure that compounds would not enter the CM and LM atmospheres and reach levels toxic to the astronauts. Spacecraft cabin materials were selected on the basis of their off-gassing characteristics. Animal toxicologic studies were made with off-gassed compounds from materials. The atmospheres of Apollo 7 and 8 CM's and the Apollo 9 LM were analysed for off-gassed compounds during altitude chamber tests at Cape Kennedy. Also, charcoal from the environmental control systems on the Apollo spacecraft was analysed postflight.

Although approximately 50 compounds have been identified in the spacecraft cabin atmosphere, their concentrations have been too low to be of toxicologic significance, even when these compounds were grouped according to their primary modes of action. Of greatest significance was the presence of relatively large concentrations of halocarbons, such as methanol, ethanol, propanol, isopropanol, methyl chloride, mesitylene and N-octane. Since halocarbons can react with lithium hydroxide, which is used for carbon dioxide absorption in spacecraft, to produce highly toxic compounds, action is being taken to reduce halocarbon concentrations still further on future flights. A review of the contaminants in the spacecraft cabin atmosphere did not identify the cause of a very minor degree of methemoglobinemia observed in the astronauts postflight. Although offensive odors were detected in the Apollo 9 and 11 spacecraft, their cause, nature and potential effects remain undetermined. Atmospheric sampling has been proposed for future flights.

7. Weightlessness

As in the Gemini missions, Apollo crews have reported an initial feeling of fullness in the head after attaining weightless flight. This sensation has lasted for a varying duration during the first day. There is also an awareness of the lack of weight of objects and clothing.

The capability to impart minimal velocities to objects in the weightless environment has been utilized repeatedly while living and working in the spacecraft. Minimal effort has been required in moving about the spacecraft, frequently in a swimming manner. A number of acrobatic maneuvers, such as rolling, tumbling and spinning, have been accomplished without difficulty. It appears that movement in the weightless environment requires much less work than in the unit gravity environment.

Some soreness in the costo-vertebral area has been reported. Crews have related this to body position and have frequently assumed the fetal position while resting in the weightless environment. It has been of no serious consequence.

In conclusion, the astronauts have generally adapted well to the weightless environment, finding it pleasant and of assistance to them in accomplishing inflight activities. Particular problem areas encountered in weightless flight will be discussed below.

8. Nutrition

Freeze-dehydrated, rehydratable and bite-sized foods similar to those used in the Gemini Program were utilized in the first two Apollo missions. One exception was the introduction of 'wet-pack' turkey bites and gravy on the Apollo 8 mission.

For several reasons, extensive changes in types of food and packaging were implemented over the six-month period of the Apollo 9, 10 and 11 missions (Figure 7). It was found that inflight food consumption was inadequate to maintain nutritional balance, even though reduced energy requirements for performance in the weightless environment were probable. Crews were reporting anorexia. Meal preparation and consumption was requiring too much time and effort. Water for reconstitution of dehydrated foods was off-flavor and contained large quantities of undissolved hydrogen and oxygen. Functional failures were occurring with rehydratable packages. There appeared to be a definite requirement to develop food which was more familiar in appearance, flavor and method of consumption.

New food consisted primarily of thermostabilized meat dishes of high moisture content (60 to 70% water), called 'wet-packs'. Pieces of meat were larger than previously. These foods, along with freeze-dehydrated meat and vegetables, were packaged so that they could be eaten with a spoon. Also added to the dietary provisions were some new beverage powder flavors, fruits and candy-like items of intermediate moisture (10 to 30% water) content, and sandwich spreads with 'fresh', sliced bread. The sandwich spreads were heat sterilized in a hyperbaric chamber to reduce deterioration of food texture, and packaged either in cans or flexible aluminum tubes. Of the 96 different 'space' foods available prior to the Apollo Program, about 60 were utilized in the Gemini Program. It is notable that of the 42 different foods to be provided on the forthcoming Apollo 12 mission, only 24 were on the original Apollo dietary list.

The inclusion of foods which did not require rehydration prior to consumption simplified procedures and reduced the time taken for meal preparation. This measure also circumvented problems of off-flavor and undissolved gas from the spacecraft water supply. The packaging failures which occurred in flight have now been effectively prevented through design changes and additional quality control procedures.

Inflight anorexia has led some crewmen to comment that the foods supplied would be more desirable if they were stowed in bulk units, similar to a pantry, than if stowed in nominal meal units. This would allow a crewmember to make a meal-time selection of desired foods based on appetite rather than accept a menu established a month prior to flight. Apollo 11 CM food stowage was configured in nominal meal units (45 meals, 15 man-days, or 5 mission-days) located in the lower equipment bay, and in bulk units (9 mission-days) in the left hand equipment bay and beneath the center couch. Postflight debriefing indicated that this configuration was satisfactory, but not

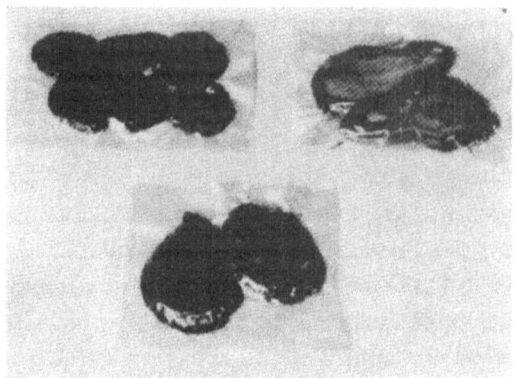

**APOLLO
FOOD**

DRIED FRUIT

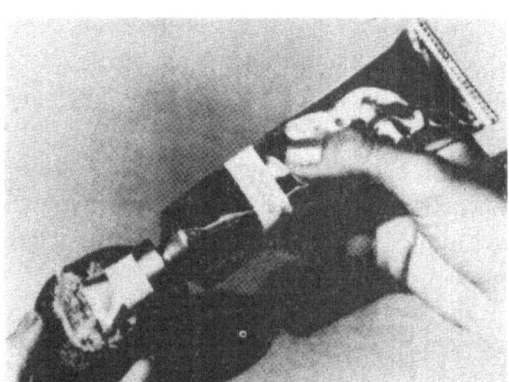

CHICKEN SALAD

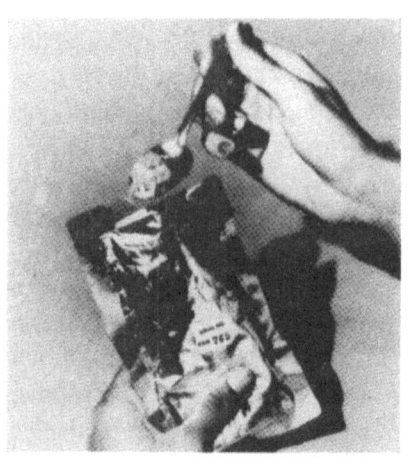

BEEF WITH VEGETABLES

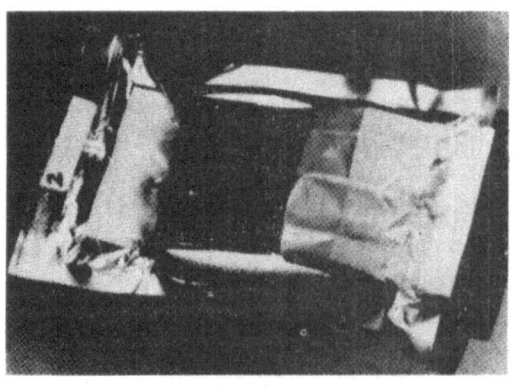

FRANKS

TURKEY WITH GRAVY

Fig. 7.   New foods and packaging for the Apollo Program.

TABLE IV

Body weights and energy intakes of astronauts of Apollo 7 through 11 missions

		Body weight (lb) Average preflight (28, 24, and 5 days before launch	Launch day	Recovery day	Day after recovery	Average daily caloric intake (kcal)
Apollo 7	Commander	195	194	188	191	1966
	CM pilot	153	157	147	151	2144
	LM pilot	157	156	148	154	1804
Apollo 8	Commander	169	169	161	163	1477
	CM pilot	169	172	164	165	1688
	LM pilot	146	142	138	139	1339
Apollo 9	Commander	161	159	154	156	1924
	CM pilot	181	178	173	181	1715
	LM pilot	164	159	153	157	1639
Apollo 10	Commander	175	171	169	171	1407
	CM pilot	169	165	160	161	1487
	LM pilot	175	173	163	165	1311
Apollo 11	Commander	173	172	164	170	5300[a]
	CM pilot	167	166	159	159	
	LM pilot	172	167	166	170	
Totals		2526	2500	2407	2453	25201
Average		168.4	166.67	160.47	163.53	1680

[a] Average total of 5300 kcal daily, estimated by the 3 astronauts.

absolutely necessary. The crew estimated that 80% of the nominal meal unit food was consumed, whereas 40% of the bulk stowage food was consumed. LM food, stowed in the LM, was provided for 4 meal periods over the scheduled 21 hours of lunar surface time. The two LM crewmembers estimated that 40% of these supplies were eaten.

Crew acceptance of all new foods and packaging has generally been quite good. Also, a much better understanding of food preference has been attained. However, it appears that the quantity of food consumed during Apollo missions did not increase, for the crews have subsisted primarily on the supply of new foods, which were intended only to supplement the nominal food supply. Although the crews of Apollo 10 and 11 spacecraft were quite pleased with the foods provided, their postflight body weights still indicated that they attained a negative nutritional balance.

Body weights and energy intakes of the Apollo crews are given in Table IV. Although there is no 'average astronaut', it is of interest to note that 15 men with an average weight of 166.6 lb were launched in the Apollo Program. At recovery, their weight averaged 160.4 lb, and one day after recovery averaged 163.5 lb. Hence, the average inflight weight loss was 6.2 lb, half of which has been attributed to water loss.

Precise measurements of changes in body mass and accurate records of food intake should provide data necessary to determine future food requirements. Such data will be vital particularly to establishing a baseline for the evaluation of the effects of space flight on the musculoskeletal system in the Apollo Applications Program flights of 28 and 56 days duration.

Finally, it should be noted that in their postflight debriefing, all Apollo crews indicated that the intensity of hunger sensations is the same as that of preflight. However, they did observe that hunger occurs less frequently and that food requirements are only two-thirds of 'normal' in space. At least one crew has reported that gastric distension precluded intake of normal quantities of food and beverage. Based on these observations and critical stowage volume, menus were designed to provide approximately 2300 kcal energy per man per day.

9. Water Management

Data indicates that water servicing procedures and the addition of disinfectant chemicals (chlorine in CM and iodine in LM) have been effective in rendering water delivered from Apollo CM and LM spacecraft systems (Figure 8) potable. The crews did complain of the chlorine taste of water during early Apollo missions. However, revised chlorination procedures eliminated this problem. Objectionable amounts of free oxygen and hydrogen were present in the Apollo 9 CM potable water supply. On the Apollo 11 flight a water/gas separator satisfactorily removed this gas. In addition to the water/gas separator, Apollo 12 will utilize a silver-palladium hydrogen separator which will further decrease the amounts of these gasses in potable water.

Rapid iodine depletion rates in the first two manned LM spacecraft made it necessary to install a microbial filter upstream of the water outlet. Alteration of the Apollo 11 LM water system servicing procedure resulted in a microbially effective iodine residual throughout flight, without having to use the microbial filter. Future LM

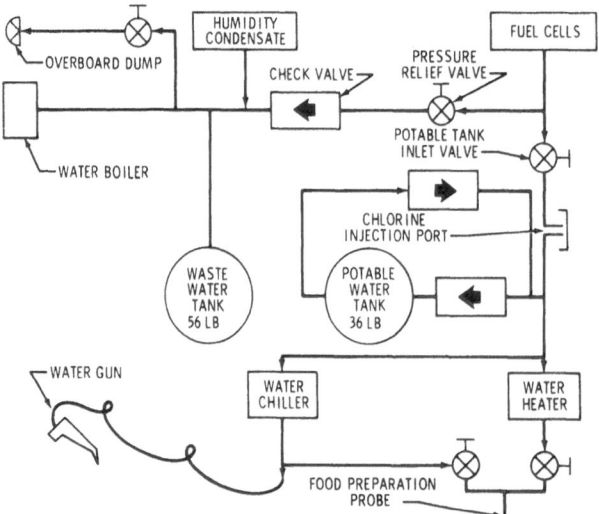

Fig. 8.   Apollo CM potable water system.

flights should not have to use this filter, although with extension of lunar surface times, revisions of the water system servicing procedure will be required to assure that an effective iodine residual is maintained in the LM water system.

10. Waste Management

Feces collection in the CM and LM is accomplished with the fecal collection system used in the Gemini Program (Figure 9). This tape-on bag is considered only marginally adequate, since its use is quite time-consuming and no provision is made to eliminate odors which accompany defecation.

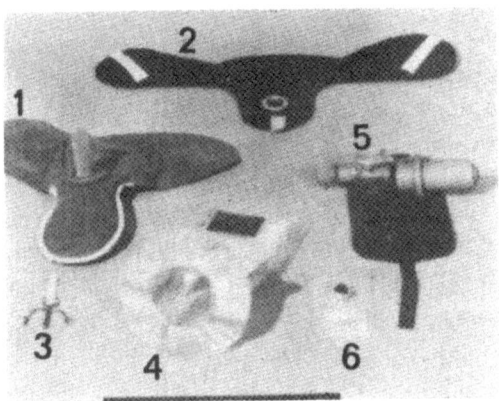

1 URINE COLLECTION DEVICE
   (GEMINI TYPE)

2 URINE COLLECTION TRANSFER ASSY

3 UCD CLAMP

4 DEFECATION COLLECTION DEVICE
   (GEMINI TYPE)

5 M5A/M7 EQUIPMENT
   (MODIFIED GEMINI TYPE)

6 URINE SAMPLE BAG
   (GEMINI TYPE)

Fig. 9.   Apollo waste management equipment.

The Gemini urine transfer assembly was improved for use in the CM (Figure 9). This device incorporates a roll-on cuff and an intermediate urine storage bag. The Apollo 12 crew will test a urine transfer assembly which eliminates direct interface of the user with the collecting portion.

Urine collection in the LM has been accomplished satisfactorily with a roll-on cuff assembly connected to a urine bag in the space suit. Its use is planned for future Apollo missions.

11. Work/Sleep Cycles

Before manned spaceflight became a reality, many in the medical community predicted that space flight would produce serious disturbances and alterations in man's sleep, ranging from narcolepsy to insomnia. Although the Mercury Program disproved these extreme forecasts, the Gemini Program clearly demonstrated that Earth-orbiting spaceflights of long duration could produce conditions which prevented adequate sleep. These conditions included cyclic noise disturbances from such events as thruster firings, communications or movement within the spacecraft, staggered sleep periods, significant alteration of the preflight diurnal cycle of crewmembers, the so-called 'command pilot syndrome', the unfamiliar sleep environment, and excitement.

The Apollo astronauts have faced the same sleep difficulties as their predecessors. Unfortunately, medical knowledge and expertise can provide little assistance in resolving this problem area, for Apollo mission plans must be highly inflexible and constraining. The astronaut must then be integrated into the fixed mission plan as best he can.

The Apollo 7 work/sleep cycles were quite irregular, and staggered sleep periods shifted considerably from the preflight (Cape Kennedy) bedtime. The crew never adapted to these cycles, reporting very poor sleep during the first 3 days of flight. One crewmember fell asleep on his watch, and on another occasion took 5 mg d-amphetamine to stay awake during his work period. The Apollo 7 Commander recommended that future flight crews evaluate their work/sleep cycles carefully.

Sleep period scheduling became a crew option on the Apollo 8 mission as confidence in spacecraft systems was gained. Also, the sedative, secobarbital, in 50 and 100 mg doses, was added to the medical kit. The Apollo 8 work/sleep cycles are shown in Figure 10. They varied greatly from Eastern Standard Time (Cape Kennedy), and had the added complication of a 20-hr loitering period in lunar orbit. Crew fatigue, particularly prior to trans-earth injection, led to minor procedural errors, and forced 'real-time' changes of the flight plan. Only the LM Pilot used secobarbital (50 mg) regularly for sleep.

On Apollo 9 all three astronauts slept simultaneously. The quantity and quality of crew sleep was definitely improved over the preceding mission experience, and the lack of postflight fatigue was evident during medical examination of the crew on the recovery day.

Sleep periods occurred simultaneously during the Apollo 10 mission and deviated little from the normal diurnal rhythm of the crew. One exception was when the Commander and LM Pilot flew during the lunar orbit phase.

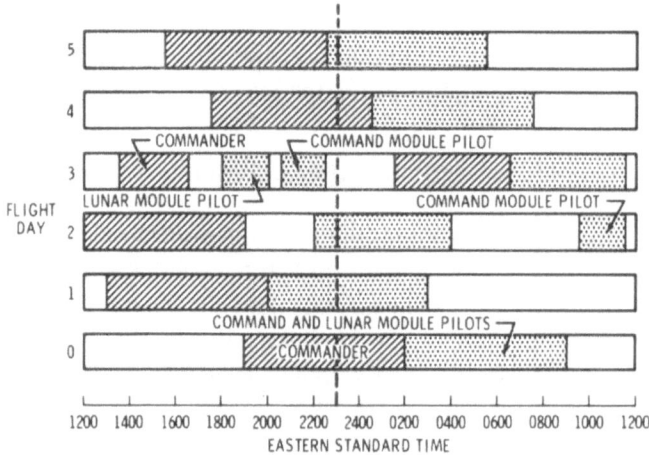

Fig. 10.   Crew rest cycles during Apollo 8 mission.

On the Apollo 11 lunar landing flight the work/sleep cycles of the crew, as shown in Figure 11, were actually quite ideal prior to lunar orbit insertion. Table V lists quantitative sleep estimates during the first four days of flight from the study of telemetered heart and respiratory rates, and from the crew's reports. Limitations in estimating sleep durations from heart and respiratory rates must be recognized. Nonetheless, the amount of sleep was adequate enough by either method of estimation to approve medically earlier extravehicular activity on the lunar surface than was originally planned.

During their lunar stay neither the Commander nor the LM Pilot slept well. The LM environment was too noisy and the space suit too cold for adequate sleep. In addition, accommodations for sleeping in the LM were quite poor. The Commander estimated that he had little, if any, sleep in the LM. The LM Pilot had about 2 hr sleep. On the return flight, the crew slept very well during the three trans-earth sleep periods.

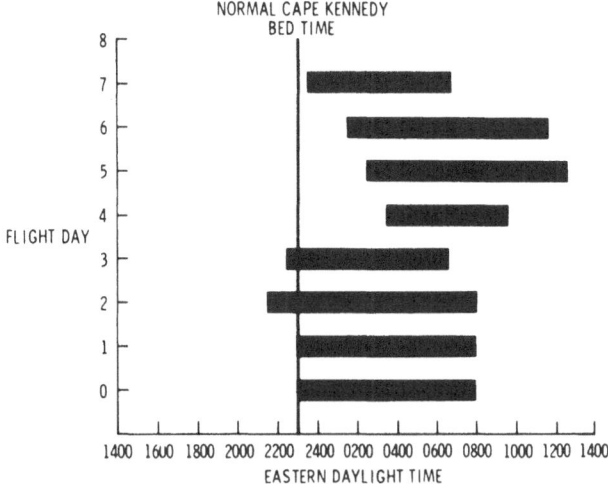

Fig. 11.   Crew sleep periods during Apollo 11 mission.

TABLE V

Estimated sleep periods of Apollo 11 crewmembers before lunar landing

| Flight day | Estimated sleep | | | | | |
| | Telemetry | | | Crew report | | |
	Commander	CM pilot	LM pilot	Commander	CM pilot	LM pilot
July 1, 1969	10:25	10:10	8:30	7:00	7:00	5:30
July 2, 1969	9:40	10:10	9:15	8:00	9:00	8:00
July 3, 1969	9:35	Not available	9:20	7:30	7:30	6:30
July 4, 1969	6:30	6:30	5:30	6:30	6:30	5:30
Totals	36:10	–	32:35	29:00	30:00	25:30

In summation, efforts must be continued with flight planners to maintain the work-day in flight at about 12 hr, and allowing 8 hr for sleep, and 4 hr for leisure. Better tools, such as the electroencephalogram are required for more detailed assessment of sleep in future space programs.

12. Medical Kit

Contents of the Apollo CM (Figure 12) and LM medical kits are listed in Tables VI and VII. Table VI also indicates the number of items used during the missions. Flight experience has dictated some changes in the types and numbers of drug items carried. On one flight Benadryl and Tylenol were replacements due to drug sensitivity in one

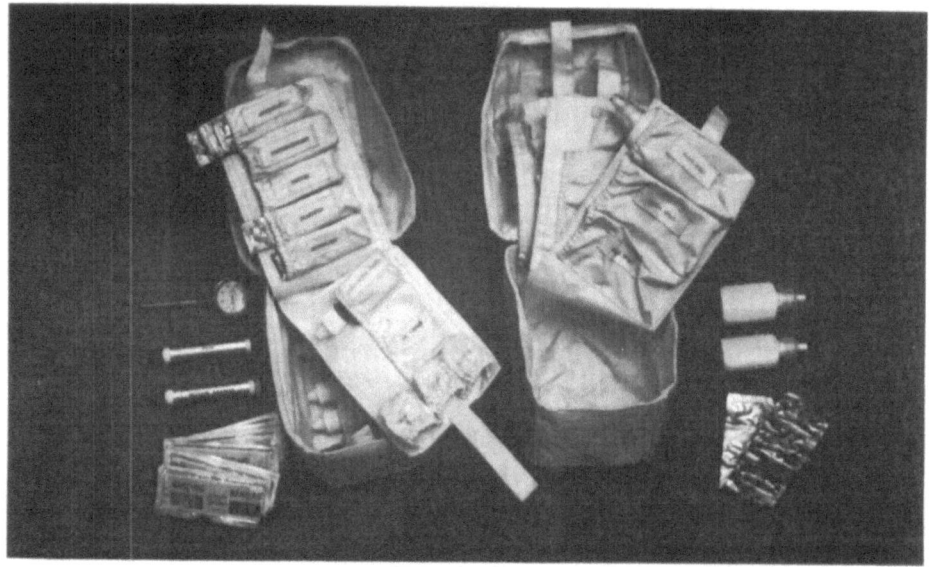

Fig. 12.   Apollo medical kit.

of the crewmen. Added to the Apollo 11 CM medical kit were a Scopolamine-Dexe-drine combination for the treatment of motion sickness and Mylicon to reduce gastrointestinal gas bubble size.

All astronauts are tested for sensitivity and response to each of the medications carried in their medical kit. Particular interest has been focused on performance from 1 to 4 hr after the ingestion of Seconal. Flight related performance tests have been satisfactory after use of this drug.

13. Bioinstrumentation

Difficulties encountered with bioinstrumentation on the Apollo 7 flight have been detailed in a previous report (Berry, 1969a). No difficulties were encountered in re-

TABLE VI

Apollo CM medical kit contents (quantity per mission)

	Mission number									
	7		8		9		10		11	
	Stowed	Used	Stowed	Used	Stowed	Used	Stowed	Used	Stowed	Used
Compress bandage	2	0	2	0	2	0	2	0	2	(Quan-
Band aid	12	2	12	0	12	0	12	0	12	tity un-
Antibiotic oint.	1	1	1	0	1	0	1	0	1	known)
Skin cream	1	0	1	1	1	1	1	0	1	
Demerol injector	3	0	3	0	3	0	3	0	3	
Marezine injectors	3	0	3	0	3	0	3	0	3	
Marezine tab	24	3	24	1	24	4	12	0	0	
Dexedrine tab	12	1	12	0	12	0	12	0	12	
Darvon cmp cap	12	2	18[a]	0	18	0	18	0	18	
Actified tab	24	24	60	0	60	12	60	2	60	
Lomotil tab	24	8	24	3	24	1	24	13	24	2
Nasal emollient	1	1	2	1	3	3	1	0	3	
Aspirin tab	72	48	72	8	72	2	72	16	72	
Achromycin tab	24	0	24	0	24	0	15	0	15	
Ampicillin tab	0	0	60	0	60	0	45	0	45	
Seconal, 100 mg cap	0	0	21	1	21	10	21	0	21	
Seconal, 50 mg cap	0	0	12	7	0	0	0	0	0	
Nasal spray (Afrin)	0	0	3	0	3	1	3	0	3	
Benadryl cap	0	0	8	0	0	0	0	0	0	
Tylenol cap	0	0	14	7	0	0	0	0	0	
Eye drops ($\frac{1}{4}$% methyl-cellulose soln.)	2	1	2	2	2	0	0	0	0	
Eye drops (1% methyl-cellulose soln.)	0	0	0	0	1	0	2	0	2	
Bacitracin ophthalmic oint.	0	0	0	0	1	0	0	0	0	
Scopolamine-dexedrine cap	0	0	0	0	0	0	0	0	12	6
Mylicon tab	0	0	0	0	0	0	0	0	20	

[a] plain.

TABLE VII

Apollo LM medical kit contents (quantity per mission) (no usage of kit through the Apollo 11 mission)

Lomotil tab	8
Dexedrine tab	4
Aspirin	12
Seconal cap	2
Methylcellulose, 1% soln.	1
Compress bandage	2

cording biomedical data following redesign of the bioinstrumentation harness for the Apollo 8 mission. Subsequent Apollo mission bioinstrumentation has also performed satisfactorily. Crews have been briefed preflight concerning sensor application and temperature to be expected in the DC-to-DC converter and signal conditioners. Drying of electrode paste has caused some degradation of electrocardiographic data at times, necessitating replacement of the sensor, which then operated satisfactorily. Biomedical data recorded during the Apollo missions are reported elsewhere in this paper.

14. Preventive Medicine and Inflight Disease

The preventive medicine program was detailed in the Medical Requirements Document. Following the experience with preflight, inflight and postflight illnesses on the Apollo 7 mission, space crews have maintained modified isolation during the 21-day preflight period. Their food, water and air have been controlled as best as possible, and their contacts with other individuals have been kept to a minimum compatible with mission success. This has required great cooperation on the part of both the astronauts and supporting personnel.

Several factors dictate the need for an isolation period lasting at least 21 days. In flights of greater than a week in duration it is quite possible for disease to occur in flight without being evident in preflight medical examinations. One must be maximally sure that illness in the crew will not cause a launch delay, especially when the spacecraft must enter a particular launch 'window' in lunar missions. Possible consequences of crew illness during lunar surface time are readily apparent. Moreover, on the Apollo 11 mission the 21-day postflight quarantine period made the preflight preventive medicine period assume great importance.

Details of the preflight and inflight upper respiratory illnesses which occurred on the Apollo 7 mission, and the gastrointestinal disturbance which occurred on the Apollo 8 mission have been reported elsewhere (Berry, 1969a). Table VIII summarizes

TABLE VIII

Preflight medical problems in Apollo 7 to 11 crews

Problem	Cause	Incidence
Mild upper respiratory infection	Undetermined	3
Rhinitis and pharyngitis	Herpes simplex	2
Gastroenteritis	? Salmonellosis (walnut meats)	2
Gastroenteritis	Undetermined	3
Facial rash	Seborrhea	2
Folliculitis (abdomen)	Undetermined	1
Ringworm (arm)	Microsporum canis	1
Tinea crura	Undetermined	1
Tinea pedis	Undetermined	1
Pulpitis, tooth No. 31	Previous restoration and caries	1
Influenza syndrome	Undetermined	2

medical problems identified in the preflight phase of the Apollo 7 to 11 missions. Rhinitis and pharyngitis caused a delay of the Apollo 9 mission. Although none of these conditions was severe, such common, mild viral infections as upper respiratory infections and gastroenteritis in the preflight phase must be viewed with great concern with respect to their possible effects on astronaut performance, and hence mission success.

TABLE IX

Inflight medical problems in Apollo 7 to 11 crews

Problem	Cause	Incidence
Coryza	Undetermined	3
Stomatitis	Apthous ulcers	1
Nausea and vomiting	Undetermined	1
Nausea and vomiting	Labyrinthine	1
Stomach awareness	Labyrinthine	5
Recurrence of facial rash	? Contact dermatitis	1
Respiratory irritation	Fiberglass	1
Eye irritation	Fiberglass	1
Skin irritation	Fiberglass	2

Inflight medical problems in the Apollo 7 to 11 missions are listed in Table IX. The three cases of coryza occurred on the Apollo 7 mission. One episode of nausea and vomiting, probably due to viral gastroenteritis, and the apthous ulcers were reported on the flight of Apollo 8. The fiberglass irritation occurred on the Apollo 10 mission.

Five of the 6 crewmen on the Apollo 8 and 9 missions reported symptoms of motion sickness ranging from mild stomach awareness with head and body motion in the weightless environment, to nausea and vomiting in one crewman. These symptoms lasted from 2 hr to 5 days, after which adaptation allowed movement without symptoms occurring. One Apollo 10 crewman also had stomach awareness lasting 2 days, again indicating that adaptation to the weightless environment takes place. Anti-motion sickness medication was used in 3 of the 6 episodes reported.

It should be noted that prior to the Apollo 10 mission the crew had been instructed to carry out programmed head movements during the first two flight days to hasten the adaptive process. The crewman reporting stomach awareness noted an increase in the severity of this symptom after one minute of head movement. When attempted on the 7th flight day, these head movements produced stomach awareness after 5 minutes.

The Apollo 11 astronauts were briefed about the head movement program, the availability of medication for the prevention and control of motion sickness symptoms, and the use of cautious movement in the spacecraft during the adaptive period. No symptoms were noted nor were the special preventive measures used.

It appears that the opportunity to move about more freely in the Apollo cabin than in previous spacecraft is a factor producing the motion sickness problem. Sensory inputs from the semicircular canals to the central nervous system during head movements in space are thought to be enhanced due to altered activity of the otolith organs in the weightless state. This is a significant problem which must receive continued attention in the space program, for it can markedly affect astronaut performance.

A number of medical problems, listed in Table X, have occurred in the postflight period. Again, viral illnesses predominated.

TABLE X

Postflight medical problems in Apollo 7 to 11 missions

Problem	Cause	Incidence
Gastroenteritis	Possible food poisoning	1
Mild upper respiratory infection	Undetermined	1
Rhinitis, pharyngitis	Influenza B	1
Flu syndrome	Influenza B	1
Flu syndrome	Undetermined	1
Pulpitis, tooth No. 7	Influenza A_2	1
Congestive prostatitis	Undetermined	1
Unilateral nasal discharge	Undetermined	1
Serous otitis media (very mild)	Undetermined	1

The lack of illnesses in the Apollo 10 and 11 missions has been gratifying. A number of factors might have contributed to this. The disease incidence in the general population was less at mission times. Attempts were made to assure adequate rest in the preflight periods. Contact of crews with other individuals was restricted as dictated by the preventive medicine program discussed above.

15. Medical Evaluation

The medical monitoring program for each Apollo mission began 30 days prior to launch with a crew briefing on medical examinations to be performed and biomedical findings on previous missions. Concerns relating to the particular flight were also discussed, and the first physical examination and collection of specimens for laboratory analysis completed. Detailed medical examinations were conducted at 14 and 5 days in the preflight period. A brief physical examination was performed on the launch day, except for the Apollo 11 mission, before which the crewmen were examined daily for 5 days. Postflight medical examinations were conducted as soon as possible and at 24 hours after recovery. The Apollo 11 crew was examined daily during their 21-day quarantine period.

Other than those observations to be discussed below, there has been no evidence of deterioration of body system function. Medical problems occurring in the Apollo missions were discussed above.

A. CARDIOVASCULAR EVALUATION

It has been well documented in the literature that orthostatic tolerance can be diminished by inactivity, by such earth-based simulations of weightlessness as water immersion or recumbency and, indeed, by the flight environment itself. Potential problems from cardiovascular deconditioning had been predicted long before man first ventured into space. Cardiovascular deconditioning, as evidenced by diminished orthostatic tolerance, was consistently demonstrated in early postflight periods in the Mercury and Gemini Programs. However, this phenomenon appeared to pose no serious problems following flights of 14 days in duration in Earth orbit, nor was it thought that it would have a detrimental effect on the astronauts during ascent from the lunar surface, even though they would be standing in the erect position during launch. In fact, one might expect that exposure to $\frac{1}{6}$ g while on the lunar surface might reverse somewhat the cardiovascular deconditioning which occurred during the early phase of the Apollo 11 mission.

Pre- and postflight cardiovascular evaluations were performed on all Apollo crewmembers and on suitable control subjects, to assess the effects of the mission profiles on orthostatic tolerance. Table XI lists the test methods used. The use of lower body

TABLE XI

Methods for evaluation of orthostatic tolerance in Apollo program

A. Provocative tests of the anti-gravity responses of the cardiovascular system
  1. Lower body negative pressure (LBNP) by incremental differential pressure (Apollo 7, 8, and 9 missions)
  2. 90° Passive standing (Apollo 9, 10, and 11 missions)
     Both tests were preceded by 5 min of supine control measurements. LBNP test was followed by 5 min of recovery measurements

B. Pre- and postflight collection of timed physiologic measurements
  1. Heart rate
  2. Blood pressure (systolic pressure, diastolic pressure, mean blood pressure, pulse pressure)
  3. Change in leg volume
  4. Other related data (weight, blood volume, vasoactive hormones, exercise capacity)

negative pressure (LBNP) was precluded by quarantine constraints on Apollo 11. Physiologic measurements obtained during each orthostatic test were heart rate, blood pressure and calf circumference. Other data utilized in evaluating test results included body weight, blood volume, exercise capacity and vasoreactive hormone level. Representative data plots for LBNP and 90° passive standing, tests are detailed in Figures 13 and 14 respectively.

Whatever may be the factors causing cardiovascular deconditioning, heart rate remains the most sensitive index of orthostatic tolerance at this time. Table XII summarizes the heart rate responses to orthostatic testing of Apollo 7 through 11 crewmembers. Notably, only 9 (60%) of the 15 astronauts exhibited significant postflight elevations in their supine heart rates, whereas 7 (77%) of the 9 stressed by LBNP, and all of the 9 stressed by 90° passive standing revealed significantly elevated pulse rates. Therefore, it appears that provocative cardiovascular testing reveals a cardiovascular response which might otherwise not be detected merely by observation of a resting individual. Finally, it should be noted that nearly all crewmembers have returned to their preflight response levels, as measured by pulse-rate changes during repeated provocative cardiovascular testing, within 30 to 50 hr after recovery. This period of recovery time was also observed after missions of longer duration in the Gemini

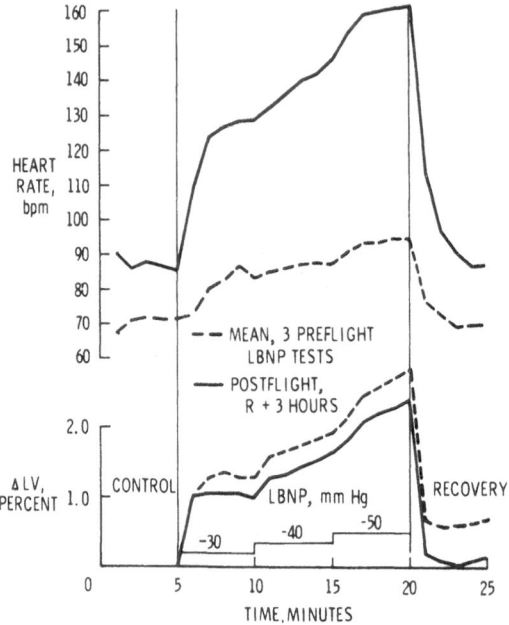

Fig. 13.   Representative changes of heart rate and calf circumference (ΔLV) during lower body negative pressure (LBNP) testing, preflight and postflight (3 hr after recovery).

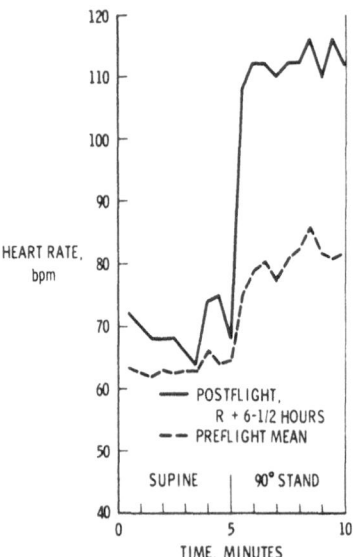

Fig. 14.   Representative changes of heart rate during 90° passive standing, preflight and postflight (6½ hr after recovery).

TABLE XII

Postflight heart rate responses to orthostatic testing of Apollo 7 through 11 crewmembers, compared to mean responses of 3 tests taken preflight

Test day	Orthostatic test	No. of subjects	Number of subjects postflight with heart rates			Range of postflight heart rates minus preflight average
			>2 S.D. preflight average	No significant change	<2 S.D. preflight average	
			Apollo crewmembers			
Day of recovery	Resting supine	15	9	4	2	−7 to +22
	LBNP	9	7	2	—	+13 to +66
	90° passive standing	9	9	—	—	+13 to +47
Day after recovery	Resting supine	15	5	9	1	−7 to +9
	LBNP	9	5	4	—	−3 to +38
	90° passive standing	9	6	3	—	+1 to +35
Two days after recovery	Resting supine	6	2	3	1	−7 to +10
	LBNP	6	1	5	—	−11 to +19
	90° passive standing	3	1	2	—	−4 to +18

Return of postflight heart rate responses to preflight values during orthostatic testing generally by 30 to 50 hr after recovery

			Control population			
Day before recovery	Resting supine	13	2	11	—	−8 to +11
	LBNP	7	1	5	1	−15 to +9
	90° passive standing	7	1	6	—	−2 to +11

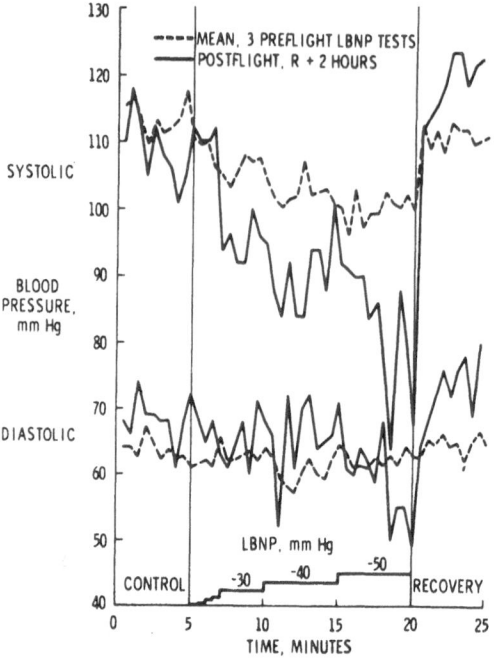

Fig. 15. Representative changes of blood pressure during lower body negative pressure (LBNP) testing, preflight and postflight (2 hr after recovery).

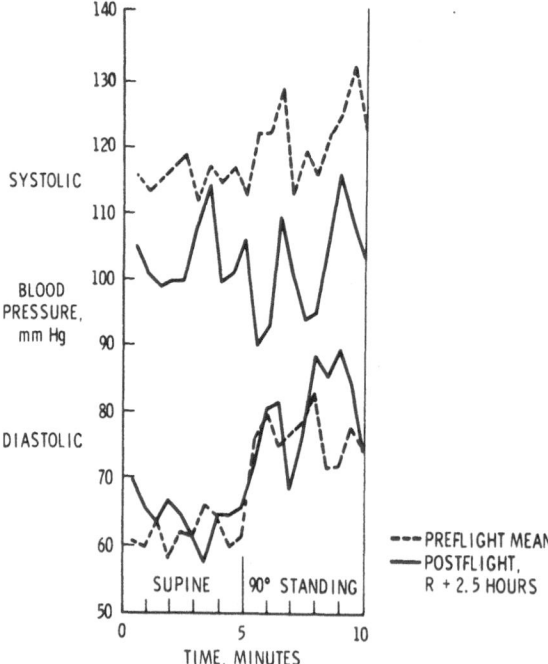

Fig. 16. Representative changes of blood pressure during 90° passive standing, preflight and postflight (2½ hr after recovery).

Program. Calf circumference changes were measured during LBNP testing in the 9 crewmembers from the Apollo 7 through 9 missions. This measurement increased significantly ($P<0.05$) in 2 cases, decreased significantly ($P<0.05$) in 3 cases, and was variable in the remainder. This finding suggests that the postflight heart rate response is a much better index of cardiovascular deconditioning than changes in calf circumference, or degree of lower extremity blood pooling, during LBNP.

One would think that changes in blood pressure would reflect consistently the effects of actual and simulated gravity on the cardiovascular system. However, as shown in Figures 15 and 16, blood pressure responses to LBNP and 90° passive standing pre- and postflight were quite variable. This was generally also true for pulse pressure changes. Although pulse pressures taken in the supine position were decreased in the postflight period in 13 of the 15 crewmembers, this change was significant ($P<0.05$) in only 4 cases. The pulse pressure decrease during LBNP was greater postflight than preflight in 9 astronauts tested, but only to a significant degree ($P<0.05$) in 5 cases. Interestingly, 3 crewmembers experienced pre-syncope during postflight LBNP testing. The pulse pressure decrease during 90° passive standing was greater postflight than preflight in 7 of the 9 astronauts tested, but only to a significant degree ($P<0.05$) in 3 cases. Finally, it should be noted that blood pressures of the crewmen have been found quite labile up to 3 days after recovery.

All 15 Apollo Program astronauts lost weight during their respective missions. Their weight data is recorded in Tables IV and XIII. Their mean weight loss was 5.6

TABLE XIII

Body weights of Apollo astronauts (lb)

Mission	Astronaut	Launch day	Recovery day	Difference
Apollo 7 (11 days)	Schirra	194.3	188.0	− 6.3
	Eisele	157.0	147.0	− 10.0
	Cunningham	156.0	148.0	− 8.0
Apollo 8 (8 days)	Borman	169.25	160.5	− 8.75
	Lovell	171.8	164.0	− 7.8
	Anders	142.0	138.0	− 4.0
Apollo 9 (10 days)	McDivitt	158.75	153.5	− 5.25
	Scott	178.25	172.5	− 5.75
	Schweickart	159.12	153.0	− 6.12
Apollo 10 (8 days)	Stafford	170.5	168.5	− 2.0
	Young	165.25	159.5	− 5.75
	Cernan	172.5	163.0	− 9.5
Apollo 11 (8 days)	Armstrong	171.5	164	− 7.5
	Collins	166.0	159	− 6.0
	Aldrin	167.25	166	− 1.25

Average weight loss = − 5.6 lb (range = − 1.25 to 10.0 lb).

1b (range 1.25 to 10 lb) over periods of 8 to 11 days in space. Fluid and associated electrolyte losses have been implicated as responsible for most of the weight change. Alterations in body fluid compartments would therefore account to a degree for the altered cardiovascular responses to orthostatic tests, discussed above, during the postflight periods. Finally, preliminary data indicates that altered vasoactive and adrenocortical hormone production postflight may be responsible for these cardiovascular responses.

B. HEMATOLOGICAL AND BIOCHEMICAL EVALUATIONS

Essential hematological and biochemical studies have been performed pre- and postflight in the Apollo Program. Although initially broad in spectrum, these studies were curtailed somewhat in the Apollo 10 and 11 missions by quarantine and other operational constraints.

Changes in the routine hematological profiles during the Apollo missions (pre- vs. immediate postflight periods) are summarized in Table XIV. As in the Gemini Program, a leucocytosis, associated with an absolute neutrophilia and an absolute lymphopenia, has been observed in the immediate postflight periods. These changes were transient, the total and differential white blood cell counts always reverting to preflight levels within 24 hr postflight. They are probably a consequence of increased blood epinephrine and steroid levels associated with mission stresses.

Data on the red cell fraction of the blood have been of particular interest in the Apollo Program in the light of the consistent loss of red cell mass, to a maximum of 20%, observed in the Gemini Program. A favored hypothesis for this phenomenon is a lysing effect of the pure oxygen, 5 psia atmosphere, used in the Gemini spacecraft, on

TABLE XIV

Changes in routine hematological profile during Apollo missions (pre- vs. immediate postflight periods)

Parameter	Mission					
	Apollo 7	Apollo 8	Apollo 9	Apollo 10	Apollo 11	AOA[a]
Red blood cells	0	↑↑	↓↓	↑↑	0	0
Hematocrit	0	↑↑	0	↑↑	0	0
Hemoglobin	0	↑↑	↑↑	0	0	
Reticulocytes	0	0		0	0	
White blood cells	↑↑↑	↑↑↑	0	↑↑	↑↑↑	↑↑↑
Neutrophils	↑↑	↑↑	0	↑↑↑	↑↑↑	↑↑
Lymphocytes	↓↓	↓↓	0	↑↑	↓↓	↓↓
Monocytes	0	↓↓	0	0	↓↓	↓↓
Eosinophils				↓↓	↓↓	↓
Basophils				↓↓	↓↓	0
Platelets	0	0	0	0	0	0

[a] Apollo over all.
Legend: 0 no occurrence; ↑ significant trend (positive); ↑↑ +2σ (σ represents standard deviation); ↑↑↑ +3σ; ↓ significant trend (negative); ↓↓ −2σ; ↓↓↓ −3σ; ND not done; + occurrence; TF data to follow.

TABLE XV

Summary of changes in hematology data during Apollo missions (pre- vs. immediate postflight periods)

Parameter	Mission				
	Apollo 7	Apollo 8	Apollo 9	Apollo 10	Apollo 11
Red cell mass	0	0	Decrease	ND	ND
Plasma volume	0	Decrease	Decrease	ND	ND
Ferrokinetics	Decrease	Decrease	ND	ND	ND
^{14}C-glycine survival	0	0	0	ND	ND
^{51}Cr survival	0	0	Decrease	ND	ND
Passive red blood cell Na$^+$-K$^+$ flux	ND	ND	0[a]	0[a]	ND
Active red blood cell Na$^+$-K$^+$ flux	ND	ND	Decrease	0	ND
Plasma vitamin E	0	Decrease	Decrease	TF	ND
Red blood cell vitamin E	0	0	0	TF	ND
Plasma vitamin A	ND	ND	Decrease	TF	ND
Red blood cell membrane lipids	0	0	Decrease	TF	ND
Phosphofructokinase	0	Decrease	0	ND	ND
Hexokinase	Increase	0	0	ND	ND
Phosphoglyceric kinase	Increase	0	Decrease	ND	ND
Glucose-3-phosphate dehydrogenase	0	Decrease	Increase	ND	ND
Glutathion (reduced form)	Decrease	0	Increase	ND	ND
ATP content in red blood cells	0	Increase	0	ND	ND
H$_2$O$_2$ sensitivity	Increase	0	Increase	ND	ND
Methemoglobin formation	0	Increase	0	ND	TF
Red blood cell morphologic changes (wet preparation)	0	0	Increase	ND	ND

[a] Technically unsatisfactory.
ND – not done.
TF – data to follow.

red blood cells. As shown in Table XV, there was essentially no change in red cell mass in Apollo 7 and 8 crewmembers. This might be due to the fact 5 to 7% nitrogen remained in the space cabins from the original prelaunch atmosphere (Figure 1) and had an inhibitory effect on red cell lysis. Yet, using an identical simulation of atmospheric exposure in an 11-day test, 3 crewmembers showed a mean decrease of 4.4% in red cell mass.

A significant loss of red cell mass occurred in the Apollo 9 mission. The space cabin atmosphere in this mission was different from that in the Apollo 7 and 8 spacecraft, since early in the flight. LM activation and extravehicular activity required depressurization of the CM cabin to a vacuum, followed by repressurization with pure oxygen. Thus, there was no residual nitrogen in the spacecraft cabin for 7 days of the 10-day Apollo 9 mission. This finding therefore lends further support to the hypothesis that pure oxygen space cabin atmospheres have been a major factor in producing the red cell mass losses observed in space flights, and that perhaps even small quantities of diluent gas (nitrogen) may exert a protective or modifying effect on oxygen toxicity as evidenced by loss of red cell mass.

As shown in Table XV, mean plasma volumes were essentially unchanged (decreased 4%) in the Apollo 7 mission and decreased (13%) in the Apollo 8 mission. The plasma volume also decreased (8%) somewhat during the Apollo 9 mission. A battery of additional hematological tests performed on both the plasma and red blood cells is also summarized qualitatively in Table XV.

Results of a great number of biochemical studies performed on the blood of Apollo Program crews are summarized in Table XVI. The consistently occurring transient postflight hyperglycemia is a probable result of an increased output of catecholamines and steroids secondary to the 'stress' of reentry. The decline of serum cholesterol and uric acid levels during flight is probably due to altered diet of the crewmembers. A transient decrease in fractions 3-, 4- and 5-lactic dehydrogenase were often observed. However, no other biochemical changes supporting liver or other disease have been noted.

TABLE XVI

Summary of changes in blood biochemistry data during Apollo missions
(pre- vs. immediate postflight periods)

Parameter	Mission					
	Apollo 7	Apollo 8	Apollo 9	Apollo 10	Apollo 11	AOA[a]
Glucose	↑↑↑	↑↑	↑	↑↑↑		↑↑
Cholesterol	↓	↓↓	↑	↓		↓
Serum glutamic-oxalacetic transaminase						
Blood urea nitrogen				↑↑		
Uric acid	↓	↓↓	↓	↓↓	↓↓	↓
Alkaline phosphatase			↑↑↑			
Ca						
Mg				↓↓	↓↓	
Inorganic phosphate		↑↑	↑↑↑	↑↑	↓↓	
Total bilirubin		↑		↑↑	↑↑	
Creatinine	↑↑					↑↑
Creatinine phosphokinase		↑↑	↓↓			
Lactic dehydrogenase (LDH)	↑↑		↓↓	↓↓	↓↓	
English nomenclature — LDH1 / LDH2 heart fraction		↑↑	↑↑↑	↓↓	↓↓	
LDH3			↓↓		↓↓	↓↓
LDH4		↓↓	↓↓		↑↑↑	↑↑
LDH5 – liver fraction				↑↑		
Na	↑↑	↓	↓↓	↓↓	↑↑	
K	↓↓	↓				
Cl	↑	↓		↓↓		
Osmolality	↓↓	↓↓	↑↑	↓↓	↓↓	
Total protein			↑↑	↑	↑↑	
Albumin			↑↑	↑		
Alpha 1			↑↑	↑↑		
Alpha 2	↑		↑↑	↑↑	↑↑	
Beta				↑↑		
Gamma				↑↑		

[a] Apollo over all.

Legend: see Table XIV.

TABLE XVII

Summary of changes in urine chemistry data during Apollo missions
(pre- vs. immediate postflight periods)

Parameter	Mission					
	Apollo 7	Apollo 8	Apollo 9	Apollo 10	Apollo 11	AOA[a]
Urine volume					↓ ↓	
Specific gravity	↑ ↑					
Hydroxyproline	↑ ↑	↑				↑ ↑ ↑
Uric acid	↑ ↑	↑			↓ ↓	
Creatinine	↑ ↑	↑		↓ ↓		
Inorganic phosphate	↑ ↑	↑			↓ ↓	
Na		↓		↓ ↓	↓ ↓	↓
K		↓		↓ ↓	↓	↓
Ca	↓ ↓	↑ ↑		↓ ↓	↓ ↓	
Mg	↓ ↓				↓ ↓	
Cl	↓		↓ ↓	↓ ↓	↓ ↓	↓ ↓

a Apollo over all.
Legend: see TABLE XIV.

TABLE XVIII

Summary of changes in humoral immunology data during Apollo missions
(pre- vs. immediate postflight periods)

Parameter	Mission					
	Apollo 7	Apollo 8	Apollo 9	Apollo 10	Apollo 11	AOA[a]
Immune globulin G				↑ ↑	↑	↑ ↑
Immune globulin M						
Immune globulin A			↑ ↑	↑ ↑ ↑	↑	↑
Haptoglobin			↑ ↑	↑ ↑	↑	↑ ↑
Ceruloplasmin			↑ ↑	↑ ↑ ↑		
Transferrin				↓ ↓		
Alpha-1 antitrypsin				↑ ↑		
Alpha-1 acid glycoprotein						
Alpha-2 macroglobulin				↑ ↑	↑ ↑ ↑	↑ ↑
C-reactive protein						
Beta-1 alpha globulin (third fraction of complement)			↑ ↑	↑ ↑	↑	

a Apollo over all.
Legend: see TABLE XIV.

Findings of urine chemistry studies during Apollo missions are summarized in Table XVII. It is noted that the postflight urinary excretion of hydroxyproline was increased over preflight basal levels and that there were consistently diminished excretions of sodium, potassium and chloride in the immediate postflight periods.

C. IMMUNOLOGICAL EVALUATION

A great number of immunologic studies, summarized in Table XVIII, have been conducted in the Apollo Program. The postflight increases in C-reactive protein levels observed in two Apollo 7 crewmembers were consistent with their inflight illnesses, as reported above. Later Apollo flights revealed significant postflight increases of immune globulins G and A, and haptoglobulin, ceruloplasmin and alpha-2 globulin concentrations. Increases in the immonuglobulins are probably related to the episodes of clinical illnesses reported above, and increases in the haptoglobulin and ceruloplasmin portions are probably due to the moderate generalized stress reaction of the crewmen.

D. MICROBIOLOGICAL EVALUATION

Microbiological studies in the Apollo Program have fallen into the realms of bacteriology, mycology, virology, parasitology, and protozoology. The prime objective of these studies is to define 'normal' (preflight) and 'spaceflight-adjusted' (postflight) microbiota of each crewmember, both qualitatively and quantitatively. Swab specimens from eight body areas and specimens of urine, feces and a throat-mouth gargle were collected 30 and 14 days preflight, 8 hr prior to lift-off, and immediately after recovery. The results of comprehensive microbiological analyses of such specimens would allow the early recognition and treatment of infectious diseases or other potential problems during the preflight phase and the prediction of possible qualitative contamination of returned lunar samples, so lessening the impact of such contaminants on procedures for bioassay and the release of lunar samples from quarantine. Such results also indicate the aggregate effects of spacecraft environmental parameters on the microbiota of each crewmember and the causative factors producing illness.

Approximately 12 data bits on some 4000 microorganisms have been collected and stored in a computer during the Apollo 7 to 11 missions. Although demanding mission schedules have not permitted a thorough analysis of these data to date, certain consistent findings may be indicative of biological trends. Man-to-man transfers of pathogenic bacteria and fungi are regular occurrences in the closed ecological environment of the Apollo spacecraft. This phenomenon is accompanied not only by a significant increase in the number of crewmembers infected, but also by an increase in the number of sites from which organisms can be isolated, per man. The appearance of certain organisms only during the postflight sampling interval suggests that microbial shifts may favor the growth of opportunist organisms. Further, certain other components of the normal flora have been isolated from aberrant sites. Taken together, these observations suggest that microflora changes occurring in the spacecraft environment may not be compatible with man's health and welfare during missions of extended duration.

No observations have been made which suggest that the spacecraft environment may predispose to viral-induced illness. Rather, the illnesses occurring in Apollo crewmembers have been correlated with the normal seasonal occurrence of upper respiratory infection in the population at large and preflight exposure of the crew.

No microorganisms with unfamiliar morphological structures or unusual physiological responses were detected in microbiological analyses following the Apollo 11 mission. Neither the preflight nor postflight phases of this mission were marred by the occurrence of viral illnesses in the crewmembers. The postflight quarantine seemed to have a protective effect on the astronauts. Despite the fact that viruses associated with upper respiratory infection and gastrointestinal upsets were isolated from personnel working in the Sample Laboratory, the astronauts and other personnel in the Crew Reception Area remained free from overt manifestations of similar illnesses.

E. EVALUATION OF EXERCISE CAPACITY

The Apollo pre- and postflight exercise capacity test utilized a bicycle ergometer programmed to maintain the heart rate at a given level. The primary purpose of this test was to determine if there were any changes in the physiological response to work which could affect the completion or monitoring of lunar surface extravehicular

TABLE XIX

Apollo exercise response test (oxygen consumption immediately postflight)

Heart rate, bpm	$\bar{X}$, percent[a]	σ	No. of subjects
120	68.6	15.2	15
140	74.5	11.6	15
160	77.8	10.8	15
180	77.0	8.1	3
Over all	73.8	12.7	48

[a] 100 percent = mean of three preflight measurements.

activity. For this test, heart rates of 120, 140, 160 and, in three subjects, 180 beats per minute, were progressively maintained at each level for 3 min. Samples of expired gas were obtained at appropriate times during each test, which was conducted 30, 14 and 4 days preflight, as soon as possible after recovery, and within 24 to 36 hr after recovery.

In immediate postflight periods 12 of the Apollo crewmen have demonstrated a significant decrease in work performed and in oxygen consumed at submaximal heart rate levels, as compared to data taken preflight. The 3 crewmen tested at the maximal heart rate level of 180 beats per min exhibited similar decrements as shown in Table XIX. Except for one individual who showed identical responses to exercise before and after the Apollo 8 mission, all crewmen returned to preflight response levels within 24 to 36 hr after recovery. Supplementary supporting data indicated that decrements in work performance were not due to altered pulmonary function or to diminished ability of the crewmen to extract oxygen from the atmosphere. The physiologic mechanisms responsible for changes observed in the exercise response test following space missions remain to be identified through further investigation.

16. Lunar Surface Activity

Planning and training for extravehicular activity on the lunar surface had to take into consideration that, as previous Apollo missions had shown, there would be some effect on the crew of exposure for 3 days to weightlessness, probably manifesting as a heart rate increase due to cardiovascular deconditioning, and decrease in exercise capacity. Fortunately, decrease in red cell mass, and possible consequences thereof, appeared unlikely.

The Apollo 11 crew was appropriately monitored during 3 preflight simulations – under-water immersion conditions, in the altitude chamber and while duplicating the lunar surface timeline on a simulated lunar surface. Although none of these simulations exactly reproduced the lunar conditions to be encountered, such as $\frac{1}{6}$ g, motion and surface friction, physiological information obtained during these simulations was still used for the predictions of the energy cost of lunar surface activity. These predictions and their comparison with the actual mission estimates are listed for both the commander (CDR) and the lunar module pilot (LMP) in Table XX. Predictions were quite close for the LMP, yet quite at variance for the CDR.

Three methods were used for real-time metabolic monitoring while the astronauts were extravehicular on the lunar surface. The heart rate was compared to that on an energy cost (BTU) calibration curve obtained preflight by bicycle ergometry. Oxygen usage from the portable life support system (PLSS) was measured. Differences in the inlet and outlet temperatures in the water-cooled undergarment (LCG) were recorded. Accumulated data obtained by these methods and an integrated estimate of energy cost for the Apollo 11 CDR and LMP during extravehicular activity are summarized in Figures 17 and 18. These data showed that the oxygen usage and LCG methods

TABLE XX

Predictions of energy cost of extravehicular activity on lunar surface and their comparison with actual Apollo 11 mission estimates

Predictions	Commander (CDR)		Lunar module pilot (LMP)	
	A.H.T. BTU[a]	Percentage of variation[b]	A.H.T. BTU	Percentage variation
From under-water immersion simulation study	775	–	800	–
From altitude chamber simulation study	1050	+17	1300	+8
From lunar surface simulation study	1850	+106	1375	+15
Premission predictions	1350	+50	1275	+6
Actual mission estimates	900	–	1200	–

[a] Average hourly total BTU.
[b] From actual mission estimate.

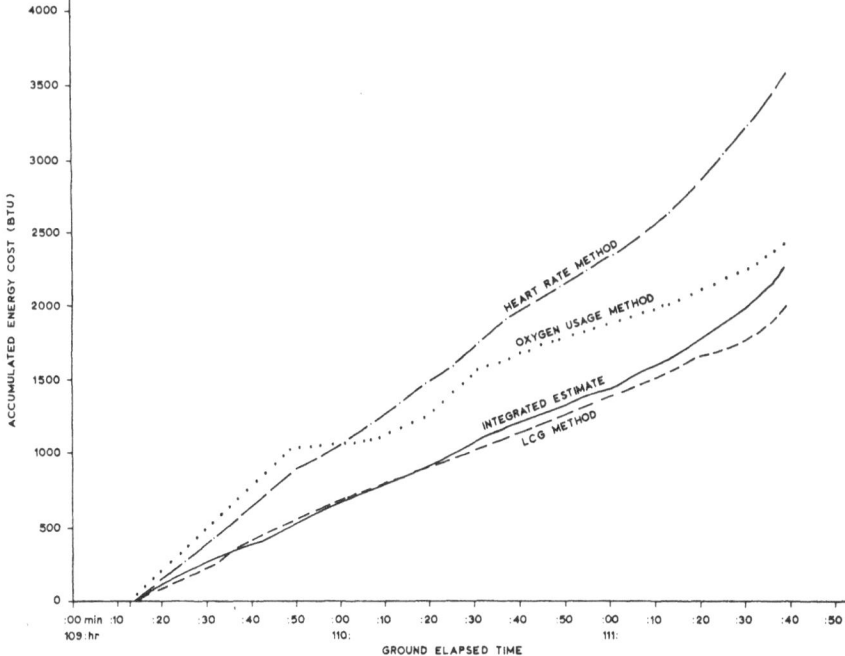

Fig. 17. Accumulated data on energy cost of the Apollo 11 commander during extravehicular lunar surface activity, using three methods of metabolic assessment, and an integrated estimate of the energy cost of this activity.

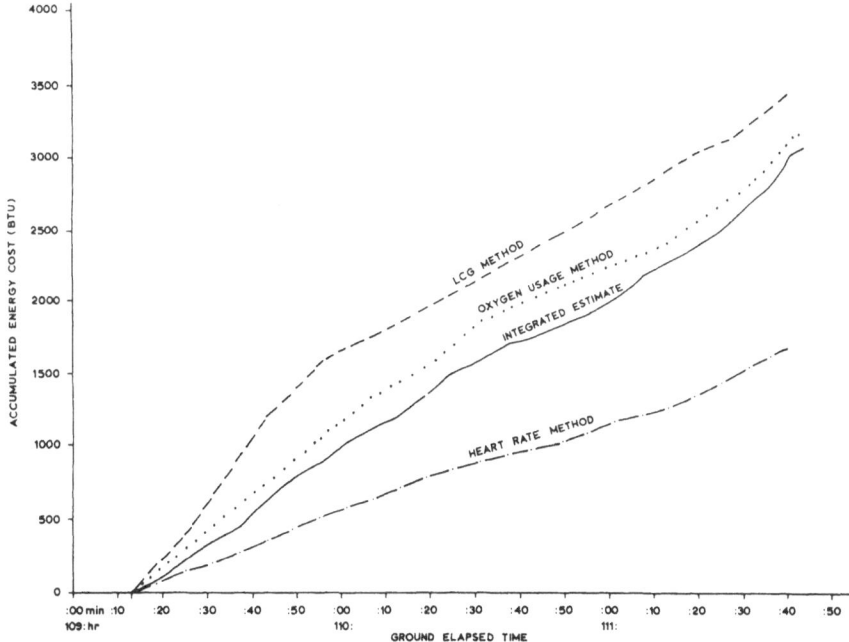

Fig. 18. Accumulated data on energy cost of the Apollo 11 lunar module pilot during extravehicular lunar surface activity, using three methods of metabolic assessment, and an integrated estimate of the energy cost of this activity.

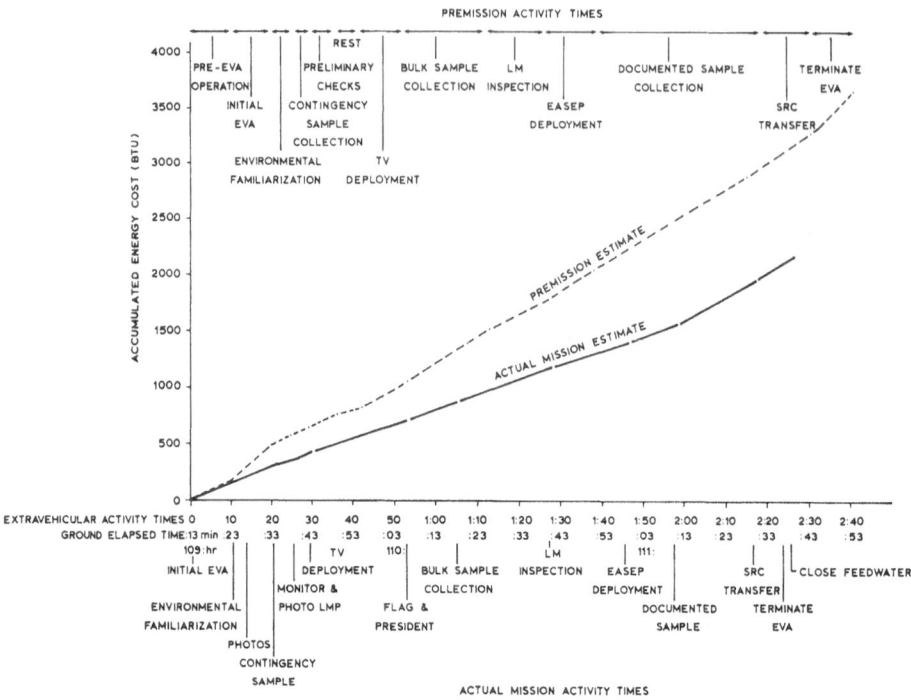

Fig. 19.   Accumulated premission and actual mission estimates of energy cost of extravehicular activity on the lunar surface for the Apollo 11 commander.

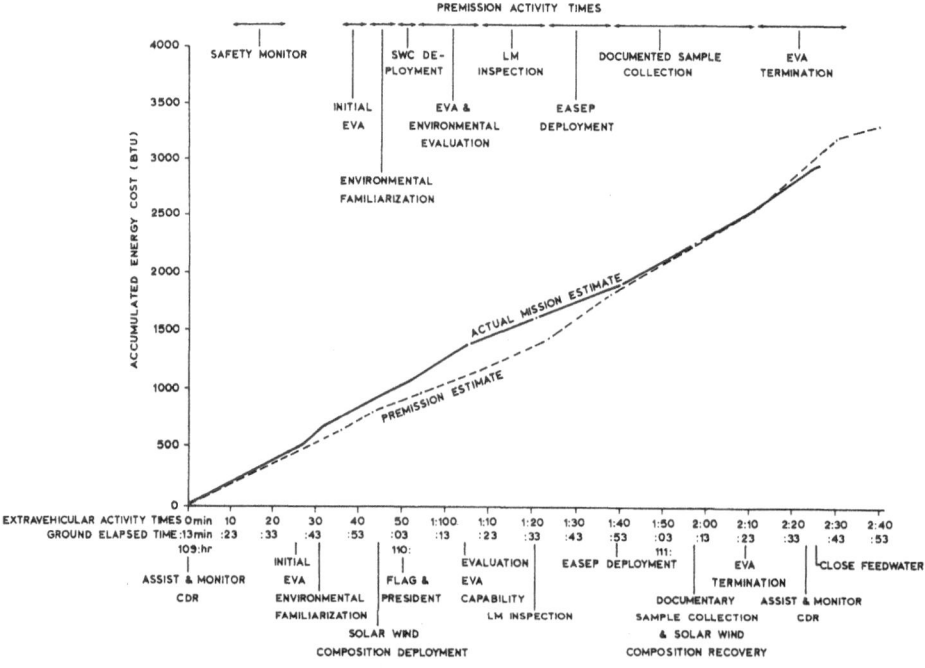

Fig. 20.   Accumulated premission and actual mission estimates of energy cost of extravehicular activity on the lunar surface for the Apollo 11 LM pilot.

gave energy cost levels 61% below those estimated by the heart rate method in the CDR and 81% above those estimated by the heart rate method in the LMP. The oxygen usage and LCG methods not only yielded similar data, but also reflected well the physical activity observed by television monitoring. The loss in accuracy in the heart rate method might be attributed to many causes, including psychological, heat storage, and cardiovascular deconditioning effects on the heart rate, and poor correlation of slow heart rates with energy cost.

Figures 19 and 20 show the accumulated premission and actual mission estimates of the energy costs of extravehicular activity on the lunar surface for the Apollo 10 CDR and LMP. These estimates compare favorably and appear to be well within the calculated margins for expendable (water and oxygen) usage. The integrated energy costs during extravehicular activity of the Apollo 11 LMP on the lunar surface is further detailed in terms of BTU production while performing specific tasks in Table XXI.

TABLE XXI

Integrated energy costs of extravehicular activity of the Apollo 11 LMP
on the lunar surface

Events EVA – lunar surface	Time		Integrated BTU production		
	G.E.T.[a] (hr:min)	Interval (min)	Rate (BTU/hr)	Total BTU for interval	BTU accumulated
Assist and monitor CDR	109:13	26	1200	500	
Inittal EVA	109:39	5	1950	163	683
Environmental familiarization (television cable deployment)	109:44	14	1200	280	963
Solar wind composition deployment	109:58	6	1275	128	1091
Flag and presidential message	110:04	14	1350	315	2270
Evaluation EVA capability (environment)	110:18	16	850	227	1633
Lunar module inspection	110:34	19	875	277	1910
EASEP deployment	110:53	18	1200	360	2270
'Documentary' sample collection (solar wind composition recovery)	111:11	12	1450	290	2560
EVA termination (ingress) (sample return container)	111:23	14	1650	385	2945
Assist and monitor CDR	111:37	2	1100	37	2982
Close Feedwater	111:39				
Total		146 min			2982 BTU

[a] Ground-elapsed time.

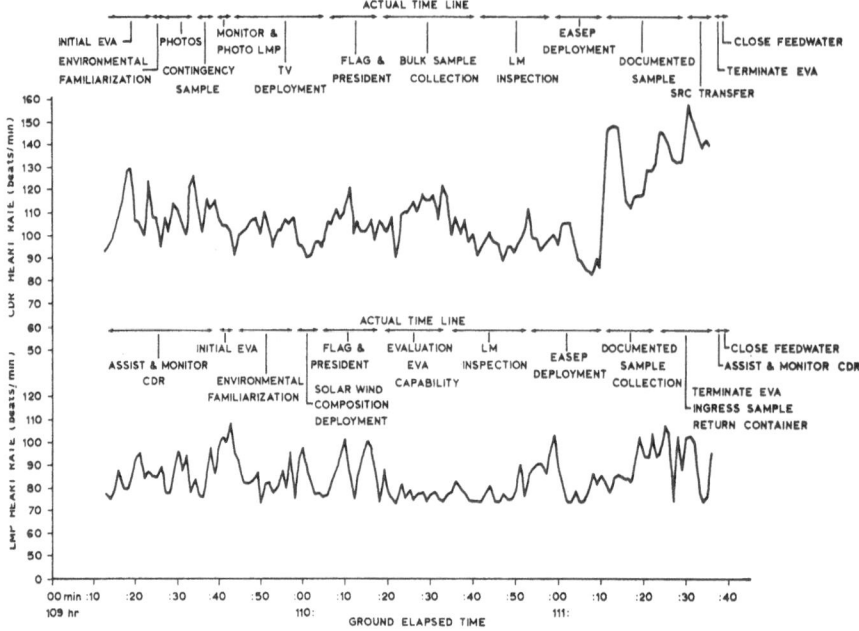

Fig. 21.   Apollo 11 CDR and LMP heart rates during extravehicular activity on the lunar surface.

The heart rates for each Apollo 11 crewman during his extravehicular activity on the lunar surface is shown in Figure 21. The highest heart rates recorded were from 140 to 160 beats per min in the CDR during lunar sample collection and transfer of the sample box to the LM.

In summary, it has been found that even though the energy cost of performing a given task differs among crewmen, the average hourly total energy cost for the crewmen was still 900 to 1200 BTU. The LCG method appears best for estimating energy cost of work for use in consummable calculations. On the other hand, the heart rate method is a valuable relative indicator, but a poor absolute indicator of the energy cost of work. Apollo 11 data indicate that extravehicular activity for 4 to 5 hr on the lunar surface is not outside man's physiological limits and the limits of the present support equipment. These data were utilized in planning the Apollo 12 extravehicular activity.

17. Quarantine

Approximately three years before the Apollo 11 mission, a decision was made to conduct a quarantine operation to preclude the possibility, even though remote, of contaminating the Earth's biosphere with lunar organisms. This decision was based on a National Academy of Sciences Report which stated that there was a remote possibility of such contamination and recommended a quarantine. The quarantine was to start at closure of the LM hatch on the lunar surface and continue for a 21-day period. Although this was an arbitrary time period, not covering all disease incubation periods, it covered most of the virulent contagious diseases. A series of procedures were developed for crew action through recovery and placement in the Mobile Quarantine Facility (MQF) for transport to the Lunar Receiving Laboratory quarantine facility at Houston, Texas.

The crew kicked lunar dust off their boots on the LM ladder and used a brush attachment to the suit hoses to vacuum the surfaces of the lunar rock box and film containers. There was considerable dust on the legs and arms of the suit and free in the LM. It was described as a fine, slippery, dark grey, talcum powder material which smeared and adhered and smelled like wet fireworks.

The astronauts got this material on their skin, under their fingernails, and apparently inadvertently inhaled and ingested it. The rock boxes and film packs were repackaged after vacuuming, so that little dust was transferred from CM to LM. The space suits were doffed and packaged in the CM and the cabin air constantly filtered during return to Earth by the lithium hydroxide cannisters. Thus, no dust should have been present on landing.

The actual recovery involved protecting the swimmers with SCUBA gear and one swimmer with a biological isolation garment. This swimmer scrubbed the hatch area and postlanding vent with an iodine preparation. He opened the hatch and gave biological isolation garments to the crew who donned them and egressed into the raft. The hatch was closed and again decontaminated, as were the crewmen and swimmer, with the same iodine solution. The astronauts then transferred to the helicopter to the recovery ship, and thence into the Mobile Quarantine Facility (MQF). The microbial sampling and initial examination were completed in the MQF and the biological samples transferred to the outside through a tank containing a sodium hypochlorite solution.

The crew, a physician and a recovery technician remained in the MQF during the three days of transit time ship and aircraft to Houston where the MQF was moved to the Lunar Receiving Laboratory. There the five individuals transferred to the Crew Reception Area (CRA). Daily examinations were conducted on all CRA personnel, and blood and microbiological samples for analysis were obtained at intervals. The crew quarantine period was remarkable for the lack of positive medical findings. No evidence of infectious disease was found in the examination of crew or similarly quarantined personnel. Careful evaluation of the microbiological samples and immunological studies revealed no evidence of bacterial, viral or fungal growth not noted preflight.

Cultures taken of the lunar dust from the space suit showed no growth. One-half of each core tube was used as a prime biological sample and placed in five viral tissue cultures, on a number of bacterial and fungal media and injected intraperitoneally into mice. No evidence of growth or adverse effect was noted. Consultation with the Interagency Committee on Back Contamination gave approval for crew release on the twenty-first day. Continued surveillance will be maintained for one year. To date, there has been no infection, disease or illness of any type in the crew. Surely the crew will develop some of the common infections which plague man. These will be identified by laboratory methods to be assured that they are of terrestrial origin.

The quarantine of the lunar samples continued until 50 days after recovery. Representative chips of the samples were then pulverized and placed in solution. Detailed bacteriological, viral and fungal studies were performed. Groups of plants, insects (cockroach, moth and fly), fish, shrimp, oyster, quail and mice were exposed to the material. In each instance one group was kept in an identical environment but not exposed to lunar sample, one group was exposed to sterilized lunar sample, and the third group to the regular lunar sample. While some animal deaths have occurred during the quarantine period, they were principally in the control groups.

18. Summary

The 3105 hr of exposing man to space-flight during the Apollo Program have added greatly to knowledge of man's response to space travel. The spacecraft cabin environment has been suitably maintained for the crew. The radiation environment has been benign, no solar flares occurring during the Apollo Program missions. Crews have generally adapted well to weightlessness and have learned to utilize it to their advantage. Improvements have been made in inflight food, with the addition of moisturized packs and such items as sandwiches and dried fruit. The body weight losses which continue to occur during space missions are not entirely due to body fluid loss. The supplying of potable water to the crews has been effective, and great strides have been made in removing gas bubbles in the water. Work/sleep cycles have been improved somewhat by having all crewmembers sleep at the same time and by having cycles closer related to those during training.

The medical kit has been adequate on all missions since the Apollo 7 mission, medications being added as the needs arose. Bioinstrumentation has continued to function well. Although a preflight preventive medicine program has been difficult to conduct, it has been effective in the later Apollo missions in reducing pre-, in-, and postflight illnesses, which had occurred in all flight phases and were usually viral upper respiratory and gastrointestinal infections. Although crews have reported motion sickness to a varying degree of severity, all crews adapted to their motion environment. This area will require continuing attention.

Cardiovascular deconditioning has been identified postflight with both lower body negative pressure and 90° passive standing techniques. This phenomenon has been of a similar degree and has lasted for the same periods as that following the Gemini missions.

A significant decrement in work capacity has been noted in the immediate period postflight. This condition usually lasts from 24 to 36 hr postflight.

As in the Gemini Program a postflight neutrophilia has been observed after crew recovery. The loss of red cell mass observed in the Gemini program occurred only during the Apollo 9 mission. This finding indicates that hyperoxia is the important factor responsible for this loss, and that even a small amount of nitrogen in the atmosphere may protect the red cell from the lytic action of oxygen.

Microbiological studies have shown that organisms transfer between crewmembers.

Moreover, the growth of opportunist organisms appears to be favored by these shifts.

Extravehicular activity on the lunar surface during the Apollo 11 mission was conducted within expected energy costs, at an average of 1200 BTU per hr. The liquid-cooled garment temperature method of energy cost estimation is the most suitable. It appears that lunar surface time can be extended safely.

The Apollo 11 quarantine was a demanding operation, conducted very successfully.

References

Anon: 1966, NASA-TM-X-60589, National Aeronautics and Space Administration, Washington, D.C.

Berry, C. A.: 1967, *J.A.M.A.* **201**, 232.

Berry, C. A.: 1968, in *Life Sciences and Space Research*, Vol. VI (ed. by A. H. Brown and F. G. Favorite), North Holland Publ. Co., Amsterdam, pp. 1–19.

Berry, C. A.: 1969a, *Aerospace Med.* **40**, 245.

Berry, C. A.: 1969b, *Aerospace Med.* **40**, 762.

Berry, C. A.: 1969c, *Sci. Journal* **5**, 103.

Berry, C. A. and Catterson, A. D.: 1967, NASA-SP-138, National Aeronautics and Space Administration, Washington, D.C., pp. 197–218.

Berry, C. A., Coons, D. O., Catterson, A. D., and Kelly, G. C. F.: 1966, NASA-SP-121, National Aeronautics and Space Administration, Washington, D.C., pp. 235–61.

Fischer, C. L., Johnson, P. C., and Berry, C. A.: 1967, *J.A.M.A.* **200**, 579.

Gooch, P. C. and Berry, C. A.: 1969, *Aerospace Med.* **40**, 610.

Graybiel, A., Miller, E. F., and Billingham, J. *et al.*: 1967, *Aerospace Med.* **38**, 360.

Kelly, G. F. and Coons, D. O.: 1967, NASA-SP-138, National Aeronautics and Space Administration, Washington, D.C., pp. 107–125.

PHYSIOLOGICAL INFORMATION MONITORING TECHNIQUES
FOR THE SOYUZ SPACECRAFT

L. I. KAKURIN, I. S. SHADRINTSEV, and A. G. ZERENIN

Academy of Medical Sciences, Moscow, U.S.S.R.

The acquisition of biomedical information from astronauts flying space missions is one of the most complicated yet extremely important problems of aerospace medicine. Even elementary physiological studies, let alone on-board data recording of various physiological parameters are seriously hindered by spaceflight conditions. Therefore, most of the well-known recording techniques used clinically or in physiological work could not be utilized under spaceflight conditions without adequate modifications.

The development of reliable physiological instrumentation that would function without failure when exposed to different spaceflight factors, as well as adequate fixation of this instrumentation to the human body, present considerable difficulties. As a rule, physiological sensors are to be placed at some specific points of body surface. Any inaccuracy in a sensor fixation permitting its displacement or weakening of its pressure on the body can produce disturbances and an attenuation of signals (*i.e.*, a distortion of the recording).

Fixed physiological sensing equipment can cause disconfort in astronauts, especially over a long period of time. It can also restrain their movements and interfere with their performance.

There are several well-known techniques of applying physiological sensors:

(1) fixation with straps;

(2) sewing into under-garments;

(3) pasting on to the skin;

(4) inserting into a natural body opening, such as the mouth cavity, an external ear canal, nostrils, etc.;

(5) insertion into the digestive tract (including radio-probing);

(6) implantation into tissue (subcutaneous, intravascular or implantation into the myocardium).

Some of these methods are at the present time completely useless on a spacecraft. Others cannot ensure the required degree of electrode securing, or interfere too much with astronauts' work. This leaves only a few methods that can be used successfully.

The list of physiological parameters to be monitored is usually determined on the basis of mission program requirements and the crew work schedule, and is to a large degree dependent on the current level of knowledge of body response to space flight stresses. The latter is acquired from laboratory simulations of some of the stresses (acceleration, vibration, movement restriction, confinement, short time weightlessness obtained by means of Keplerian trajectory, etc., and, to a great degree from the medical investigations during preceding manned spaceflights.

D. E. Busby (ed.), Recent Advances in Aerospace Medicine, 42–44. All Rights Reserved.
Copyright © 1970 by D. Reidel Publishing Company, Dordrecht-Holland.

On the basis of the data obtained from preceding investigations and space missions medical control equipment developed for Soyuz spacecraft ensured:

(1) recording and telemetering by short wave radio to the ground monitoring centers pulse rate data of each astronaut over the entire duration of the mission;

(2) amplifying and telemetering to the ground monitoring centers, in zones of direct radio visibility, electrocardiogram (ECG), seismocardiogram (SCG), pneumogram (PG) and pulse rate data from each astronaut;

(3) recording, on the on-board autonomous system, electrocardiogram and pneumogram data during specific stages of the mission, including spacecraft descent to Earth;

(4) recording on the medical control panel the pulse rate and body temperature data from astronauts when preparing to get out of the spacecraft and during actual transition to the other spacecraft.

Biomedical monitoring was carried out by means of a unified sensor system. It comprised seismocardiographic (SCG) and pneumographic (PG) sensors, two sets of silver electrocardiographic (ECG) electrodes and cloth straps to hold the sensors in place on the body. The fixation system utilized provided a reliable securing of the biosensors in place. No restriction of the astronauts' movement or any feeling of discomfort were registered.

In medical control equipment development the main problem was to find the optimum way of prompt evaluation of the health condition of astronauts during their passage from one space vehicle to another. Since some stages of the transition program are performed when the spacecraft is outside radio visibility zones of the ground monitoring centers and, of all physiological functions, only the pulse rate is monitored, it was found expedient to transfer the medical control at such times to the crew commanders. Being properly prepared, informed and instructed they appeared to be quite able to make necessary decisions when astronauts showed some changes in their cardiac cycles or body temperature in excess of established limits during transition.

During ground simulator tests of the transition program, it was found that the space suit heat rejection system was quite adequate. Nevertheless, an autonomous medical control system was introduced that provided assessment of the physiologic state of the two astronauts on the basis of pulse rate and body temperature measuring. This was done because of the insufficient information acquired so far on energy cost during activity in orbital flight, which may differ considerably from the energy cost for the same type of activity in ground conditions. Such a difference in energy cost during performance in flight and on the Earth could be associated with a number of factors. Most important of them are:

(1) lack of a firmly established stereotype for performing under weightless conditions

(2) working under emotional stress caused by the sense of responsibility for the accomplishment of the mission program and by the unfamiliar space environment

The autonomous medical control equipment included a medical control panel with data-indicating devices and body temperature probes with fixation systems.

Pulse rate was indicated by a pointer instrument placed on the medical control panel. The main problem in body temperature monitoring was the selection of the most suitable place to position the probe with the object of obtaining the most reliable information on the astronaut's body temperature during task performance envisaged in the mission program. Rectal temperature measuring was found to be optimum since the rectal temperature is as close as possible to the aortic blood temperature. Body temperature was indicated on the medical control panel by means of light signals with two different luminescence conditions according to two different thresholds of the measured data.

When body temperature of an astronaut reached the first threshold, a light signal appeared reporting the existence of a surplus body heat not yet dangerous but still requiring a continuous control. If body temperature data reached the second threshold, a light signal then meant that measures must be taken in order to ensure the safe accomplishment of the work program.

The physiological equipment and techniques described above provided an adequate monitoring of cardiovascular and respiratory activities and body temperature during all mission stages, including transition from spacecraft Soyuz IV to Soyuz III by the astronauts in space suits.

PECULIARITIES OF RESPONSES OF THE ACOUSTIC ANALYZER
OF MAN EXPOSED TO PROLONGED NOISE EFFECTS DURING
A YEAR-LONG MEDICO-ENGINEERING EXPERIMENT

T. N. KRUPINA, E. I. MATSNEV, I. YA. YAKOVLEVA,
M. A. VYTCHIKOVA, V. YA. LEVANOV

Academy of Medical Sciences, Moscow, U.S.S.R.

Noise in the spacecraft cabin, aggravated by other flight factors, may have an adverse effect on a cosmonaut's hearing, even during a mission of short duration (Yuganov *et al.*, 1965; Henry, 1966; Lott, 1965). According to Berry (1969), noise effects combined with the weightless state and circadian disturbances annoyed astronauts during the space flights of Apollos VII and VIII. In space missions of long duration, continuous exposure to noise will be of greater significance. Therefore, investigation and development of well-substantiated parameters of an optimal acoustic environment in space cabins are required. This communication summarizes studies on the functional state of the acoustic analyzer of humans continuously exposed to noise during a year-long, medico-engineering experiment.

Employing latest achievements in biology, engineering and other branches of science and technology, the Soviet Union has developed an integrative life support system provided with up-to-date research and control equipment. Three young test subjects – physician, biologist and technician – lived a year in a chamber of limited size consisting of living and green-house modules. They were sustained by water and oxygen regenerated from human wastes and dehydrated food. Reviews of the experiment were published in Soviet periodicals in 1968-1969.

The functional state of the acoustic analyzer was evaluated using the methods of threshold and supra-threshold pure tone, speech and noise audiometry. Hearing acuity was measured before and during the experiment at intervals of two weeks; after the accomplishment of the experiment the study continued until the normalization of the acoustic parameters. Experimental data obtained were treated statistically.

Hearing parameters studied during the experiment were hearing threshold in the range from 125 to 8000 Hz (air and bone conduction), differential thresholds of sound intensity and frequency using the Lüscher test. Measurements were taken at the same time of the day with the aid of a Soviet acoustic apparatus. The good quality and stability of audiometer performance were provided by means of oscillograph-aided, regular calibrations of audiometer output voltage.

Every audiometric measurement was preceded by determinations of spectral and amplitude characteristics of noise and vibration in the chamber. The monitoring system included a sound-level meter, filter and vibration meter. Noise was produced by fans and pumps. The noise level was measured in the living and green-house modules.

The total sound level in the chamber was within the range of 87 to 96 dB, the sound energy of 31.5 to 250 Hz prevailing. At certain stages of the experiment a high-frequency component (500, 1000, 4000 Hz) also appeared. The vibration level remained within the permissible limits approved in the U.S.S.R. in 1966.

Prior to the experiment all test subjects displayed no abnormalities in their hearing. During the experiment they complained of various uncomfortable sensations due to noise. The noise effect annoyed them, especially at rest. Beginning with the third to fourth days of the experiment the physician reported ear blockage and hearing loss which he observed during auscultation and arterial blood pressure measurements.

By the second month of the experiment, the test subjects developed a kind of adjustment; however, they failed to adapt completely to the noise effects until the very end of the experiment. It is interesting to note that an insignificant increase of the sound level to which the test subjects had adapted was perceived as a sharp elevation of the loudness level.

In the course of the experiment all parameters studied varied significantly. Masking thresholds were in the range from 35 to 65 dB, air conduction, and from 35 to 50 dB, bone conduction. Hearing variations changed distinctly from individual to individual. The masking thresholds, air conduction, were about 35 to 40 dB in the most stable test subject and about 50 to 65 dB in the least stable one. The three subjects displayed a positive recruitment phenomenon. According to the audiometry data, the year-long experiment can be conditionally divided into three periods:

First period (2 months) – characterized by an increase of the masking thresholds and differential thresholds of sound intensity and frequency.

Second period (3.5 months) – characterized by a relative increase of the masking thresholds, a decrease of differential thresholds and a relative stabilization of these parameters.

Third period (6.5 months) – characterized by a marked increase of the masking thresholds and a drastic decrease of differential thresholds.

Between the first to fifth days following the experiment, the test subjects reported unpleasant sensations of ear plugging, noise and ringing in the ears and head which caused unsound sleep and sleeplessness. The test subjects recovered their normal hearing sensitivity at different intervals. Two recovered it on the seventh and twenty-fifth days after the experiment. The third subject, who subjectively reported hearing loss and objectively displayed greatest variations of all the parameters tested, did not show normal hearing during 7 months of observation after the experiment. Dynamic audiometric measurements indicated a hearing loss of up to 50 dB in the 4000 Hz range. He distinctly retained a positive recruitment phenomenon. The typical audiometric picture and stability of hearing disturbances were suggestive of a noise trauma of the cochleitis type. Intensive treatment of the test subject (using vitamins, biostimulators, physical methods) led to an improvement of the audiometric parameters (the hearing level at 4000 Hz was 20 to 25 dB).

Therefore, the response of the human acoustic analyzer during the year-long experiment was characterized by certain peculiarities which might be associated with cumulative effects of noise. The dynamic audiometric measurements revealed phasic changes of the acoustic analyzer. In the course of the first stages of the experiment (first and second periods), phasic variations in the central parts of the analyzer were predominant. A distinct increase of the recruitment phenomenon by the end of the experiment and a significant increase of the masking thresholds indicate the development of changes (in the cochlea) which appear to be of metabolic origin.

In accordance with data of the International Standards Organization (1963), functional changes in the acoustic analyzer observed in one of the test subjects can be referred to as a type of temporary threshold shift, since his hearing parameters rapidly returned to normal (the hearing sensitivity recovered 7 days after the experiment). Hearing variations seen in the two other subjects cannot be referred to as this type.

The long duration of the recovery period (from 25 days to 7 months) after the experiment is indicative of significant changes in the cochlea, probably involving structural damage.

Findings of this study confirm the conclusion made by Lemann (1967) that no habituation (adaptation) to noise effects can develop. These findings have revealed individual peculiarities in the noise sensitivity of the test subjects, though audiological tests applied before the study have failed to indicate any of them. Individual sensitivity to noise may be associated with many factors, including pre-test fitness of the subject, hearing thresholds, reactions to the ambient environment, and peculiarities of the nervous regulation.

Thus, this study has demonstrated that man exposed to continuous noise effects during a year-long enclosure can maintain his hearing ability. However, acoustic trauma can occur if man has an elevated hearing sensitivity. This necessitates further bioengineering research of noise effects in extended space missions. Engineering considerations include measures taken to decrease the noise level in space cabin, to develop new sound-proof materials, to devise individual protection, etc.

Biomedical investigations of noise effects involve the development of biological protection, scientific substantiation of maximally allowable limits during long-term exposure as well as methods of detecting individual sensitivity of men. Unfortunately, current audiologic methods fail to predict reliably the stability of the acoustic analyzer under the conditions of extended noise effects (Tyomkin, 1968). According to the data reported here, a comprehensive audiometric, clinical and physiological examination of humans exposed to long-term noise effects is most promising in this respect.

References

Berry, C. A.: 1969, *Aerospace Med.* **40**, 245.

Henry, J. P.: 1966, in *Biomedical Aspects of Space Flight*. Holt, Rinehart and Winston, New York.

Lemann, G.: 1967, in *Manual of Occupational Physiology, Moscow*, pp. 303–304.

Lott, B. J.: 1965, in *Physiological Problems of Space Exploration*, Charles C. Thomas, Springfield, Ill., pp. 209–230.

Tyomkin, Ya. S.: 1969, in *Occupational Diseases and Ear Trauma*, Izd-vo Meditsina, Moscow.

Yuganov, E. M., Krylov, Y. V. and Kuznetsov, V. S.: 1965, in *Proceedings XVI International Congress of Aerospace Medicine*, Athens, pp. 13–18.

EXOBIOLOGY

A. W. SCHWARTZ

Exobiology Laboratory, Catholic University, Nijmegen, The Netherlands

The Sun is really quite an ordinary star, and it is located in a very ordinary corner of a rather undistinguished galaxy. At one time it was thought that our star might be somewhat unusual in having a family of planets, but it now appears that planets may be common throughout the universe. Because the laws of physics and chemistry are quite universal, one can predict to some extent the reactions which would take place on the surface of a newly formed planet, given certain assumptions related to its mode of formation, mass, and distance from the parent star. Under many sets of circumstances, the chemical environment of this planet would be similar to the conditions which prevailed on the primordial Earth. The universe is composed predominantly of hydrogen. Following hydrogen, if one eliminates the noble gases, which are normally unreactive, the next most abundant elements are oxygen, nitrogen and carbon, the basic materials of life. During the formation of a planet, reactions between these elements would form an atmosphere, as many of the simple compounds of carbon, oxygen, nitrogen and hydrogen are gases.

It is believed that the atmosphere with which the Earth was formed, the so-called primordial atmosphere, was a mixture of methane, ammonia, water and, of course, hydrogen (Miller and Urey, 1959). During the past 16 years, the chemistry of such an atmosphere has been studied intensively. Under the influence of various sources of energy which would have been readily available on the Earth (*e.g.* ultraviolet light, heat, electric discharges), many classes of biologically important molecules have been spontaneously synthesized (Fox, 1965). The theory of the origin of life on the Earth which has emerged holds that chemical compounds and chains of reactions would have evolved in a manner analogous to the Darwinian evolution of living species; that is, by the self perpetuation of those chemical systems which were best suited to survive, either because of the availability of the starting materials, or eventually, through the emergence of autocatalysis – the ability of a molecule to take part in and catalyze its own synthesis (Calvin, 1961). These primitive systems undergoing a kind of chemical evolution would have become increasingly complex, and consequently, more unstable in the natural environment, thereby increasing the selective advantage of any new development which could partially isolate and protect the growing molecular aggregate. One of the great steps in this process must have been the emergence of a primitive kind of cellular organization, consisting of a semi-permeable membrane, or a simple boundary, which would have provided the necessary structural integrity and chemical stability.

In all probability, the development and evolution of life on other planets would follow similar lines, although there might well be expected to be differences in detail. The same basic chemical pathways would be expected to evolve wherever the geophysical conditions were favorable. As an example of this, one may consider the amino acids. These molecules, which form the backbones of proteins, are synthesized whenever energy is supplied to a mixture of methane, ammonia, hydrogen and water (Miller, 1953). Moreover, the amino acids which are formed are precisely the ones found in proteins, and they are produced with great ease. Therefore, wherever in the universe similar conditions prevail, the same amino acids would be expected to form, and proteins would probably play a similar role in an alien life form as they play in terrestrial organisms. Similar arguments can be made for other classes of biological compounds.

The situation is not really so simple as this, however, because there is considerable debate as to whether the initial chemical reactions which began the long chain of pre-

TABLE I

Characteristics of the planets (all data based on Earth = 1)

Planet	Average distance from Sun	Solar radiation received	Mass	Density
Mercury	0.39	7	0.05	0.97
Venus	0.72	2	0.81	0.93
Earth	1.00	1.00	1.00	1.00
Mars	1.52	0.4	0.11	0.72
Jupiter	5.20	0.04	317	0.24
Saturn	9.54	0.01	95	0.13
Uranus	19.2	0.003	14	0.28
Neptune	30.1	0.001	18	0.45
Pluto	39.5	0.0006	?	?

biological evolution can be traced back to the Earth's primordial atmosphere, or to a later period in geological history, when the Earth had lost most of its initial abundance of hydrogen (Abelson, 1966). The planets of the solar system may be divided roughly into two groups, those which have retained primordial atmospheres, and those which have not (Table I). In the former category are all the giant planets – Jupiter, Saturn, Uranus and Neptune, whose orbits lie beyond the orbit of Mars. Their atmospheres are largely hydrogen and helium, with smaller proportions of methane and ammonia. Water is not detectable, but is probably frozen out of the atmospheres. These giant planets have apparently retained their primordial atmospheres because of their great distance from the Sun, and consequent low temperatures. On the other hand, the inner planets are much smaller and more dense, having lost their primordial abundance of hydrogen which, being the lightest of all elements, readily escapes into space at a rate which is proportional to temperature.

Mercury has very little, if any, atmosphere left, and is, of course, very hot. Venus is something of an enigma. Its very dense nitrogen and carbon dioxide atmosphere may have been produced by melting of the crust, or by volcanic activity. A similar process may have occurred on the Earth, and carbon oxides and nitrogen, rather than methane and ammonia, could have prevailed at some period (Rubey, 1951). Chemical studies on such model atmospheres have generally produced many less biological products than are obtained from methane-ammonia mixtures, a fact which has been used as an argument for the relevancy of the latter system. In certain cases, however, the opposite has been true, suggesting the possibility that both epochs may have contributed significantly to the eventual appearance of life on the Earth (Ponnamperuma and Gable, 1968).

Because Venus has probably never been cool enough, and the giant planets, with the possible exception of Jupiter, never warm enough, Mars remains as the only other body in our solar system on which life may have had a good opportunity to evolve. At the present period in its history, however, Mars is a borderline case. Its very thin atmosphere (about 1% of Earth's and primarily composed of carbon dioxide) contains only traces of water. However, studies with simulated Martian environments, or 'Mars Jars' have demonstrated that common terrestrial microorganisms can survive, and even grow under such conditions. The Mariner IV photographs of the cratered surface of the planet produced some initial disappointment, although it has long been appreciated that the thin atmosphere would provide little protection to the surface, and little weathering to erase the marks of the inevitable meteorite impacts. Perhaps the disappointment was the subconscious result of Percival Lowell's theories of Martian canals, and the fiction of Edgar Rice Burroughs and H. G. Wells. Actually, however, subsequent analysis of the Mariner photographs has led to the conclusion that there are many fewer craters observable than would be expected on the basis of the expected infall rate for meteorites over the total history of the planet. This could be explained if the surface were geologically young, and if a considerably denser atmosphere has existed at an earlier period in Martian history. This possibility, of course, makes the presence of life on Mars much more likely (Anders and Arnold, 1965). Although it is difficult to imagine life evolving under the present conditions, life could have developed in an earlier, more favorable period, and may still survive.

The one piece of observational evidence which tends to support the theory of Martian life is the so-called 'wave of darkening' (Figure 1). Although Mars is an extremely difficult object to observe, it has long been clear that there are definite dark areas on the surface, and that these areas become progressively darker at certain times of the year (Tombaugh, 1968). The darkening appears to begin near the retreating polar cap in spring, and proceeds toward the equator. It has been calculated that this wave progresses at about the rate which would be expected for diffusion of water vapor away from a shrinking ice cap. The accelerated growth of organisms produced by the yearly arrival of water vapor could be responsible for the darkening. A related observation which tends to support this theory is the re-emergence of dark areas which have been lightened by dust storms, as if organisms were overgrowing the deposited light dust. Of course, nonbiological processes could be responsible for all of these observations, but the possibility of life on Mars is real enough to warrant extreme precautions in protecting the surface of the planet from biological contamination, and of course, the possibility of accidentally bringing back pathogenic organ-

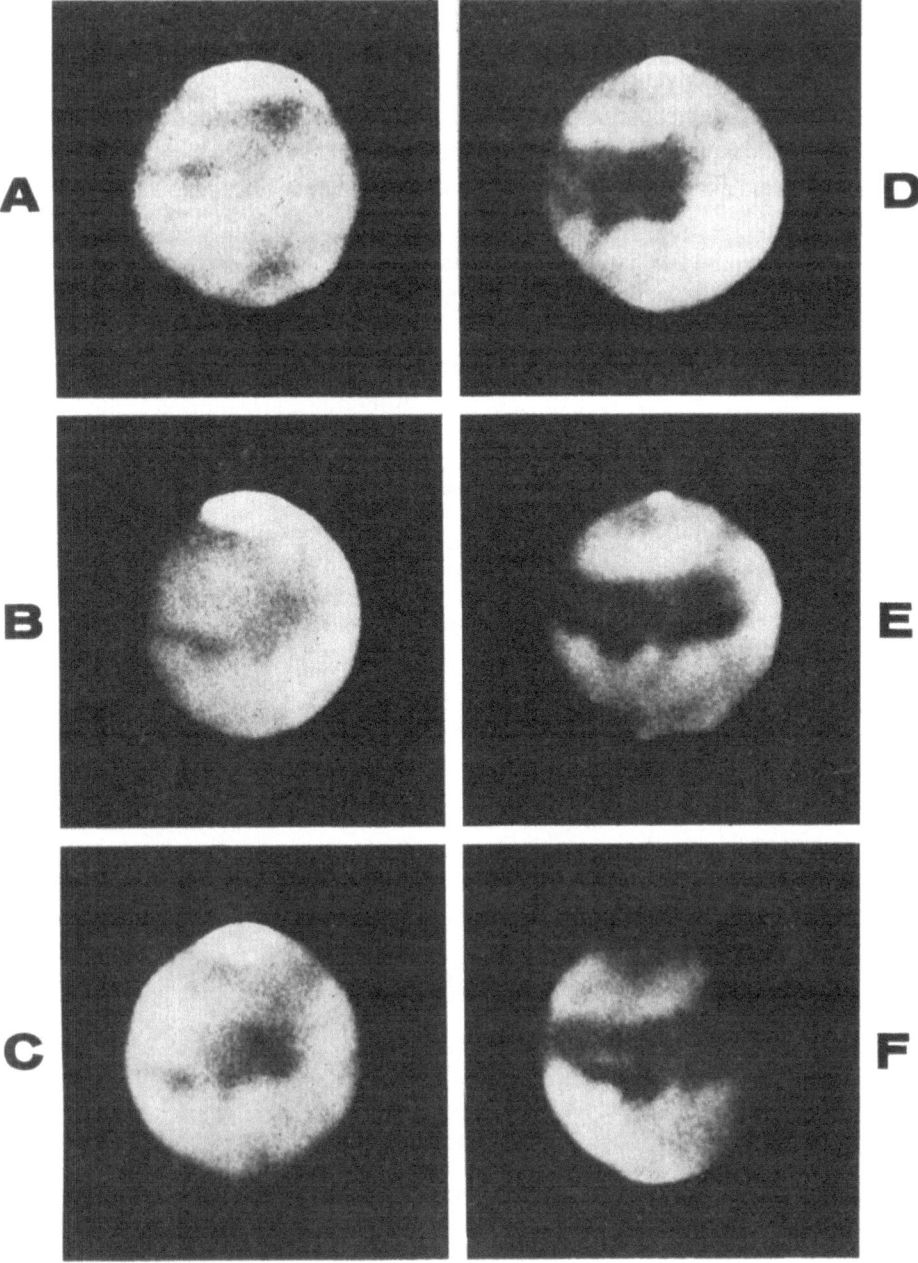

Fig. 1.   The wave of darkening on Mars. A to F, Martian dates March 10, May 11, May 30, June 23
August 1, and August 22 (from Slipher, 1962).

isms to Earth must also be guarded against. In this respect, the lunar quarantine program can be regarded as a valuable 'dress rehearsal' for Mars.

In 1975, the biological exploration of Mars will begin with the aid of instruments, designed to detect microbial metabolism. The first of these devices will perform very specific tasks. More advanced concepts may be equipped with computers and logic systems to design new experiments on the spot, in response to the results of initial exploratory tests. However ingenious the design of such robots, the final biological exploration of Mars must be conducted by that most versatile of all instruments – Man.

Positive responses received from a series of unmanned probes would, of course, eventually be followed by a complete ecological study of the planet, and the beginnings of a comparative Martian biochemistry. Even if no living organisms are detectable, the possibility of an extinct Martian biology must be investigated. This will require extensive geological study, a process which will, in any case, increase our understanding of the history of the solar system, and of the formation and evolution of the planets.

References

Abelson, P. H.: 1966, *Proc. Nat. Acad. Sci. U.S.* **55**, 1365.
Anders, E., and Arnold, J. R.: 1965, *Science* **149**, 1494.
Calvin, M.: 1961, *Chemical Evolution*, University of Oregon Press, Eugene, Oregon.
Fox, S. W. (ed.): 1965, *The Origins of Prebiological Systems*, Academic Press, New York.
Miller, S. L.: 1953, *Science* **117**, 528.
Miller, S. L. and Urey, H. C.: 1959, *Science* **130**, 245.
Ponnamperuma, C. and Gable, N. W.: 1968, *Space Life Sci.* **1**, 64.
Rubey, W. W.: 1951, *Bull. Geolog. Soc. Am.* **62**, 1111.
Slipher, E. C.: 1962, *The Photographic Story of Mars*. Sky Publishing Corp., Cambridge, Mass.
Tombaugh, C. W.: 1968, *Icarus* **8**, 227.

SECTION II

CLINICAL AVIATION MEDICINE

CORONARY RISK FACTORS AND PREVENTION

H. BLACKBURN

Laboratory of Physiological Hygiene, University of Minnesota, Minneapolis, Minn., U.S.A.

1. Introduction

The concept of coronary risk and the practical application of this concept among those men at excess risk is important for a number of reasons.

(1) A significant fraction of Coronary Heart Disease (CHD) cases is beyond any help from therapeutic medicine at the time the disease first becomes manifest (for example, those who die suddenly or unexpectedly).

(2) Another significant fraction of CHD cases dies of reinfarction or from sudden death in the first year after onset.

(3) Another significant fraction is not amenable to full rehabilitation, due to impaired coronary blood supply or poor ventricular mechanics.

(4) In the remainder, that is the fraction of CHD cases having a full functional recovery, the risk of death or reinfarction remains permanently elevated.

(5) CHD is the central and leading cause of death and disability among men of middle age leading affluent lives.

(6) Elements of risk can be identified and modified. It is demonstrated that characteristics related to risk in CHD may be simply and reliably measured, and that probability estimates may be made for the individual who is still in apparently good health, so that preventive measures can be concentrated among those at highest risk.

(7) It is possible to reduce significantly the characteristics of risk by simple, safe, palatable and hygienic approaches to more balanced living.

(8) It is likely that CHD risk can be safely reduced. The circumstantial evidence is strong. From the early experimental evidence available the chances appear good that reducing these risk factors will also reduce the risk of CHD.

(9) Recognition of excess risk can lead to constructive action toward leading more reasonable lives.

The concept is important in aerospace medicine because almost no CHD cases are re-entered into flight-related activities. Most are simply discharged from the industry and their vast experience is never again exploited.

2. The Essentiality of Prevention

Physicians in the United States are overwhelmed with the care of sick people, including many coronary patients. They are often unappreciative of the necessity of a preventive approach to reduce the overall CHD problem. In this country the mainstream of medical research effort in CHD goes into progressively more dramatic patchwork. This involves surgical revascularization, plastic arterial grafts, electronic pacemakers,

D. E. Busby (ed.), Recent Advances in Aerospace Medicine, 55–67. All Rights Reserved.

resection of poorly functioning ventricular myocardium and heroic experiments with mechanical pumps and cardiac transplants.

One can look at the best experience in the therapeutic approach to CHD, in terms of its overall impact on death from CHD. In Table I are 'guesstimates' based on current experience in the United States. At least 15% of the total mortality the first year after an initial myocardial infarction occurs in the first two hours after onset when little or no medical attention ever reaches the patient.

TABLE I

Estimated one year prognosis of coronary heart disease

Period	Per cent deaths		
	No coronary care unit	With coronary care unit	With mobile coronary service
0–2 hr	15	15	12
2 hr–4 weeks	20	13	13
4 weeks–1 yr	15	15	15
First year mortality	50%	43%	40%

Prior to establishing Coronary Care Units (CCU), the mortality in the first month of survivors who reach the better hospitals in the United States was and still is on the order of 20%. The mortality in the rest of the first year, among those who survive to leave the hospital, remains very high, about 15%, giving a 50% first-year mortality after infarction.

The best CCU experience in the second column of Table I has reduced the hospital mortality to the order of 13%, mostly from the control and therapy of serious cardiac arrhythmias. The CCU has not reduced the mortality from sudden death or among 1-month survivors leaving the hospital. The estimate here is generous in that it assumes the mortality rate of those surviving their attack because of the new and effective management of a CCU is the same as those surviving in institutions with no special coronary care. However, it is more likely that CCU survivors do somewhat less well than those who survive their hospital stay without CCU care. So, at best, special CCU in hospitals in the United States have reduced the first-year mortality after infarction from 50 to 43%; this is a highly significant reduction for those saved, and an important therapeutic advance, but is not a great lessening of the overall burden of CHD in the population.

In the last column of Table I, we speculate that skilled Mobile Coronary Services, and an associated educational program in their use, among the public and physicians, might eventually reduce by 20% the present mortality of the first 2 hours. An expert closer to the problem gives a much less optimistic appraisal (Lown et al., 1969). The overall first year CHD mortality might one day level off at 40% instead of 50%. This is a great step for a Man, but hardly a giant stride for Mankind.

TABLE II

Coronary heart disease mortality: survivorship after first infarction,
ages 45–54, compared to standard insureds (Lew, 1967)

	Survivorship rates		
	1 year	5 years	10 years
Standard	99%	98%	94%
Employed	93%	75%	55%
Disabled	93%	73%	48%
	Mortality ratios		
Standard	100%	100%	100%
Employed	1250%	650%	357%
Disabled	1750%	1000%	450%
	Life expectancy		
Standard	30 years		
Employed	18 years		
Disabled	13 years		

In Table II are some data among insured employees who survived a first myocardial infarct and, after a time, had a sufficiently good functional recovery to return to full-time employment (Lew, 1967). Their survival is compared to standard insurance experience in healthy employees and to the survival of those who remained disabled from CHD and were not re-employed.

It is clear that even in the most favorable cases of CHD, those who returned to work, the mortality rate, as the inverse of the survivorship given here, was 7% the first year, 25% the first 5 years, and 45% the first 10 years, compared to a mortality of 1, 2, and 6% in the standard employed population of men aged 45 to 54.

In the next portion of Table II, the relative risk of dying among those with CHD is given as a ratio to the rate found in standard lives. It is seen to be 12.5 times normal the first year after return to work, and 6.5 times normal the first 5 years. Even in men who survive up to 10 years there is still a three and one-half fold excess mortality post-infarction than among the normal population.

Thus the excess risk in survivors of infarction persists for years, probably permanently; the first year and immediate death rates are high, and the disability among survivors is great. Therapeutic medicine can palliate but not significantly reduce CHD, the most important disease burden of middle-aged affluent men.

3. Evidence for the Influence or the Predictive Power of So-called CHD Risk Factors

In studies such as those at Minnesota, Framingham, Albany, Ann Arbor, Chicago and Los Angeles, men were examined and classified in their apparently healthy state. Their subsequent CHD experience was related to their pre-disease physical characteristics at entry into the study. The data are generally consistent between the independently conducted U.S. studies. There is nothing new about these risk factors of hypertension and hyperlipemia. Mankind has had an 'excess of humors' since Greek medicine. Gluttony and sloth have been present since pre-history. Few physicians think smoking, elevated blood pressure or serum cholesterol are good for the individual. On the other hand, few physicians are constructively involved in the reduction of these factors. Such studies of individual risk characteristics have shown no consistent relationship of CHD incidence to height. Nor is total CHD rate significantly related to increasing class of relative weight or obesity, until one gets to the heaviest and fattest 20% of the population, where angina and intermediate episodes are significantly in excess. Infarction and CHD death are not related to measures of body build and composition.

Trends of CHD incidence or risk are clear and significant according to increasing levels of blood pressure and of serum cholesterol. The risk ratios for those in the highest 20% of the population values for these traits are on the order of 2 to 4. In other words, they have 2 to 4 times excess CHD risk compared to men with values in the lowest 20% of the population.

The same holds true for cigarette smoking. All these traits have crude predictive power even in the United States, where most men have high serum cholesterol levels and smoke.

Table III summarizes evidence on serum cholesterol levels from all major American follow-up studies relating entry serum cholesterol level to subsequent CHD incidence.

TABLE III

Relative incidence CHD in major U.S. studies by entry serum cholesterol level
(100 = age-specific rate for all men) (Keys, 1969)

Cholesterol, mg%	Under 200	200–219	220–239	240–259	260+
Coronary heart disease incidence	47	60	93	134	202

The standard rate of 100 is the rate of all groups combined, and matched by age. The standard rate for the group as a whole occurs at a cholesterol level near 240 mg% for American men. The rate for men 260 mg% or above is 4 times that of men with levels under 200 mg%. This difference is found despite the fact that the entire distribution of serum cholesterol is high in American men compared to many other countries. In that sense, the entire population is at greater risk.

Data being made available indicate that glucose intolerance, in the range under that of frank diabetes, is associated with increased CHD risk, and that the mechanisms involved may hold clues to the etiology of atherosclerosis.

Thus elevated blood pressure and blood lipids, and cigarette smoking are the major individual and most simply measurable factors related to CHD risk in otherwise healthy men followed over several years. These readily measurable, individual traits allow crude quantitative estimates of the probability of future CHD, in absolute terms over the periods studied (5 to 12 years), and in relative terms in comparing those men with elevated risk traits to those without them.

4. Combinations of Risk Factors

Next one can consider the evidence for CHD prediction from combinations of these risk factors in the same individual, and whether or not the risk is a multiple function of these traits. Table IV summarizes data from four major follow-up studies in the Unites States, listed in the left column. Different risk combinations are analyzed in the different studies. Men having all risk factors high are compared to those having all risk factors low. In the right hand column it is evident that simple measurement of traits such as blood pressure, blood cholesterol, body weight, and the cigarette smoking habit allow separation of men into classes with vastly different CHD risk probabilities, with risk differences on the order of from 4 to 13 times.

TABLE IV

Combined risk factors and coronary heart disease among men

Study	Risk factors	Men with all factors, %		'High'/ 'low' risk ratio
		'high'	'low'	
Albany-Framingham	Cholesterol Blood pressure Smoking	18	9	6.9
Western Elec. Co. Chicago	Cholesterol Blood pressure Smoking	6	25	4.1
Utility Co., Chicago	Cholesterol Blood pressure Smoking Weight	3	7	13.5
Civil servants, Los Angeles	Cholesterol Blood pressure Weight	14	17	4.4

Table V presents another evidence of the use of risk factors, here using data on seven risk factors among Framingham men (Kannel and McNamara, 1969). An arbitrary numerical value was assigned to each of the risk factors listed and a risk score computed for each man at the time of entry into the study. The entire distribution of these risk scores was laid out by decile classes from the lowest 10% of scores to the highest 10%. The multiple logistic combinations yielded high level predictions; no new CHD cases happened in those 10% (220) of men with the lowest risk scores, compared to 82 new cases among the 220 men with the highest risk scores.

The CHD incidence in these middle-aged men was 12%, or directly at the American average of 1% per year among 40–59 year old men. However, the CHD rates weer

TABLE V

Twelve-year incidence of coronary heart disease according
to decile of risk using multiple logistic function
(Kannel and McNamara, 1969)

Decile of risk*	2187 Men obs. cases	Observed 12-year incid/1000
10	82	375
9	44	201
8	31	142
7	33	151
6	22	101
5	20	91
4	13	59
3	10	34
2	3	14
1	0	0
Total	258	118

* Deciles of risk according to level of all following: age,
SPB, rel. wt., hb., no. cigs., ECG abn., chol.

quite different according to risk scores, even in a culture where the overall incidence
is high. Zero to 14/1000 was the rate in the lowest 20% of scores and 201 to 375 in the
highest 20%, better than one man in 3 for the highest 10% of the scores.

Table VI is the last approach presented here to analyses by CHD risk factors. It is
from the calculations of Dr. Epstein on American follow-up data and again is concerned with the efficiency of risk factors in identifying risk. Combinations of three
risk factors are involved (Epstein, 1967). The presence of two or more of them allows
prediction, over the subsequent 10 years, of 28 out of the 120 new events actually

TABLE VI

Predicting coronary heart disease (CHD) by means of two or three risk factors[a]
in men 40 to 59 years of age[b] (Epstein, 1967)

		Test results		
		Positive	Negative	Total
New events of CHD in 10 years	Yes (+)	28	92	120
(estimated)	No (−)	52	828	880
Total		80	920	1000

Sensitivity = $(28/120) \times 100 = 23\%$ Predictive value (+) = $(28/80) \times 100 = 35\%$

Specificity = $(828/880) \times 100 = 94\%$ Predictive value (−) = $(92/920) \times 100 = 10\%$

Risk ratio = $35/10 = 3.5$

[a] Positive test result: two of the following three – serum cholesterol more than 250 mg%; blood
pressure 'abnormal' (WHO criteria); left ventricular hypertrophy on electrocardiogram.
[b] Based on 8-year incidence data from the Framingham population.

occurring in that period, or 23% sensitivity of the criterion. At 23% sensitivity, 94% were identified of those who would remain free of the CHD during that 10-year period (specificity), or only 6% 'false positive' tests. The risk factor concept is a useful but not yet sufficiently sensitive approach to risk prediction. The nature of CHD, and of human biology is such that an ideal test, highly sensitive and specific, is not likely. One must apply the knowledge we have as long as its application is reasonable, safe and hygienic. Improvement may be eventually expected from the multiple-logistic approach to analysis and of course, from the addition over time of refined tests related to the fundamental defects of atherogenesis, thrombosis, myocardial ischemia and damage.

5. What is the Evidence that Reducing These Factors of Risk Makes Any Difference?

There are two general types of evidence available about the potential benefit of reducing CHD risk factors. One may be called circumstantial evidence; it is made from observations in natural experiments, examining the CHD incidence in men who live in different cultures and have different habits and risk characteristics. The other is from experimental evidence of the effect on CHD incidence of directly modifying certain risk attributes.

A. OBSERVATIONAL STUDIES

Table VII gives the results of systematically observed, documented CHD deaths in a 5-year follow-up of 12770 men (over 60000 man-years of observation). These are total populations of men in their communities, aged 40–59, from four contrasting geographic areas; the 'expected' number of deaths is calculated on the basis of rates in American vital statistics, by 5-year-age groups. The American groups observed and the Finnish populations experienced a 5-year CHD death rate similar to the expected rate for all American men. Two sizeable groups of men in the Mediterranean Basin experienced about one-tenth of this CHD death rate, though in the nature of circumstantial evidence, it is clear these men live under different natural experiences (Keys, 1969).

Table VIII shows the differences in measured, pre-disease characteristics for the same four populations. The American men are significantly heavier and more sedentary in occupation. The proportions of heavy smokers are not significantly different.

TABLE VII

Deaths from coronary heart disease among cohorts of men aged 40–59 followed for 5 years. The deaths 'expected' are calculated from 1962 death rates of U.S. white men age-matched by quinquennia
(Keys, 1969)

Cohort	No. of men	Number of deaths		
		Observed	Expected	O/E
U.S. railroad men	2576	66	59.7	1.11
East Finland	814	17	17.7	0.96
Dalmatia	669	1	18.0	0.06
Crete and Corfu	1212	4	27.7	0.14

Table IX shows the significant differences in mean serum cholesterol and frequency of blood pressure elevation. The American and Nordic men have significantly higher risk values than the Mediterranean men.

Table X shows that the habitual dietary consumption of saturated fatty acids is two to three times greater in the American and Finnish groups. Clearly men in free-living populations having different levels of measured risk characteristics have different CHD incidence.

B. WHAT IS THE EXPERIMENTAL EVIDENCE OF BENEFIT FROM MODIFICATION OF RISK TRAITS?

Table XI is a summary of the study of Leren in Oslo (Leren, 1966) among 412 post-infarct patients, randomized into a control group on a usual diet and an experimental

TABLE VIII

Characteristics of the cohorts of men (Keys, 1969)

Cohort	Mean relative body weight	% Heavy smokers	% Relatively sedentary
U.S. railroad men	104	22	52
East Finland	93	31	11
Dalmatia	91	23	8
Crete and Corfu	91	27	17

TABLE IX

Median serum cholesterol concentration, mg%, and percentage of men with high blood pressure (100 or more in diastole in rest) (Keys, 1969)

Cohort	Serum cholesterol	High blood pressure
U.S. railroad men	236	14%
East Finland	265	21%
Dalmatia	186	8%
Crete and Corfu	201	6%

TABLE X

Average percentage of total calories provided by total fats and by saturated (S) and polyunsaturated (P) fatty acids in the diets of the men (Keys, 1969)

Cohort	% Calories from			Median serum cholesterol, mg%
	Fat	S	P	
East Finland	39.2	22.1	2.9	265
U.S. railroad*	40	18	6	236
Dalmatia	29.5	9.3	6.7	186
Crete	40.3	7.7	2.5	203
Corfu	32.7	5.4	3.5	198

* Chemical composition estimated from tables of food composition.

group on a cholesterol reducing diet regimen of 39% fat calories; 9% of total calories was saturated fat, very close to the habitual Mediterranean diets. The average serum lipid level was unchanged in the control group, and fell 18% in the experimental group. The reinfarction and new angina rate was significantly reduced in the experimental group at ages under 60, but not among those over 60 years of age.

TABLE XI

Five-year incidence of coronary heart disease in men after first infarction (ages 30–69) in a controlled diet experiment in Norway (Leren, 1969)

	Diet	Control
No. of men at entry	206	206
Fatal relapse (fatal infarct + sudden death)	37	50
Non-fatal reinfarct	24	31
Major CHD relapse	61 ($P = 0.05$)	81
All cardiovascular deaths	38 ($P = 0.09$)	52

Table XII summarizes the data of Turpeinen (Turpeinen *et al.*, 1969) from an interesting population experiment in Helsinki. The 6-year CHD incidence was compared among healthy subjects in Mental Hospital K, kept on a usual Finnish diet, with that of Mental Hospital N in which the saturated fat intake of the diet was decreased one-half and the unsaturated fat intake increased 3 fold. An average difference of 50 mg% in serum cholesterol level was attained between the two hospitals and maintained for 6 years. The annual incidence of ECG-documented CHD and deaths from CHD was significantly different in the two institutions. A unique aspect of this study is that in 1965 the hospital diets were switched and a 6-year continuation goes on now in a cross-over design (Turpeinen *et al.*, 1969).

Several other dietary studies, including those on older men by Dayton in Veterans Administration Hospital domiciliary patients, of Christakis and Rinzler in New York, Bierenbaum in New Jersey, and Stamler in Chicago are less well controlled but show similar reductions in middle-aged and older subjects, post-infarction or at high risk.

Data on reduction of CHD by lowering of hypertension (115–129 mm Hg diastolic)

TABLE XII

Six-year incidence of coronary heart disease in a controlled closed population study in Finland (Turpeinen *et al.*, 1969)

	Hospital	
	N	K
Patients at risk	313	241
CHD: ECG or death	17	30
Annual incidence per 1000	14.4	33.0

Significance of difference:
$X^2 = 7.75$ $P < 0.01$

are available from the study of Freis in Veterans Administration Hospital patients, and are now becoming available for lesser elevations of blood pressure. In 21 months there were 27 severe cardiovascular events among the untreated experimental groups of hypertensives *versus* 2 in the treated group. The study was stopped (Freis, 1967).

6. Constructive Guidelines to CHD Risk and Coronary Prevention

The evidence is clear that simple measurements will identify men at excess risk of future CHD and death. The evidence is also clear that characteristics of risk can be modified. The evidence is suggestive that modification of risk is desirable and that actual CHD risk is thereby reduced.

How is this information handled in the worlds of medical practice and industrial medicine? It is largely ignored. The physician accustomed to deal with the ill characteristically believes that people and disease are highly variable, that this sort of prediction applied to the individual is equivalent to the prognostication of gypsies, and that there is no causal proof in these relationships; so he takes no action. This understandable but unfortunate attitude results in a loss of many positive opportunities, for example, in aeromedicine, to direct young people at highest risk away from flight operations early. This laissez-faire attitude avoids action of a safe and constructive nature to modify risk and improve the living pattern of those at excess risk; it prevents a responsible look by industry at its major health problem, including that among flight personnel.

But one of the first problems, if reasonable measures are undertaken, is the one of where, along the curve of risk, does one decide to take action? All are aware of the arbitrariness of such decisions about risk; the most obvious example is at what age to retire men from flying. The group curve of risk by age is generally a smooth one with no very sharp bend above which the accident or death rate is great, or below which it is negligible. The same is true with risk related to serum cholesterol and blood pressure and to overall risk scores. Of course, there is an intimate relationship between the curves of age, these risk factors, and frequency of CHD.

A. 'EXCESSIVE' RISK

'Excessive' CHD risk may be considered that on the order of 4 times (400%) the expected value. This risk is found in about 5% of middle-aged American men who are apparently healthy and productive, but in fact have risk equivalent to the risk encountered with serious manifest diseases. Generally, individuals at this level of risk, according to age, should be treated the same as individuals with serious chronic diseases of the brain, lung, kidney, gastrointestinal tract, *etcetera*.

If risk levels of this order are found at the time of pre-employment examination, they probably should exclude the applicant from flight operations. The alternative is to give a postponed status until the excessive risk is confirmed on later examination and favorably modified over a trial period.

If excessive risk is found in periodic examinations of flight personnel, these individuals probably should be grounded until the excessive risk status is confirmed and favorably modified over a trial period.

B. 'AVERAGE' RISK

For individuals with average, or somewhat above average risk (up to 2 times the expected risk), it is appropriate to recommend a general preventive program with positive educational efforts made toward hygienic, balanced living. No special attention and advice or follow-up is given but an educational program of energy balance, elimination of cigarette smoking, and prompt management of any hypertensive or diabetic tendencies is proposed. This leaves a sizeable and important group at 'Intermediate' levels of excess CHD risk.

C. 'INTERMEDIATE' RISK

CHD risk on the order of twice expected up to 4-fold risk, is an arbitrary but convenient class below which only the general hygienic principles mentioned are encouraged. But in this class definitive action should be required and programs provided. Table XIII gives the minimum criteria for this level of risk for the American Heart Association risk recommendations. This action should consist of a distinct confrontation

TABLE XIII

American Heart Association recommended
treatment levels of risk factors*

Cholesterol	> 260 mg%
Triglycerides	> 250 mg%
Blood pressure	> 160/95 mm Hg
Body weight	> 130%
Uric acid	> 7.5 mg%
Glucose intolerance	Any
ECG Abnormalities	Any
Cigarette smoking	Habitual

* Levels represent approximately double risk of CHD, compared to those with lower values, among U.S. middle-aged men.

between the individual employee and the industrial physician, an explanation of the risk concept as separate from the disease concept, information about the general level of excess risk involved, and education, resources and encouragement given toward a positive hygienic approach. Visits should then be regular for instructions, for checking progress, and for reinforcement. Group efforts are highly applicable in this class of risk. Elements of a program are:

(1) Diet – the American Heart Association recommended diet is good for hyperlipidemias, the obese, the hypertensive, diabetic and their families.

(2) Smoking – stop permanently.

(3) Blood pressure therapy, adequate and permanent.

(4) Exercise – a rational and cautious approach is indicated until more is known, but starting people moving again (walking) is advised.

(5) Drugs are not a major part of the solution to the CHD problem. They attack only one factor at a time and are not a solution to a vast problem of social origins. They are used in extreme cases of risk or in failure of a hygienic program to favorably modify the elevated factor.

Much material is available from the American Heart Association, including a recent summary of experience in preventive programs of diet, exercise, blood pressure and smoking, in a Symposium on Prevention in Cardiology available from that association at 44 East 23rd Street, New York City. The general principles of prevention of cardiovascular disease, and specific advice, are well summarized in the *Lectures in Preventive Cardiology* by Jeremiah Stamler (published by Grune and Stratton, 1967).

Finally, when responsible flight personnel are demonstrated to be at excess CHD risk, the preventive program should be made clear. There should be no failure on the medical side to provide the best of information and most positive of advice. Flight safety and personal hygiene would then both depend on the maturity of the pilot.

A well-informed pilot, knowing his excessive risk status but engaged in an active prevention program, and who is disciplined to observe himself and to relinquish control of his aircraft at any moment of malaise, is a considerably better relative risk than his usual senior pilot counterpart who is uninformed. The latter individual often denies or accepts fatalistically the excess risk of his way of life without constructive action. He, like the captain of a sailing ship, would not consider turning over the controls of his aircraft if there were a breath of life left in him. He is increasingly harried, sedentary, tobacco- and alcohol-dependent, and lives on an affluent high-saturated fat diet. He is very much like some of us, his physicians.

7. Summary of the force of Risk Factors and the Argument for CHD prevention

Therapeutic medicine cannot control the modern problem of atherosclerosis and its complications, because the disease is advanced when it becomes manifest, and because it is an epidemic largely of a social nature, related to our way of life. It therefore requires a social-medical approach to its elimination.

Serum cholesterol and serum triglyceride levels, based on an average of two determinations, allow adequate classification of the risk due to elevated lipids. These data identify those most amenable to diet change, and those who may require more vigorous therapy. Serum lipids are a major and largely correctable risk factor in CHD mortality.

The arterial pressure level, based on an average of several determinations, allows adequate classification of the risk due to elevated pressure. It identifies those requiring special anti-hypertensive therapy. Systolic pressure is as good a predictor of CHD as is the diastolic pressure. Elevated blood pressure is a major risk factor in CHD and generally is susceptible to correction. Much or most of the risk of future CHD can be accounted for by measuring serum lipids and blood pressure.

The cigarette smoking habit provides important information about future risk of myocardial infarction and mortality; this information is additive to that obtained from serum lipids and blood pressure. It also is amenable to favorable modification.

Body weight is a poor predictor of CHD risk, and relative body weight is a weak predictor of risk throughout most of the range of values. Skin-fold measurement is slightly superior, but is a relatively weak risk factor, being poorly related to CHD risk through most of the distribution of values. Individuals in the upper 10% to 20% of the distribution are at slightly excess risk, and are more likely to have elevated blood pressure and decreased glucose tolerance. The obesity problem is correctable.

Physical activity habits are a weak predictor of future CHD risk. Long-term activity affords little protection from CHD in areas with unfavorable dietary habits. Survival may be improved, and activity can be important in reducing other risk factors, so correction of sedentary habits is possible and recommended.

Family history of CHD provides little information about future CHD risk which is not available from measureable, inherited characteristics of blood lipids, glucose and blood pressure. This does not rule out a familial or hereditary effect, but it is largely disguised and overwhelmed by the environmentally determined risk influences.

The electrocardiogram is not a risk factor itself but rather a risk predictor which represents myocardial involvement and an increased likelihood of greater, later involvement. It is a weak predictor in terms of the yield, but when any of a number of distinct ECG findings are present their prognostic significance is strong and largely independent of information from other risk measures.

The addition of multiple-factor analytical programs and eventually of more specific tests, such as hormonal assays, immunological reactions and enzyme deficiency tests, should improve increasingly the quantitative characterization of risk now based on crude risk traits.

Knowledge available indicates that it is possible, safe and desirable to modify elevated CHD risk factors.

Acknowledgments

Data provided here are from studies supported in part by grants as follows: to Professor Ancel Keys (USPHS HE-04697 and the American Heart Association); to Professor Henry Taylor (USPHS HE-03088); and to Professor Henry Blackburn through the Cardiovascular Center Grant (USPHS HE-06314).

References

Epstein, F. H.: 1967, *J.A.M.A.* **201**, 795.
Freis, E. D.: 1967, *J.A.M.A.* **202**, 1028.
Kannel, W. B. and McNamara, D. M.: 1969, *Minnesota Med.* **52**, 1197.
Keys, A.: 1969, *Minnesota Med.* **52**, 1191.
Leren, P.: 1966, *Acta Med. Scand.*, Suppl. 466.
Lew, E. A.: 1967, *Amer. J. Publ. Health* **57**, 118.
Lown, B., Klein, M. D., and Hershberg, P. I.: 1969, *Amer. J. Med.* **46**, 705.
Turpeinen, O., Miettinen, M., Karvonen, M. J. *et al.*: 1969, *Minnesota Med.* **52**, 124 7.

EXPERTISE CARDIOLOGIQUE ET PERSONNEL NAVIGANT: SES PRINCIPALES DIFFICULTÉS

R. CARRÉ, J. C. RICHART, J. SALVAGNIAC et F. PLAS

C.P.E.M.P.N. Ministère de l'Air, Boulevard Victor, Paris 15, France

1. Introduction

L'aptitude aux emplois du personnel navigant requiert l'intégrité absolue, organique et fonctionnelle, de l'appareil circulatoire. Cette étude analyse les principales difficultés cardiologiques rencontrées dans l'expertise du personnel navigant.

2. Anomalies électrocardiographiques

(a) En l'absence de tout signe clinique évocateur, il est difficile devant une atypie du segment ST ou de l'onde T, de poser un diagnostic, car le diagnostic de l'intégrité coronarienne est un des problèmes les plus importants posés aux médecins experts. Avant 1946, ces atypies de la repolarisation étaient considérées comme des manifestations de coronarite. Mais depuis cette date, ce diagnostic a été remis en cause tant en France où Plas (1950) observe ces atypies chez les navigants et les sportifs, qu'à l'étranger où Wendkers et Logue (1946) étudient ces altérations dans leurs rapports avec l'asthénie neuro-circulatoire. Les atypies de la repolarisation bénignes, d'étiologie indéterminée, ont en commun un certain nombre de caractères:

(1) Localisation quasi élective sur D2, D3, VF et les précordiales gauches V5 à V7.

(2) Leur instabilité dans le temps. Ces atypies varient d'une heure à l'autre, d'un jour à l'autre, sans qu'il soit possible de déterminer le facteur causal de cette variation. Cette variation dans le temps n'est pas constante. Certains sujets ont des altérations durables pendant des semaines ou des mois; chez d'autres, on constate des variabilités fantaisistes avec one onde T négative le matin, positive l'après-midi, sans que rien n'explique cette variabilité.

(3) Leur labilité sous l'influence de diverses épreuves fonctionnelles ou pharmaco-dynamiques (Tableau I).

(a) Epreuve d'effort: Nous pratiquons soit une épreuve d'effort de 150 watts pendant 5 min à la bicyclette ergométrique, soit une épreuve de Martinet (20 flexions sur les jambes). Au cours de cette épreuve d'effort les tracés peuvent s'améliorer ou se normaliser et le diagnostic 'd'asthénie neuro-circulatoire' est facilement porté. Mais le diagnostic 'avec ischémie coronarienne' est plus délicat quant au cours d'une épreuve d'effort l'onde T, d'abord plate, se creuse surtout en D2, D3. Rappelons qu'un aplatissement de T2 ou une inversion de T3 est une constatation banale sur un tracé enregistré au cours du travail musculaire est, de ce fait, et bien connu en médecine sportive.

(b) Epreuve d'anoxémie en caisson à dépression (palier de 20 min à l'altitude de

TABLEAU I

Épreuves pratiquées chez les sujets porteurs d'atypies de la repolarisation bénignes, d'étiologie indéterminée

Épreuves	Nombre d'épreuves pratiquées	Tracés améliorés ou normalisés	Tracés aggravés	Tracés non influencés
Épreuve d'effort (Martinet)	61	35	10	16
Épreuve du caisson (20 min à 5000 m)	59	16	24	19
Surcharge-potassique (6 g de KCl)	54	20	6	28
Gynergène (0.5 mg)	39	23	3	13

8000 m dont le point d'impact n'est pas forcément, comme on le croyait, une anoxémie myocardique mais plus vraisemblablement une hypoxie des cellules nerveuses dont l'effort se fait sentir sur le myocarde par l'intermédiaire du sympathique).

(c) Injection sous cutanée de 0.8 mg de tartrate d'ergotamine.

(d) Ingestion de 6 g de chlorure de potassium.

Il existe des discordances dans les résultats de ces quatre épreuves. Lorsque l'électrocardiogramme est amélioré ou normalisé par une de ces épreuves, on pense qu'il s'agit d'altérations bénignes. Mais il est plus difficile de conclure lorsque ces tracés sont ou aggravés ou non influencés. Tabusse et Pannier (1965) ont rapporté deux observations trompeuses et montrent qu'il faut être prudents dans l'interprétation isolée de la repolarisation. En définitive, les enseignements que l'on peut espérer obtenir des diverses épreuves d'effort, d'anoxie, ou pharmacodynamiques, ne nous permettent pas une conclusion.

Devant les anomalies de la repolarisation, nous appliquons la règle suivante:

(1) A l'admission: lorsque ces anomalies de la repolarisation sont patentes et non corrigibles par les épreuves envisagées ci-dessus, la décision prise est une décision de prudence; l'inaptitude temporaire, au besoin de quelques mois, est prononcée donnant à l'expert un recul suffisant.

(2) Aux examens révisionnels: inaptitude si le moindre doute plane sur l'intégrité coronarienne. Aptitude, ou inaptitude temporaire, lorsque rien ne permet d'évoquer une altération coronarienne.

(b) Les aspects de bloc droit incomplet fréquemment rencontrés nous paraissent compatibles avec l'aviation si la durée totale de QRS ne dépasse pas 0.12 sec, si l'aspect de bloc en V1, du type rSr', reste immuable ou disparaît lors de l'épreuve de Flack, ou endurance test, à 40 mm Hg. En effet, une étude statistique faite au Centre Principal d'Expertise Médicale du Personnel Navigant de Paris a montré que ces aspects de bloc droit incomplet étaient retrouvés chez 12% des candidats à l'admission;

que cette fréquence était d'autant plus grande que le groupe des sujets examinés était jeune. Aussi peut-on considérer que, très souvent, ces aspects de bloc droit incomplet susceptibles de disparaître sous l'influence de la rotation du cœur malgré l'hyperpression ventriculaire droite provoquée par la manœuvre de Flack, ne sont qu'un aspect purement physiologique de l'électrocardiogramme juvénile. Il serait donc abusif d'éliminer automatiquement les sujets porteurs de ces aspects.

(c) Le syndrome de Wolff-Parkinson-White a été défini par ces auteurs, en 1930, comme une anomalie électrocardiographique comportant: rythme sinusal, intervalle PR court, inférieur à 0.11 sec, existence d'une onde delta, et élargissement du complexe QRS supérieur à 0.08 sec. Nous trouvons que sa prévalence est du même ordre que celle des auteurs de l'U.S. Air Force, de l'ordre de 1.5/1000 (Averill *et al.*, 1960). Nous avons réuni 40 observations de Wolff-Parkinson-White, dont 8 sont intermittents. Mais notre opinion diverge des auteurs anglo-saxons sur l'aptitude au vol. Nous éliminons les candidats porteurs de cette anomalie, en raison:

(1) du risque non négligeable de tachycardie paroxystique;

(2) la possibilité de coexistence de cardiopathies de diagnostic parfois difficile, telles que cardiomégalie familiale ou cardiomyopathie obstructive;

(3) une observation privilégiée de Wolff-Parkinson-White intermittent a permis, grâce aux enregistrements mécanographiques, de montrer que l'intervalle electro-mécanique (Q-pied d'apexogramme) était allongé tandis que les temps de contraction pré-isométrique et isométrique étaient normaux, mettant ainsi en évidence in allongement du temps de conduction dans ce syndrome.

3. Difficulté dans l'interprétation des souffles systoliques

Nous avions déjà exposé au Congrès International de Lisbonne ce problème et nous voudrions simplement en rapporter les points essentiels. L'auscultation cardiaque aidée des examens complémentaires que sont l'électrocardiogramme et la radiographie cardiaque suffisent, dans la majorité des cas, à affirmer l'organicité ou l'anorganicité d'un souffle systolique. Dans quelques cas, la clinique se trouve en défaut; dans ces cas vu l'importance du diagnostic d'organicité pour la détermination de l'aptitude au personnel navigant, il paraît utile de s'aider de techniques non sanglantes que sont les mécanogrammes cardiaques (Tableaux II et III).

Les techniques mécanographiques que nous employons sont les suivantes:

(1) Phonocardiogramme, avec quatre bandes de fréquence, pris au niveau d'auscultation du souffle systolique.

(2) L'étude du carotidogramme porte sur deux éléments: étude de la morphologie du tracé, et étude des chronologies des divers accidents de la courbe: temps d'ascension, temps de $\frac{1}{2}$ ascension, et durée de l'éjection ventriculaire gauche.

(3) Apexogramme.

(4) Epreuves dynamiques, comprenant:

(a) La manœuvre de Valsalva qui permet d'affirmer que le souffle est gauche ou

TABLEAU II

Mécanogrammes des souffles systoliques anorganiques.

	Souffles systoliques anorganiques		
	Souffle infundibulo-pulmonaire	Souffle cardio-pulmonaire	Souffle anorganique aortique
Phonocardiogramme	Souffle d'ejection droit	Variabilité	Souffle d'ejection gauche
Carotidogramme	N	N	Anacrotisme
Apexogramme	N	N	N

TABLEAU III

Mécanogrammes des souffles systoliques organiques

	Souffles systoliques organiques					
	R.A.	C.M.O.	Insuffisance mitrale	C.I.A.	C.I.V.	Coarctation aortique
Phono-cardiogramme	Souffle d'éjection gauche	Souffle d'éjection gauche	Souffle de régurgita-tion gauche	Souffle d'éjection droit	Souffle de régurgita-tion gauche	Souffle d'éjection gauche
Carotidogramme	(1) Anomalies morpholo-giques (2) Anomalies chronolo-giques	(1) Type I Bulge (2) Type II	N	N	N	N
Apexogramme	Onde A	(1) Bifidité (2) Onde A	Onde E	N	N	N

droit. Dans le souffle d'origine droite, le souffle prend à la fin de l'épreuve son intensité maximum; alors, qu'à l'inverse pour le souffle d'origine gauche, il ne devient maximum que cinq systoles suivant l'arrêt de l'épreuve.

(b) Epreuves pharmacodynamiques avec prise de tracés après: épreuve au nitrite d'amyle ou l'isuprel, complétée par les épreuves aux substances vaso-pressives (aramine, methoxamine). Les tracés phonocardiographiques permettent de reconnaître si le souffle systolique est d'éjection ou de régurgitation.

A la suite des travaux de Leatham, on peut, en effet, opposer point pour point ces deux souffles. Le souffle d'éjection est losangique, naît à distance de B1, n'atteint pas B2, est renforcé après pause extrasystolique, l'épreuve au nitrite d'amyle ou l'isuprel et est diminué par l'aramine ou methoxamine. A l'inverse, le souffle de regurgitation est rectangulaire, holosystolique, va de B1 à B2, n'est pas renforcé après pause extrasystolique, est diminué par l'épreuve au nitrite d'amyle ou l'isuprel et est renforcé par l'épreuve à l'aramine ou methoxamine.

Nous étudierons les aspects mécanographiques des souffles systoliques qui posent un problème à l'expert de médecine aéronautique.

(1) Le souffle infundibulopulmonaire – ou souffle de Tripier-Devic, est un souffle systolique siegeant dans la région parasternale gauche à la partie interne du 2ème ou 3ème espace intercostal gauche. Le mécanisme du souffle est l'engouffrement du sang dans un orifice pulmonaire jouant le rôle de rétrécissement fonctionnel. Ce sera un souffle d'éjection droit. Du point de vue morphologique, on remarquera que le souffle est protosystolique accolé au 1er bruit, laissant libre la meso et la télésystole.

(2) Les souffles cardiopulmonaires ou souffle de Potain, ne naissent pas au niveau d'un orifice du cœur et varient considérablement avec les phases dy cycle respiratoire et la position du patient. Sur les tracés, le souffle n'a aucun caractère précis et ceci se comprend en fonction de son mécanisme. Il varie de morphologie d'une systole à l'autre et varie en fonction du cycle respiratoire. La pharmacodynamie n'apporte rien de précis.

(3) La cardiomyopathie obstructive est une affection de connaissance récente réalisant un obstacle à l'éjection ventriculaire gauche. Donc, le tracé du phonocardiogramme visualisera un souffle d'éjection, type gauche. Le carotidogramme joue un rôle essentiel dans le diagnostic.

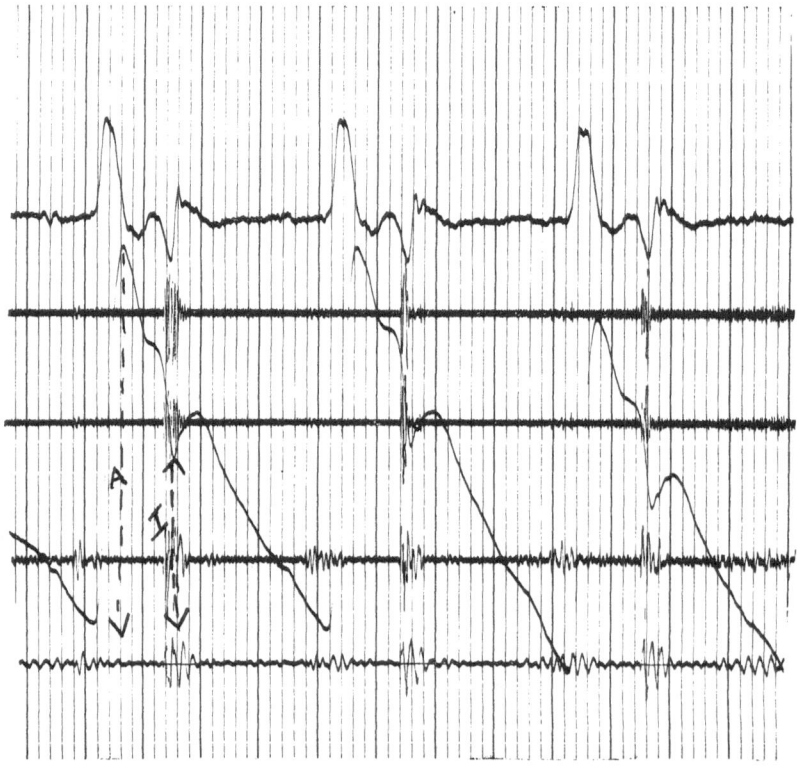

Fig. 1.   Carotidogramme d'un sujet de 20 ans. De haut en bas (1) dérivée première du carotidogramme; (2) carotidogramme; (3) 4 bandes de phonocardiogramme.

Avec Coblence *et al.* (1965) on peut distinguer deux types. Le type I comporte sur la portion descendante, après une brusque descente, suivie d'un creux, une nouvelle onde positive moins élevée que la première, surnommée par les auteurs américains, 'systolic bulge'. Ce signe n'est pas tout à fait pathognomonique puisque, avec Pernod et Kermarec nous l'avons rencontré dans 20 tracés sur les 1000 tracés pris chez les sujets normaux. Le type II présente, après une ascension accélérée, un sommet aigu suivi d'une descente très rapide à aspect concave. L'apexogramme est quelquefois bifide et peut présenter une petite onde a.

4. Étude de l'élasticité de la paroi artérielle

Dans une étude statistique portant sur une période de 12 ans, de 1955 à 1966 inclus, dans les Centres d'Expertise Médicale du Personnel Navigant, nous avions trouvé que c'est le groupe des affections cardiovasculaires qui fournit le taux d'inaptitudes le plus élevé (30%, soit presque le $\frac{1}{3}$ des inaptitudes pour maladies), et en particulier dans les tranches d'âge entre 40 et 50 ans. Ces chiffres justifient à eux seuls qu'après 40 ans l'expertise révisionnelle soit plus spécialement orientée vers le dépistage de l'athéro-sclérose. Certes, nous pratiquons un dosage de cholestérol, Kunkel phénol, Burnstein,

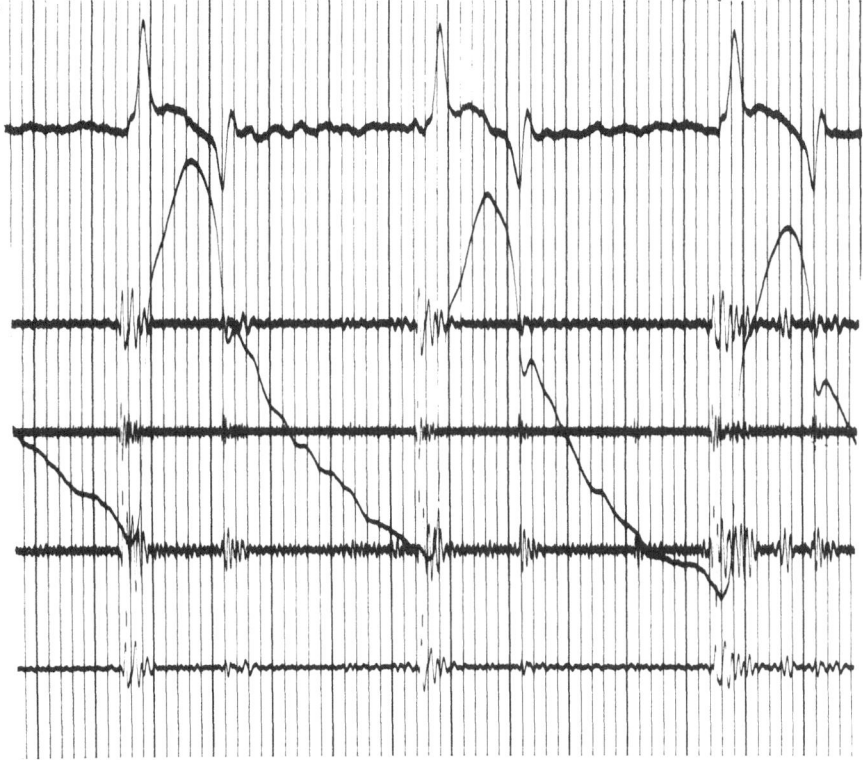

Fig. 2.   Carotidogramme du sujet de 50 ans. De haut en bas (1) dérivée première du carotidogramme; (2) carotidogramme; (3) 4 bandes de phonocardiogramme.

glycémie et acide urique, mais ces dosages ne nous apportent guère de renseignements.

Une étude statistique portant sur 1000 tracés nous avait montré que le carotido-gramme évolue avec l'âge (Figures 1 et 2); le deuxième sommet systolique progresse le long du segment descendant jusqu'à dépasser le premier sommet et aboutir au tracé de type anacrote. En même temps, nous constatons avec l'âge que le rapport hauteur de l'incisure catacrote sur amplitude de l'onde pulsatile augmente (rapport I/A augmente). Une étude faite au C.E.R.M.A. par Nogues *et al.*, 1969, a montré que ce rapport *I/A* est le reflet de la distensibilité artérielle.

Le carotidogramme, procédé non sanglant et facilement reproductible de ce fait, devrait être pratiqué systématiquement après 40 ans.

Bibliographie

Averill, K. H., Fosmoe, R. J., et Lamb, L. E.: 1960, *Amer. J. Cardiol.* **6**, 108.

Coblence, B., Gerbeaux, A., Aujuère, J., *et al.*: 1965, *Arch. des maladies du cœur et des vaisseaux* **58**, 776.

Nogues, C., Carré, R., Kermarec, J., *et al.*: 1969, *Rev. Méd. Aéro. et Spatiale* **8**, 22.

Pernod, J. Carré, R., et Vasile, N.: 1966, XVème Congrès International de Médecine Aéronautique et Cosmonautique, Prague, 1966.

Pernod, J. Carré, R., et Kermarec, J.: 1967a, *Soc. Méd. Milit. Française* **61**, 153.

Pernod, J., Coblence, B., Carré, R., *et al.*: 1967b, *Arch. des maladies du cœur et des vaisseaux* **60**, 1241.

Pernod, J., Carré, R., Vasile, N. et Kermarec, J.: 1969, *Arch. des maladies du cœur et des vaisseaux* **62**, 1941.

Plas, F.: 1950, *Presse Méd.* **58**, 285.

Tabusse, L. et Pannier, R.: 1965, *Rev. Méd. Aéro.* III,16.

Wendkers, M. H. et Logue, R. B.: 1946, *Amer. Heart J.* **31**, 711.

Wolff, L., Parkinson, J., *et* White, P. D.: 1930, *Amer. Heart J.* **5**, 685.

SYNDROME DE WOLFF-PARKINSON ET WHITE ET APTITUDE AU PERSONNEL NAVIGANT

R. CARRÉ, J. C. RICHART, J. SALVAGNIAC et F. PLAS

C.P.E.M.P.N. Ministère de l'Air, Boulevard Victor, Paris 15, France

1. Introduction

C'est sous le vocable de 'bloc de branche avec intervalle PR court chez des sujets jeunes', prédisposés aux tachycardies paroxystiques, que Wolff, Parkinson et White, en 1930, découvrent cette curiosité électrocardiographique. Dans ce travail, nous apportons un certain nombre d'observations recrutées sur une population d'adultes jeunes réputés bien portants, et nous étudierons ce syndrome sous l'angle de l'expertise médico-aéronautique.

2. Définition du syndrome de Wolff-Parkinson-White (WPW)

En dehors des crises de tachycardies paroxystiques, ce syndrome est purement électrique. Rappelons donc, brièvement, les signes électriques caractéristiques de cette affection:

(1) Existence d'ondes 'P' sinusales. Il est capital de rappeler que dans ce syndrome le pacemaker reste le nœud sinusal.

(2) Raccourcissement de l'espace PR. La majorité des auteurs s'accordent pour lui attribuer une valeur inférieure à 0.11 sec.

(3) Elargissement du complexe QRS qui devient supérieur à 0.08 sec; ce phénomène est dû à une anomalie particulière du complexe ventriculaire. Il s'agit d'un empatement de l'onde initiale ascendante plus communément nommée onde 'delta'. Cette onde delta est positive si QRS est positif et négative si QRS est négatif.

(4) L'espace PJ s'étendant du début de P à la fin de QRS reste dans les limites de la normale, soit inférieur à 0.20 sec. Cette notion permet de distinguer le WPW du bloc de branche au cours duquel cet espace est constamment allongé.

(5) Retard d'apparition de la deflexion intrinsècoïde dans les précordiales gauches si le tracé est du type B, ou dans les précordiales droites si le tracé est du type A.

(6) Enfin, existence fréquente d'anomalie du segment ST qui peut être sus ou sous dénivelé, et de troubles secondaires de la repolarisation avec opposition des axes de QRS et de T.

Mais il faut savoir que ces différentes anomalies ne sont pas constantes. Elles peuvent en effet, sur un même tracé, alterner avec des complexes normaux, parfois même de façon régulière, donnant l'impression d'un bigemminisme. L'espace PR peut croître progressivement tandis que QRS diminue de la même façon, seul l'espace PJ restant constant. Toutes ces variations peuvent survenir spontanément ou être observées sous

D. E. Busby (ed.), Recent Advances in Aerospace Medicine, 75–79. All Rights Reserved.
Copyright © 1970 by D. Reidel Publishing Company, Dordrecht-Holland.

l'influence de l'effort, de la stimulation vagale, ou de drogues telles que l'atropine, la digitaline, la quinidine ou l'ajmaline. Enfin, quelle que soit l'influence de ces différentes causes, le tracé peut redevenir strictement normal.

On distingue schématiquement deux types principaux dans le WPW syndrome.

(1) *Le Groupe A*, qui présente les caractéristiques suivantes:

(a) l'axe de QRS est dévié à droite de +30 deg et situé aux alentours de 120 deg;

(b) les complexes ventriculaires restent positifs dans toutes les dérivations précordiales;

(c) le retard à la deflexion intrinsècoïde est surtout net dans les précordiales droites;

(d) l'étude des dérivations oesophagiennes et intra-cardiaques montre que l'activation ventriculaire s'effectue de haut en bas, d'arrère en avant et de gauche à droite.

(2) *Le Groupe B*, est plus fréquent:

(a) l'axe de QRS est à gauche de +30 deg. Parfois une forte déviation axiale est responsable de l'aspect QS en D3, VF; aspect faisant penser à tort à un infarctus postéro-diaphragmatique;

(b) les complexes ventriculaires sont plus à gauche et négatifs en précordiales droites;

(c) les dérivations endo-cavitaires montrent que le processus d'activation s'effectue de droite à gauche, de bas en haut et d'avant en arrière.

Tels sont donc caractérisés les deux grands groupes les plus fréquemment observés chez les malades porteurs de ce syndrome électrique. Mais il existe un certain nombre de formes intermédiaires comme le souligne Coelibo.

Pour être complet, il faut compléter cette étude électrique par des notions de vectocardiographie. On met ainsi en évidence un rapprochement des repères chronologiques dans la partie initiale, centrifuge de la boucle QRS et une opposition de direction entre le point S et l'onde T d'une part, la boucle R d'autre part. Rappelons, enfinque le vectocardiogramme frontal montre que dans 75% des cas les premiers vecteurs anormaux se dirigent à gauche de +60 deg; dans 25% des cas à droite de +60 deg.

Telle est donc rapidement résumée la définition électrique du syndrome WPW typique. Mais en tant qu'expert en médecine aéronautique, nous voudrions insister sur les variantes cliniques et surtout sur les états frontières de ce syndrome.

Comme variantes électriques, on peut retenir:

(a) soit un syndrome associant un espace PR normal avec complexe QRS élargi et existence d'une onde delta;

(b) soit une anomalie électrique où le complexe QRS est de durée normale mais avec une onde delta;

(c) et comme état frontière, l'association de QRS normal mais espace PR court inférieur à 0.11 sec ou syndrome de Cristescu.

A l'expertise du personnel navigant, nous rencontrons fréquemment cette anomalie et la question que nous voudrions poser: doit-on retenir cette anomalie comme une variation du syndrome WPW avec ses répercussions sur l'aptitude au vol, ou comme une curiosité électrique mais physiologique?

3. Fréquence du syndrome WPW

Au Centre Principal d'Expertise Médicale du Personnel Navigant de Paris, nous avons observé 39 fois cette anomalie électrocardiographique. Neuf observations étaient de type A; 30 observations étaient de type B. Trente-deux syndromes de WPW étaient permanents, et 7 étaient intermittents. Il nous a paru interessant d'insister sur ces WPW intermittents d'abord par le nombre relativement élevé et par leur difficulté diagnostic; l'anomalie electrocardiographique disparaissait après effort et réapparaissait au repos.

Nous avons chiffré la prévalence du syndrome WPW à 1.6/1000. Nos chiffres sont comparables aux statistiques des auteurs américains. Sears et Manning (1962) étudiant 15000 membres d'équipage dans l'Aviation canadienne trouvent 46 sujets porteurs d'un WPW (soit 3.0/1000) dont deux seulement ayant eu des manifestations tachycardiques Averill *et al.* (1960) ont trouvé 188 WPW sur 67375 sujets (soit 2.8/1000) et Hiss et Lamb (1962) 184 WPW sur 122043, sujets (soit 1.5/1000). Dans l'aviation navale américaine les chiffres cités par Smith (1963) sont 27 WPW, dont 2 ayant eu des épisodes tachycardiques, sur 28295 navigants, et 5 WPW, dont 3 avec tachycardie, sur 4006 non-navigants (soit 1.3/1000).

4. Aptitude aux emplois du personnel navigant

En France les candidats porteurs de cette anomalie électrocardiographique sont déclarés inaptes à l'emploi du personnel navigant. Cette inaptitude nous paraît être justifiée par les arguments suivants:

(1) Le risque de tachycardie paroxystique est diversement apprécié suivant les auteurs et la diversité des résultats est fonction de l'origine des malades. Certaines statistiques provenant des services de cardiologie donnent des chiffres élevés. Tranchesi donne un pourcentage de 55%, Ohnell (1944) 70%, Soulie *et al.* (1963) 75%, et Hejtmancik et Hermann (1957) 55%. Tandisque les statistiques venant de résultats d'examens systématiques donnent des chiffres beaucoup plus bas, Averill (1956) donne un pourcentage de 12% (U.S.A.F.), et Smith (1963) 15% (U.S. Navy). Dans notre service, à cause de l'inaptitude nous n'avons pu suivre nos observations, mais l'interrogatoire a permis de retrouver 3 antécédents de tachycardie paroxystique.

(2) Il est bien connu que le syndrome WPW peut survenir sur des cœurs pathologiques présentant soit des cardiopathies acquises (hypertendus artériels, infarctus du myocarde, maladie de Bouillaud), soit des cardiopathies acquises ou congénitales de diverses causes. Plusieurs publications ont, en particulier, insisté sur la fréquence des WPW de type B (constants ou intermittents) dans la maladie d'Ebstein. Toutes ces affections sont de diagnostic facile et ne posent pas de problème pour l'expert; mais toutes ces observations montrent la fréquence des associations morbides avec le syndrome WPW.

Nous voudrions insister sur deux affections familiales de diagnostic souvent difficile qui peuvent être associées avec le syndrome électrique de WPW: la cardio

mégalie familiale et la cardiomyopathie obstructive. La coexistence avec la cardiomégalie familiale a été relevée par de nombreux auteurs (Campbell et Turner-Warwick,
1956; Soulie *et al.*, 1957; Schiebler *et al.*, 1959).

Braunwald *et al.*, (1964) a montré la fréquence de l'association de cardiomyopathie
obstructive avec le WPW (24 observations). Par ailleurs, nous avons, avec Pernod et
Kemarec à l'Hôpital Militaire Percy, trouvé 3 malades porteurs d'une cardiomyopathie obstructive avec un WPW (Pernod *et al.*, 1966).

(3) La pathogénie du syndrome de WPW peut être résumée à une double activation
ventriculaire; d'une part une activation qui se fait normalement par les voies physiologiques (faisceau de Hiss et ses branches) et d'autre part une activation anormale à
point de départ ventriculaire (cette seconde activation anormale débute plus précoce
ment que celle qui se fait par les voies normales). Mais la propagation de l'onde d-
dépolarisation ectopique se faisant par l'intermédiaire du myocarde indifférencié, se
fait plus lentement.

Si la préexcitation est généralement admise comme expliquant la morphologie des
tracés, il existe deux groupes d'hypothèses – soit l'hypothèse d'un faisceau aberrant
reliant oreillette et ventricule (faisceau de Kent), soit la théorie de la conduction accélérée par les voies normales. Certaines cellules du nœud auriculo-ventriculaire, à la
suite de lésion, ayant perdu la propriété de retarder la conduction de l'onde de la
dépolarisation.

Une observation privilégiée de WPW intermittent nous a permis, grâce aux enregistrements mécanographiques synchrones (électrocardiogrammes, phonocardio-
grammes, apexogrammes) de montrer que l'intervalle électromécaniqne (Q–pied
d'apexogramme) était allongé. Donc la contraction ventriculaire gauche se fait en
retard dans le cas des systoles avec WPW par rapport aux systoles normales. Les
temps de contraction pré-isométrique, isométrique et d'éjection ventriculaire gauche
sont normaux. On peut en conclure que, dans le cas du WPW le temps de conduction
nerveuse est allongé; peut-être cet allongement du temps de conduction correspond-il
au temps de passage par le faisceau de Kent?

Quoiqu'il en soit, ces sujets sont porteurs d'un trouble de l'excitabilité (pré-excita-
tion ventriculaire) et d'un trouble de conduction (allongement de l'intervalle électro-
mécanique). Ces deux constatations sont des raisons supplémentaires de conclure à
l'inaptitude à l'emploi du personnel navigant.

Bibliographie

Averill, J. H.: 1956, *Amer. Heart J.* **51**, 943.
Averill, J. H., Fosmoe, R. J., et Lamb, L. E.: 1960, *Amer. J. Cardiol.* **6**, 108.
Braunwald, E., Costas, T., Lanbrew, S. D., *et al.*: 1964, *Amer. Heart Assoc. Monograph*, No. 10, p. 3.
Campbell, M. et Turner-Warwick, M.: 1956, *Brit. Heart J.* **18**, 393.
Hejtmancik, M. R. et Herrman, G. R.: 1957, *Amer. Heart J.* **54**, 708.
Hiss, R. G. et Lamb, L. E.: 1962, *Circulation* **25**, 947.
Ohnell, R. F.: 1944, *Acta Med. Scand.*, Suppl. **152**, 118.
Pernod, J., Ferrane, J., Quinot, B., *et al.*: 1966, *La Presse Médicale* **74**, 2135.
Schiebler, G. C., Adams, P., et Anderson, R. C.: 1959, *Amer. Heart J.* **58**, 113.

Sears, G. L. et Manning, G. W.: 1962, *J. Canad. Med. Assoc.* **87**, 1213.

Smith, R. F.: 1963, U.S. Naval School of Aviation Medicine, Pensacola, Fla., U.S.A.

Soulie, P., Matteo, J. de, Abaza, A., *et al.*: 1957, *Arch. maladies du cœur* **50**, 22.

Soulie, P., Degeorges, M., et Duperrier, C.: 1963, *La semaine des hôpitaux de Paris* **30**, 1191.

Wolff, L., Parkinson, J., et White, P. D.: 1930, *Amer. Heart J.* **5**, 685.

NORMS FOR QUANTITATIVE VECTORCARDIOGRAPHY
WITH SPECIAL EMPHASIS ON THE MEDICAL EVALUATION
OF FLYING PERSONNEL

P. RIJLANT, I. RUTTKAY-NEDECKY, J. CERNOHORSKY and A. ALLARD

Physiology Laboratory, Free University of Brussels, Brussels, Belgium

Clinical vectorcardiography draws upon two sources – an accurate knowledge of the meaning of a vector display of the heart's electrical activity and an extensive experience of the relationship between pathological conditions and modified vector displays. The vectorcardiogram is the display of the relative dipole moments of a single generator, equivalent to the heart's generator system. Many different methods have been considered to provide for an adequate approximation of the moments of the equivalent generator. These quantitative methods do not claim to provide for an absolute truth but for a reasonable compromise. The general trend is the measurement, at a distance from the generator system, of potentials which will provide enough insight of the underlying current flow fed by the heart's generator system. Experiments on models have provided enough information for a statistically significant approach which considers given surface locations, utilized directly, or by feeding current into a network connecting several electrodes do provide an information that can be adequately referred to its source. Frank's, Schmitt's, MacFee's, Helm's methods are extensively used for clinical vectorcardiography. Some statistical appraisals are also available. The limits of normal vector displays are clearly recognized.

One of us (Rijlant, 1957), developed a method based on the same principles. The only difference from other quantitative methods is a more generous utilization of the available surface information – 72 regularly distributed surface locations being considered – and a more exhaustive rejection of the disturbances related to singularities in the potential distribution on the surface of the body. This rejection is provided by the transfer of the actual measurements from the surface of the body to adequate locations inside an extensive resistive network built as an isomorph of a homogeneous conducting space of non-euclidian geometry and into which 72 electrodes feed current. The method is inspired by the well known systematization of the field of current, fed by a compound generator system, when the distance between the elements of the generator and the location of the measurement is increased. This was already emphasized by Wilson. The non-euclidian characteristics of the conducting space provided by the network are needed to provide for a relative independence of the regulating action from the decay of the potential level with the increase in distance.

Several thousand recordings of vectorcardiograms have been obtained utilizing Rijlant's method. The recordings are either vector displays, or recordings on magnetic tape of the relative dipole moments for the vertical, transverse, and antero-posterior axes. The general method of recording has been the same for a 12-yr period. The skin of the torso is washed with ethyl alcohol and dried and then rubbed with a small amount of Sanborn electrocardiographic paste. An elastic vest, which carries the 72 regularly-spaced electrodes, can be fitted to individual needs. Each electrode is a 1-inch diameter silver disk enclosed in a piece of non-putrescible cloth moistened with Elema electrocardiographic liquid. The electrodes are directly connected by short wires to the 72 input nodes of the network.

Measurements inside the network are performed differentially for 3 mutually orthogonal axes; vertical, transverse and antero-posterior. The potentials are amplified and carried to an Elema 42B recorder and a Tektronix 536 X-Y oscillograph, electronically commutated on both axes and providing a simultaneous display of the frontal, sagittal and horizontal vectorcardiograms with 1000 cps synchronous time marks, and to high precision resolvers. From 1960, recording of this information on magnetic tape by frequency modulation, at 60 ips, has been a standard procedure.

In addition to these measurements, standard 12-lead electrocardiograms have been systematically recorded. Before recording on magnetic tape was available, from 1957 until 1960, resolving has been performed directly. This resulted in a variation of the vector display with respiration and time, the duration of the procedure lasting about 15 min. This also resulted in a less careful determination of the ideal reference frame.

The Y, X and Z reference frame is obtained by 3 successive rotations of the display – in site, azimuth and elevation – with angular values α, β and γ, until the new vector display has its maximal projection (R) for the Y-axis and its orthogonal maximal projection for the X-axis. In normal individuals the Z-projection is then of negligible amplitude; its magnitude is usually less than 5% of the maximal value of R (Y-axis). These small Z-components occur more frequently either during the initial (Q) or terminal (S) phases, or near the maximum of the R wave.

The resolvers utilize very accurate sine and cosine potentiometers immersed in oil baths with a resolution better than $\frac{1}{2}$ deg.

Most of the recordings utilized in this study have been obtained from a very large group of young students, male or female, the age being 17 to 35 years, without anamnestic, clinical or conventional electrocardiographic signs of cardiac pathology. Next to these a very important group of flying and ground personnel of Sabena Airlines has been examined. Smaller groups of industrial workers have also been examined and sedentary personnel of different age groups (insurance companies) has provided needed information on the evolution of the vector display with aging.

The purpose has been to define what constitutes a normal vectorcardiogram and what has to be considered as a pathological change. In this study a conventional statistical analysis is utilized. The preliminary step necessary is to find out if available information is distributed in a normal pattern. The number of attempts to look for normal distribution curves of parameters which characterize the heart's electric field is small, and the outcome of these studies has been negative, as shape and structure of the human torso provide for individual variations. As one measures the equivalent dipole moments directly in a resistive network, to cancel out the singularities of the

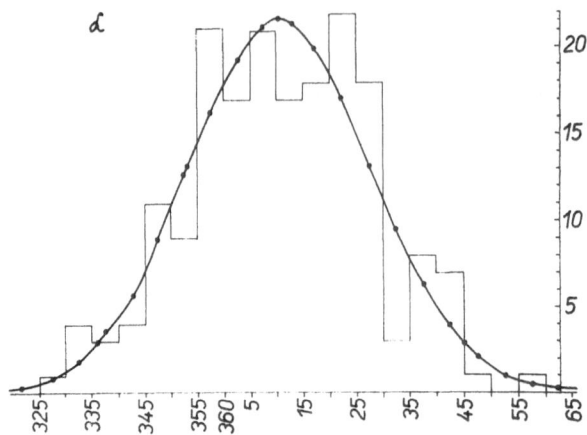

Fig. 1.   Frequency histogram of angular values of α resolver rotation. Mean 10°.6; standard deviation 17°.2; class interval 5. Estimated population variance 17°.24. Standard error of the mean 1°.26.

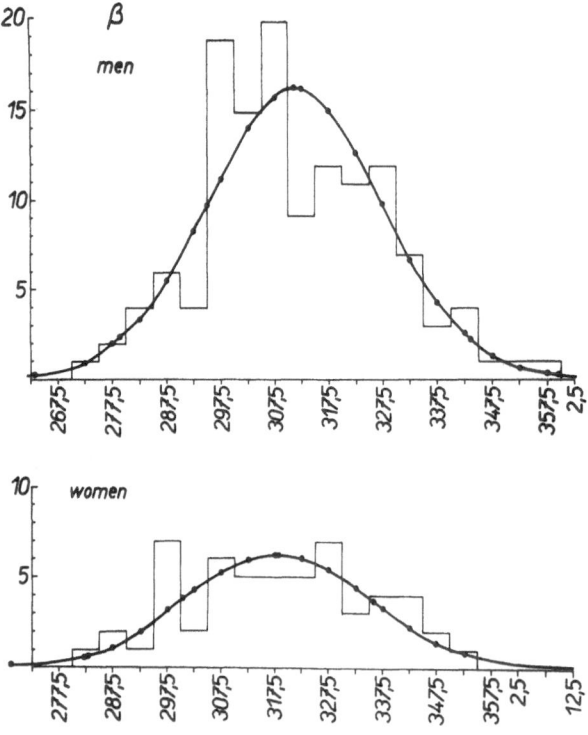

Fig. 2.   Frequency histogram and computed normal distribution curve for angular values of β resolver
rotation either for men or for women. Mean 311°.2 (men), 318°.2 (women); standard deviation 16°.1
(men), 17°.7 (women). Population variance 16°.15 (men), 17°.86 (women). Standard error of the mean
1°.42 (men), 2°.4 (women).

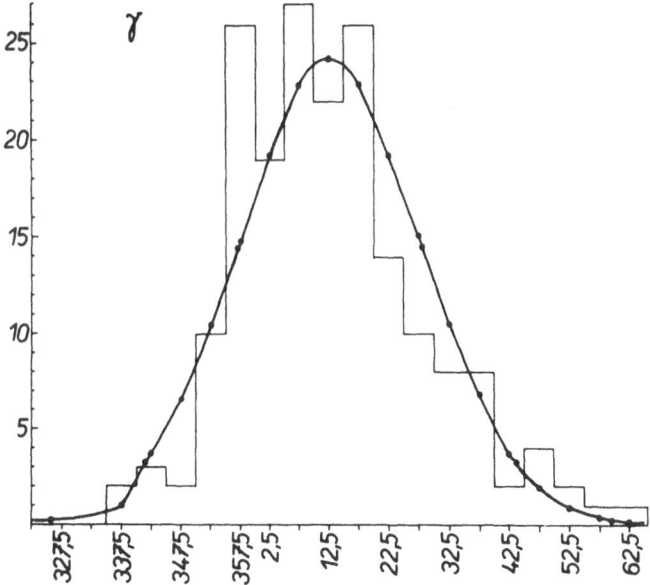

Fig. 3. Frequency histogram and computed normal distribution curve for angular values of γ resolver rotation. Mean 12°.6; standard deviation 15°.6. Estimated population variance 15°.63. Standard error of the mean 1°.56.

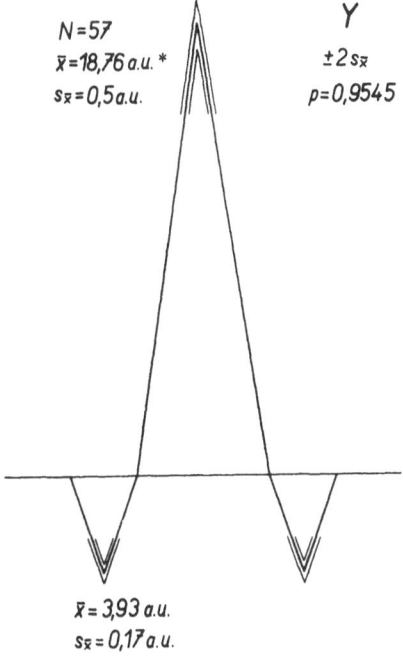

* arbitrary unit.

Fig. 4. Schematic representation of the Y lead vectorial electrocardiogram. Peaks are mean values plus and minus 2 standard deviations.

surface distribution, it is hoped for a substantial reduction of the distortions of the heart's electrical field by torso boundary conditions and intrinsic heterogeneities.

To facilitate the comparison of the findings with already available statistical data, small homogeneous groups of between 100 and 200 individuals have been selected and the α, β and γ angles measured, so providing a proper resolution. Testing by the Kolmogoroff-Smirnov test, a statistically significant deviation of the measured values from the normal distribution curve could not be found. No sex differences were discovered, except for rotations in azimuth, and this should be reconsidered on the

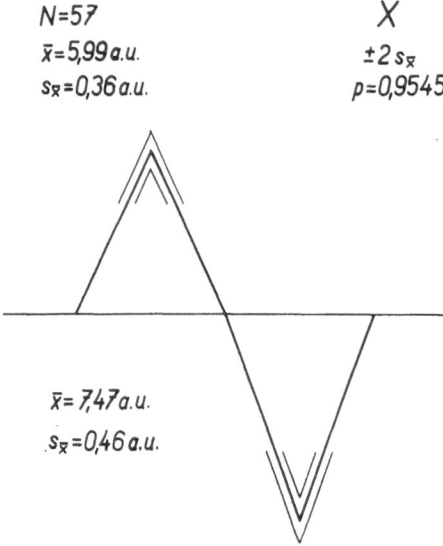

$N=57$
$\bar{x}=5{,}99\,a.u.$
$s_{\bar{x}}=0{,}36\,a.u.$

X
$\pm 2\,s_{\bar{x}}$
$p=0{,}9545$

$\bar{x}=7{,}47\,a.u.$
$s_{\bar{x}}=0{,}46\,a.u.$

Fig. 5.   Schematic representation of the X lead vectorial electrocardiogram (see Figure 4).

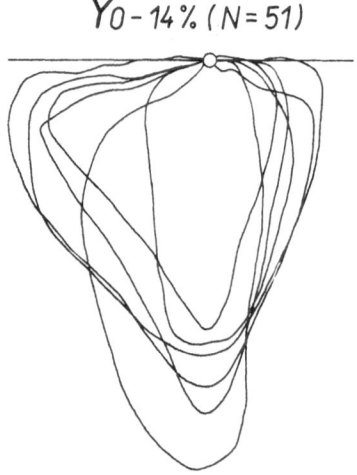

$Y_0 - 14\% \ (N = 51)$

Fig. 6.   Superposition of proper plane QRS vector loops without Q or S (14%).

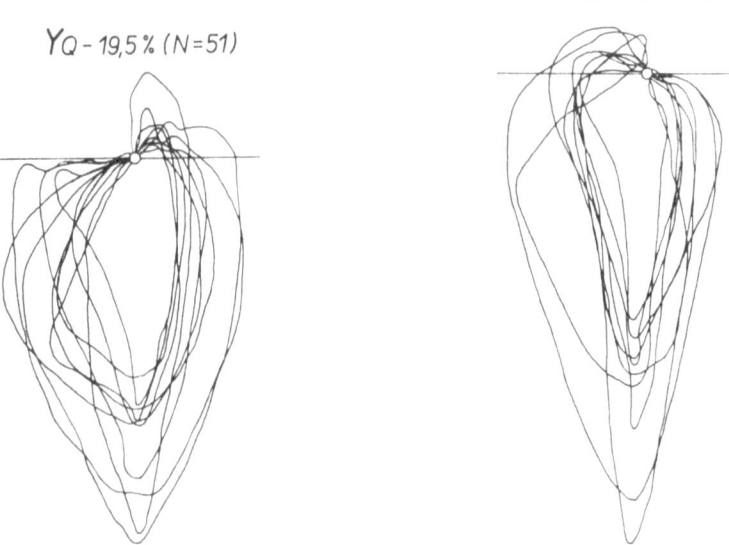

Fig. 7. *QRS* vector loops without *Q* (19.5%). Fig. 8. *QRS* vector loops without *S* (17.5%).

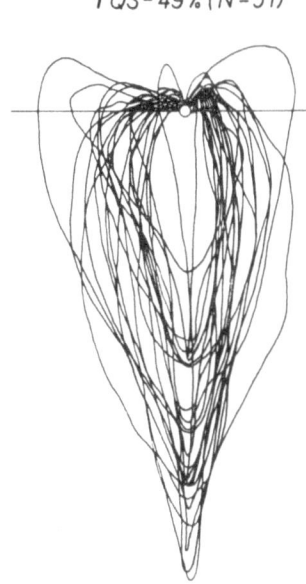

Fig. 9. *QRS* vector loops with a pronounced *Q* and *S* (49%).

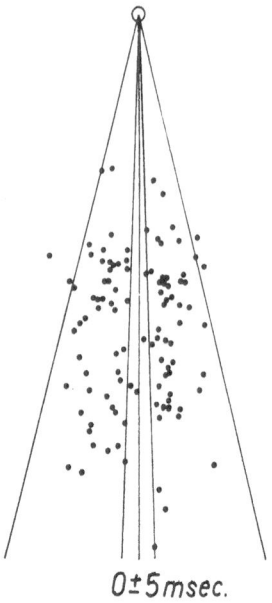

0±5msec.

Fig. 10. Dispersion of the orientation of momentaneous vectors in the proper plane exactly 5 msec before (to the right) or 5 msec after the R maximum in space. The dots represent the end points of the momentaneous vectors. The 95% range is delineated by sectors. The angular speed is very variable either before or after the maximum of R.

basis of larger samples. It is already evident that this very small difference does not play a significant role. Pipberger and Carter (1962) did not observe a normal distribution in a group of normal individuals explored by Frank's and Schmitt's methods. Figures 1, 2 and 3, show the distribution of angular values for the three rotations: α in the frontal plane (Figure 1), β in the horizontal plane (figure 2) and γ in the sagittal plane (Figure 3). The full line shows the normal distribution curve for the given sample size (men and women cumulated sample size 187; men sample size 132; women sample size 55; age 17–35 years).

As the spatial orientation of the QRS loop does fit the normal distribution curve very well in healthy young subjects, the use of classical statistical procedures for differentiation between norm and pathology is acceptable. Resolving for Q, R, and S provides for three electrocardiograms in which the QRS complex has a systematic appearance. In the Y electrocardiogram, the R wave is positive and prominent. Small Q or S waves can be present. In the X electrocardiogram, the QRS is diphasic and of the RS type. The variability of this set of leads is reduced to a minimum as is shown for its main parameters in Figures 4 and 5.

The typology of the QRS has also been studied by superposition techniques. Figures 6 to 9 group, respectively, the R type, RS type, QR type and QRS type vector loops in their proper or preferential plane (the sample size is $N=51$; the percentages are, respectively, 14, 19.5, 17.5 and 49%).

The orientation of the momentaneous vectors has been determined for 5 msec time

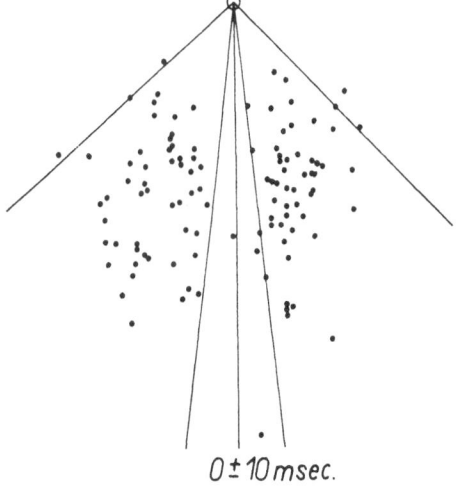

0 ± 10 msec.

Fig. 11.   Dispersion 10 msec
before or after R maximal.

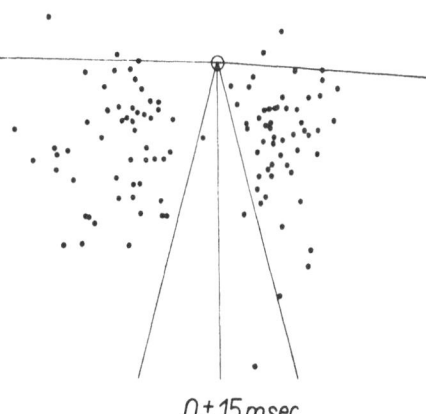

0 ± 15 msec.

Fig. 12.   Dispersion 15 msec
before or after R maximal.

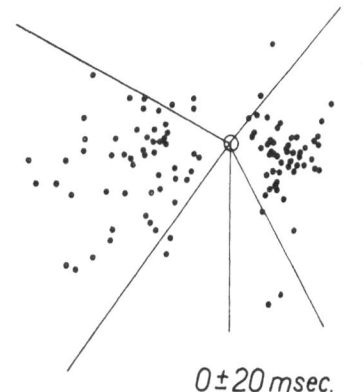

0 ± 20 msec.

Fig. 13.   Dispersion 20 msec before or after R
maximal.

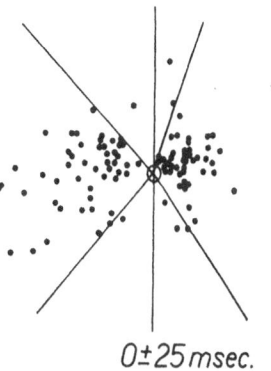

0 ± 25 msec.

Fig. 14.   Dispersion 25 msec before or after R
maximal.

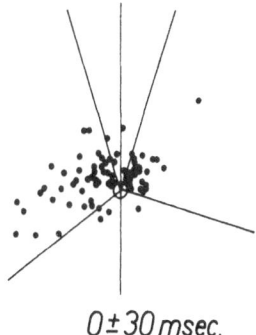

0 ± 30 msec.

Fig. 15.   Dispersion 30 msec before or after R
maximal.

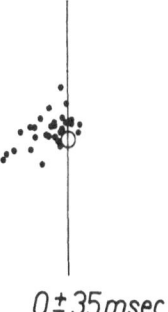

0 ± 35 msec.

Fig. 16.   Dispersion 35 msec before or after R
maximal.

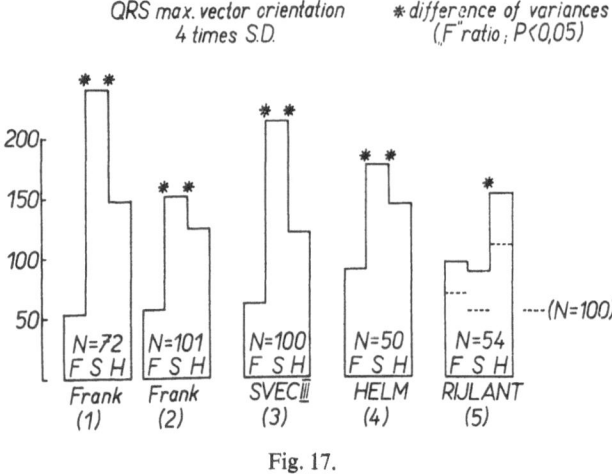

Fig. 17.

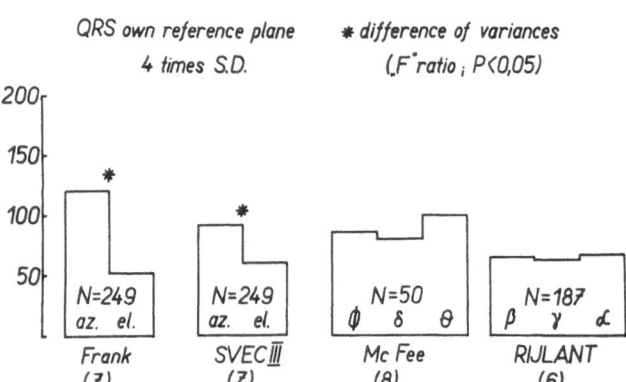

Fig. 18.

Figs. 17 and 18. Comparison of the variance (4 times the standard deviation) of *QRS* maximum vector orientation in published samples from studies with different lead systems. *F*: frontal, *S*: sagittal, *H*: horizontal. The numbers are literature references, referred in the text. Statistically significant differences of variances are marked by an asterisk. Broken lines indicate values depending on an increased sample size to 100. AZ = azimuth; el = elevation.

intervals taking the maximum of the *R* vector as the reference moment (Figures 10–16). Dots represent the end points of momentaneous vectors. The 95% range is delineated by sectors. The plus and minus sectors for the same time intervals either 5, 10, 15, 20, 25, 30 or 35 msec are represented in the same figure.

An important step has been the comparison of the total variance of the characteristic parameters for Rijlant's method with other methods (Figures 17 and 18). If the sample variance is expressed by 4 times its standard deviation and if the already published data related to Frank's, Schmitt's, MacFee's and Helm's methods are utilized, noticeable differences become evident. If the maximum vector of the *QRS* plane is considered in its relation to the frontal, sagittal and horizontal plane, the variance of its orientation has very different values for the three reference planes.

This is very evident in the schematic representation of the total variance based on the data published by (1) Bristow (1961), by (2) Sotobata *et al.* (1968) and by (7) Pipberger and Carter (1962) for Frank's method, by (4) Calhoun Witham (1966) for Helm's method, by (3) Pipberger (1958), and (7) Pipberger and Carter (1962) for Schmitt's method, and by (8) Abildskov *et al.* (1963) for MacFee's method.

It is evident that for MacFee's and Rijlant's methods, the variance is independent of the orientation and is relatively small. There is no statistically significant difference between the variances of the orientation of the horizontal, sagittal and frontal plane maximum vectors. The impact of these variance comparisons is twofold. First, it shows in which of the systems explored may be found the conditions most favorable for a discrimination between the normal and the pathological. Second, it may also be interpreted as a measure of the effectiveness of the network system in minimizing the distortion of the cardiac electric field due to individual torso boundary conditions and to non-homogeneities.

The angle of the T vector to the proper plane and in this plane the angle of the orthogonal projection of the T vector to the maximal R vector have been measured. Also measured has been the angle between the T and the maximal R vector. The ST vector has been treated the same way when of noticeable amplitude. As this work is still in progress no valid statistical analysis is yet available. The same holds for the groups of flying and ground personnel of Sabena Airlines. The normal variation of the cardiac parameters has to be clearly defined before conclusions can be drawn from the analysis of small groups. This work is in progress with a special emphasis on the modifications due to age. Most of the subjects already examined 10 to 12 yr ago are now being examined again under similar conditions to provide for a statistically valid definition of the modification of the parameters of the electrical activity of the heart by age, or eventually by special environment or working conditions.

References

Abildskov, J. A., MacFee, R., and Schecter, G.: 1963, *Am. Heart J.* **65**, 220.

Bristow, J. D.: 1961, *Am. Heart J.* **61**, 242.

Calhoum Witham, A.: 1966, *Am. Heart J.* **72**, 284.

Pipberger, H. V.: 1958, *Circulation* **17**, 1102.

Pipberger, H. V. and Carter, T. A.: 1962, *Circulation* **25**, 827.

Rijlant, P.: 1957, *Bull. Acad. Roy. Méd. Belgique* VIe Sér., **22**, 156; *Bull. Acad. Roy. Méd. Belgique* VIe Sér., **22**, 464.

Rijlant, P.: 1965, *Bull. Acad. Roy. Méd. Belgique* VIIe Sér., **5**, 457.

Sotobata, I., Richman, H., and Simonson, E.: 1968, *Circulation* **37**, 438.

THE DIAGNOSTICS OF EARLY FORMS OF ATHEROSCLEROSIS AND LATENT CORONARY INSUFFICIENCY IN FLIGHT CREWS

B. L. HELAM, I. M. PITSCHUGIN, G. L. STRONGIN,
L. I. KUZNETSOVA and A. A. SHISHOVA

Medical Department, Aeroflot, Moscow, U.S.S.R.

The importance of the early recognition and treatment of coronary atherosclerosis is dictated by the necessity of guaranteeing flight safety, and preserving the health of the highly experienced and qualified group of middle aged and aged pilots. Over the past five years, 244 flight crew members suspected of having atherosclerosis and latent coronary insufficiency were examined in the Central Clinical Hospital of Civil Aviation. Also examined were 100 healthy pilots, who served as a control group.

The medical history taken on pilots is of little importance in their medical examination, for pilots hide facts for fear of being medically grounded. Moreover, subjective manifestations of early stages of atherosclerosis may be absent.

The majority of pilots in the study group were found to have left cardiac enlargement and diminished heart sounds on physical examination. Rarely, the aortic second sound was increased and systolic murmurs were present.

Assessment of the lipid metabolism of the healthy control group of pilots made it possible to establish standards of biochemical indices of lipid metabolism for flying personnel in civil aviation. One must point out here that there is a great necessity for further study of pathways in lipid metabolism responsible for atherosclerosis.

Data showed that the serum cholesterol level is not an adequate indicator of atherosclerosis, for only 58.5% of those affected by atherosclerosis had an elevated serum cholesterol. Hyperbetalipoproteinemia was discovered in 82.2% of the study group. Also increased were serum total lipids in 71.4%, serum triglycerides in 81.4% and serum free non-esterified fatty acids in 80.4% of those in this group. Eighty-one per cent of the pilots with atherosclerosis had a decrease of their serum lipoprotein lipase. It was noted that increases of total lipids and betalipoproteins corresponded closely with decreases in lipoprotein lipase levels. The results of these studies indicate that elevated concentrations of serum betalipoproteins was the best indicator of atherosclerosis of all the biochemical blood tests of lipid metabolism performed.

Much data of interest has been obtained by studying the effects of hypoxia on lipid metabolism during hypoxic exposure. It was noted that hypoxia produces increases of the levels of serum total lipids, triglycerides and betalipoproteins. A number of those affected by atherosclerosis have developed disturbances in carbohydrate metabolism and electrolyte balance.

Chest X-rays allowed observation of changes in the cardiac configuration and examination of the thoracic segment of the aorta. These X-rays indicated the value of radiographic study of the abdominal segment of the aorta and other major arteries to identify areas of calcification in these vessels.

The recognition of coronary insufficiency was the main aim of the electrocardiographic examination. The complex of cardiac stresses applied included 15 squattings over a 30-sec period, the Double Master's Two-Step Test, riding a bicycle ergometer at 500 to 800 kg-meters/min, hypoxia produced by breathing a gas mixture containing 10% oxygen and 90% nitrogen for 20 min, and ingestion of 100 to 150 g glucose in water, fasting. A depression of the ST segment in the electrocardiographic trace in response to physical stress was considered as positive evidence of coronary insufficiency. A reversal of T-wave polarity from negative (inverted) to positive (upright) was also taken into account. Electrocardiographic recordings were taken while the subjects rode a bicycle ergometer and for 10 min after this stress. This allowed close observation of the transition of the oblique, rising portion of the ST segment, which had decreased during exercise (J-point depression) to horizontal, and *vice versa*, in a number of cases. The fact that different types of ST-segment depressions are related to coronary insufficiency makes it necessary to observe 'harmless' J-point depressions closely, especially if electrocardiographic recordings, taken after physical stress, are insufficient for monitoring recovery.

Latent coronary insufficiency was identified in 8.1% of the study group during the squatting test, 27.5% during the Double Master's Two-Step Test and in 46.7% in the bicycle ergometer test. The hypoxia test produced positive changes in 17.6% of the study group.

The glucose test has received less investigation than the physical stress and hypoxia tests. Limits of interpretation criteria have been set on the basis of 2.5% incidence of electrocardiographic changes in the control group of 58 pilots tested. Suggested criteria for positive changes are:

(1) Horizontal ST-segment reduction; the appearance of negative, two-phase and deformed T waves.

(2) T-wave reduction by more than half its height.

(3) Considerable increase of TU/TU-waves ratio (index of reaction discordance).

A positive glucose test was observed in 64.6% of the study group, with 39% having changes falling into criterion (1) above. Current data in the scientific literature, as well as this experimental data do not give any evidence as to the connection between a positive glucose tolerance and insufficient coronary blood circulation. Most probably, this finding reflects changes of myocardial metabolism due to disturbance of high energy phosphorus compound balance. Hypoxia is the cause of this disturbance in atherosclerotic patients.

The value of any functional test depends on its sensitivity, safety, comparative simplicity, adequacy for the function under study, safety, the technique of application and professional specificity. Taking these considerations into account, the squatting test is thought unnecessary. The Double Master's Two-Step Test is quite sensitive, safe, and simple; it is recommended in commissioning flying personnel. The bicycle ergometer test is the most effective in revealing coronary insufficiency. However, the complexity of equipment used and the danger of all kinds of complications during its application demand that it be used only in clinical situations.

The necessity of conducting a hypoxia test is dictated by the fact that hypoxia is still one of the main flight conditions. Therefore, improving the degree of coronary blood flow response to this stress is considered important in order to make a definitive decision.

A glucose test is a sensitive test, helping to determine disturbances of mycocardial metabolism.

The individual's age did not necessarily correlate with the outcome of these functional tests. Sixty-one per cent of those above 40 years of age in the study group did not show any disturbance of coronary blood circulation.

The heart's systolic phase has been analysed to estimate the condition of the ejection capability of the myocardium. This analysis was also performed during functional stress testing, so allowing one to obtain additional information on the compensatory capacity of the heart.

Special accidental situations were simulated during 'flight' of pilots suffering from coronary insufficiency. Ischemic ST-segment and T-wave changes were observed on the electrocardiogram. These changes were very much like those recorded in the physical stress and hypoxia tests.

The diagnostic techniques which have been applied in this study make it possible to identify atherosclerotic disease of the aorta and the coronary arteries. They also allow one to differentiate atherosclerotic changes in the cardiovascular system from disease from other causes. With such modern diagnostics, it is possible to recognize and so possibly stop the progress of atherosclerosis and coronary insufficiency by applying medical preventive methods, and achieving in a number of cases some improvement of coronary blood circulation.

MEDICAL WASTAGE OF MILITARY AND CIVIL AIRCREW IN GREAT BRITAIN 1963-68

G. BENNETT

Board of Trade, London, England, U.K.

and

P. J. O'CONNOR

Royal Air Force, London, England, U.K.

This paper compares the medical wastage of trained professional aviators in military and civil flying in the United Kingdom for the years 1963–68. The term 'medical wastage' refers to those flight deck personnel who are prevented from revalidating their flying licence by reason of ill-health or death. The Board of Trade which issues flying licences to all civilian aircrew gave the civil medical wastage. The Statistics Branch of the Royal Air Force gave details of medical wastage and strength for military aircrew. Medical wastage rates were calculated in the four age groups, under 30 years, 30 to 39, 40 to 49 and over 50 years of age. For each of these epochs the number of aircrew, who were 'grounded' was divided by the number of aviators at risk in that age group. This gives the results expressed as rates per thousand aircrew. The total wastage for the six years 1963 to 1968 was divided by six to give the wastage rate per thousand aircrew per annum.

The total medical wastage rates in military aviators and in one section of civilian flying in United Kingdom have been found to be roughly equal, at approximately one per cent per annum. Three quarters of this one per cent were due to cardiovascular disease, flying accidents and psychiatric illness. The relative proportions of the three conditions differed considerably between military and civilian aircrews, although in both cases the sum was the same (i.e., $\frac{3}{4}$ of 1% per annum). The object of this paper is to examine at greater length the different incidences of medical disabilities in military and civil commercial flying in the United Kingdom.

Figure 1 gives the age profiles for the military and civil aircrews. Almost exactly a third of military and civil aircrew are less than 30 years of age. There are fewer civilian aircrew aged 30 to 39 and more in the age group over 50 years. This is because a military aviator is rarely given a flying assignment over 47 years of age and relatively few fly regularly over the age of 43, whereas his civilian counterpart will in general fly to 55 years of age.

The following figures compare the causes of medical wastage in civil and military aircrew at comparable ages. As shown in Figure 2, cardiovascular disease is the main cause of wastage in civil flying. The annual rate of loss of licence due to cardiovascular disease is slightly higher in civil than military aircrew in the lower age groups, but above the age of 40 the preponderance of this complaint in civilian aircrew increases. Over the age of 40, civilian aircrew in general fly many more hours each year than do

D. E. Busby (ed.), Recent Advances in Aerospace Medicine, 93–99. All Rights Reserved.

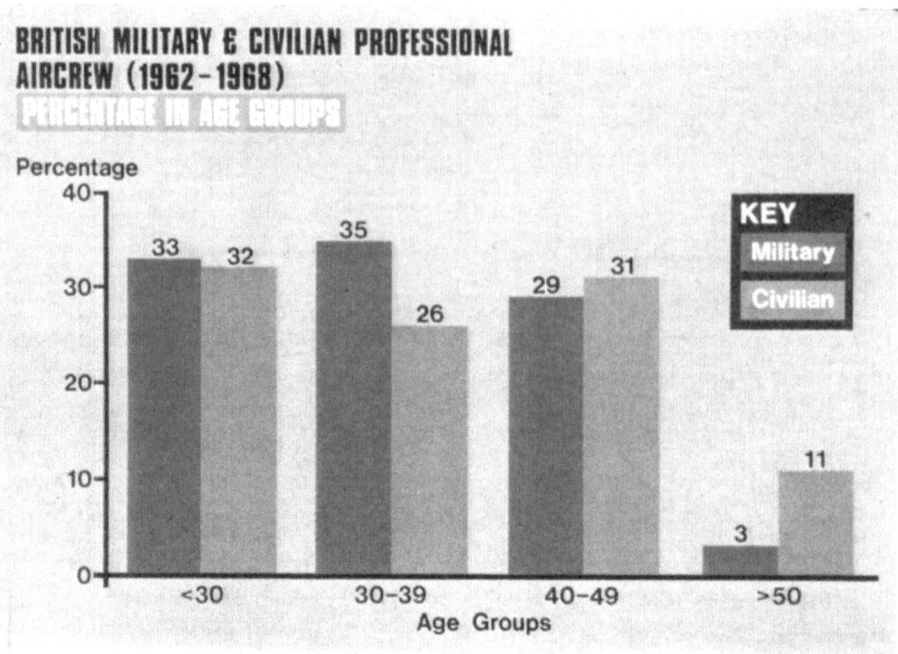

Fig. 1.   Age profiles for military and civil aircrews.

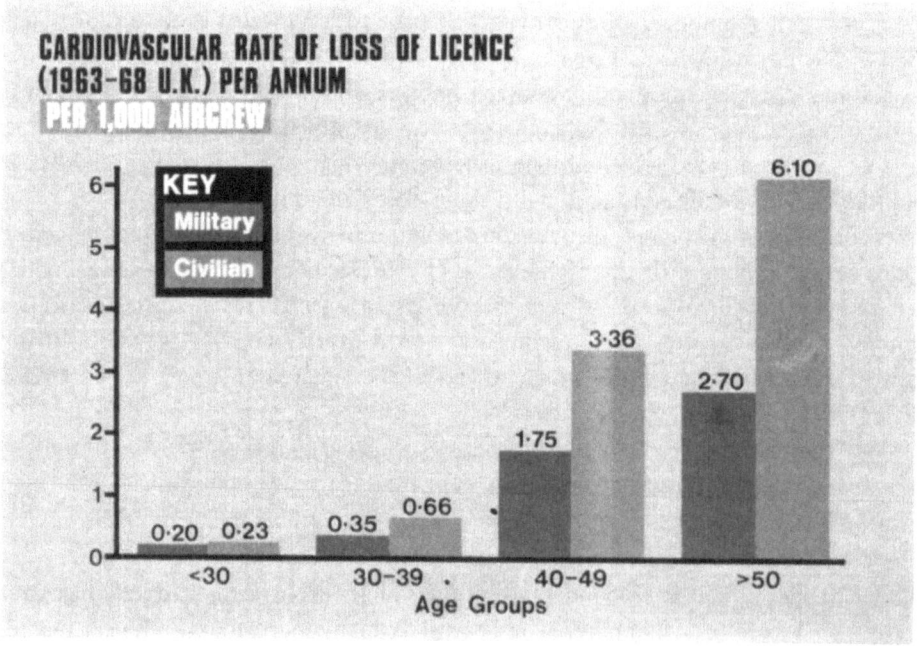

Fig. 2.   Loss of licence due to cardiovascular disease; incidence per 1000 aircrew in each age group.

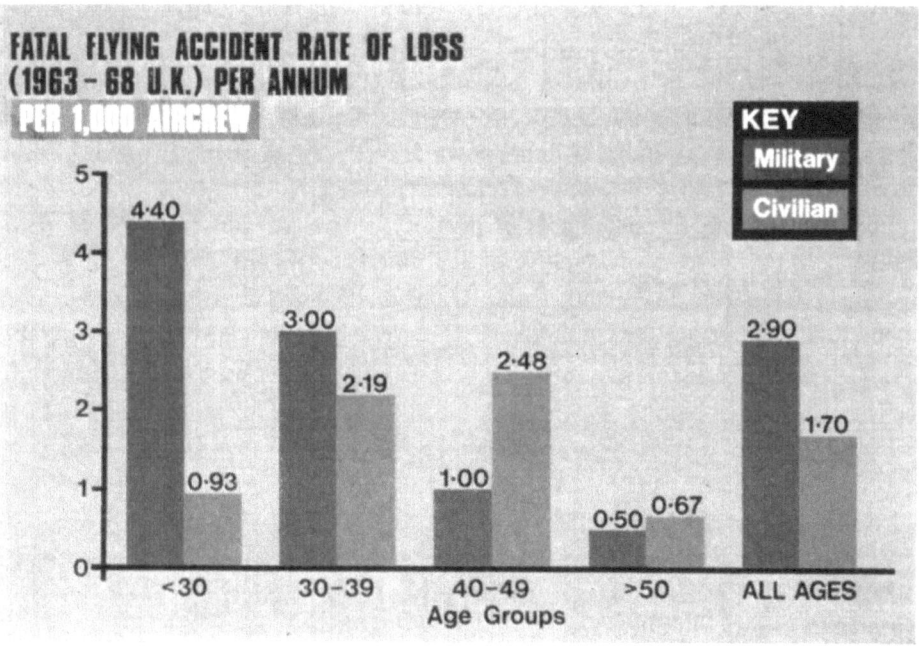

Fig. 3.   Loss of licence due to fatal flying accidents; incidence per 1000 aircrew in each age group.

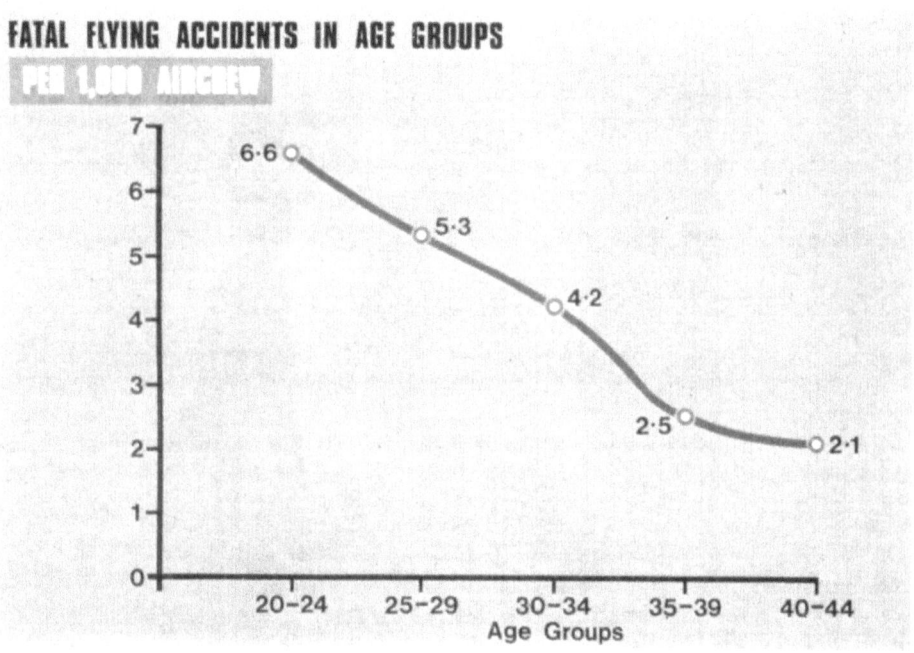

Fig. 4.   Incidence of military flying accidents per 1000 aircrew in each age group.

military aviators. In general also, by the nature of their tasks, a larger proportion of civilian aircrew lead a more sedentary and less energetic life than the serviceman. Whether or not the sharp rise in incidence of coronary artery disease in civilian aircrews, for this is the cause of 90% of loss of licence in the cardiovascular group, is directly related to the number of hours flown or to the more sedentary life or to some other cause is not known, but the discrepancy is marked.

Before examining the differences in psychiatric wastage and that due to flying accidents, one should examine some of the differences in the attitudes of the two groups towards their flying and in the nature of their flying tasks. Although both civilian and military aircrew are trained to a very high standard and considerable emphasis is laid on flight safety, the military aviator, unlike his civilian counterpart, is expected to be able to fly his aircraft to the limits of its capability in all weather, to

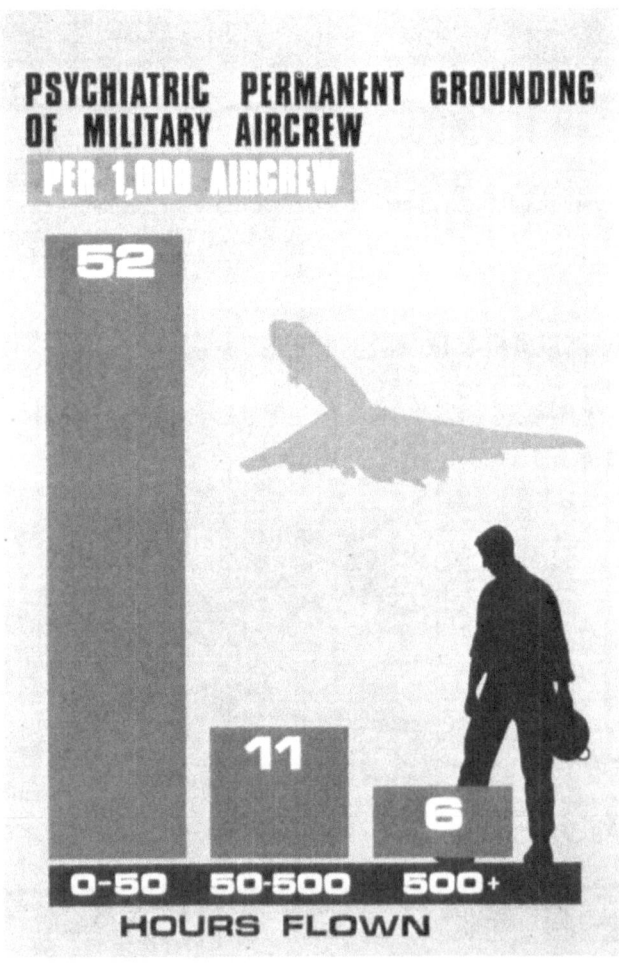

Fig. 5.   Psychiatric grounding in military aircrew related to hours flown.

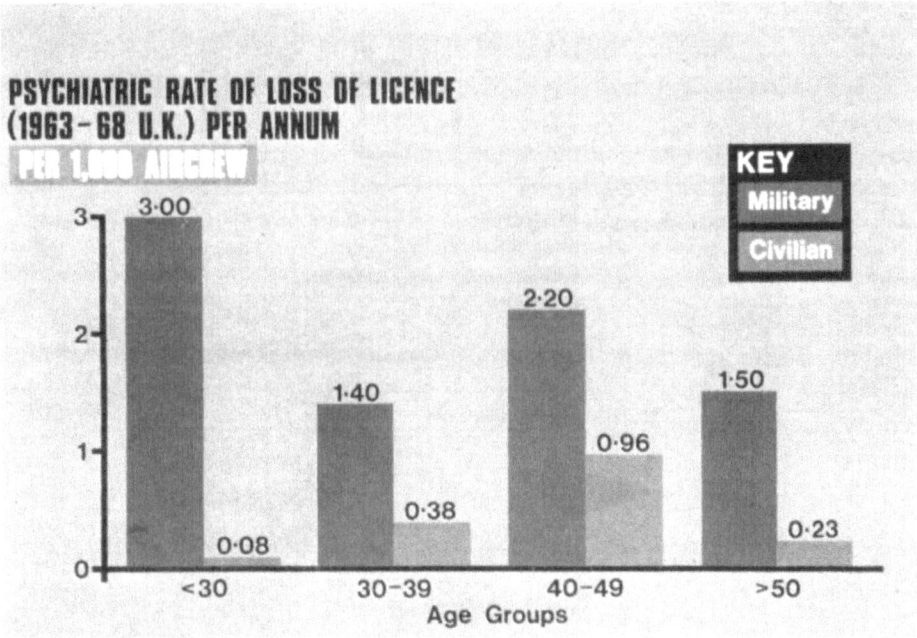

Fig. 6.   Psychiatric wastage per 1000 military and civil aircrew in each age group.

perform aerobatics and to carry out formation and combat flying; upon these skills depends his ability to press home an attack in wartime and to outwit enemy defences. Military flying therefore carries a greater risk of accident and causes more acute psychiatric stress than civil flying. There is undoubted psychiatric stress in civil flying also, but it is of a different kind. It is less acute and has its roots in the concern for the safety of passengers, in recurrent sleep disturbance and in suitcase living.

The distinction between civil and military flying is not absolute. Military aircrew in Air Support Command have a flying life very similar to civil aviation both in the long hours spent at the controls, frequent time zone changes and length of suitcase living. By and large, however, the differences outlined above obtain; the military airman flies fewer hours in a year but the flying he does, especially in his early days, is more strenuous. The civilian commercial aviator flies more hours in each year and for more years than a military aviator; his flying is less strenuous but he has responsibility for passengers, and because of his longer flying life he spends more gross time away from his family.

The social milieu of the two groups is very different. The Service flier is first and foremost a Service officer subject to Service disciplines, and has administrative and command responsibilities in relation to other duties outside the aircraft cockpit. He is subjected to moves on posting at intervals of 2 to 3 years; the type of flying or ground duties on which he is employed changes from time to time and he cannot change his job at will. The rates of pay of civilian pilots are at least twice as great as Service rates,

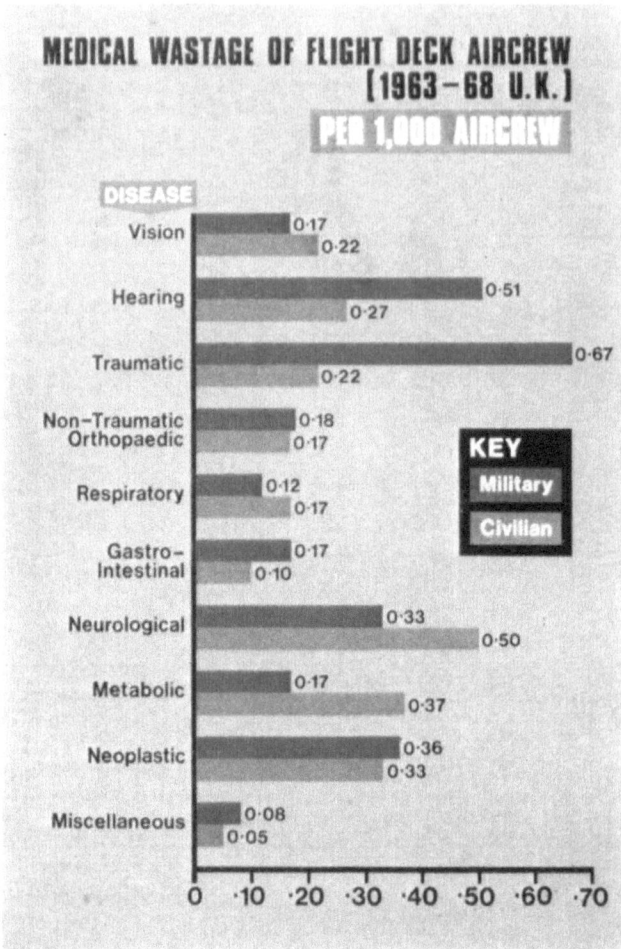

Fig. 7. Wastage rates. Causes other than cardiovascular, psychiatric, and flying accidents (number per 1000 aircrew – all ages.)

a situation succinctly epitomized by the news headline that astronaut Colonel Michael Collins' pay was less than that of a qualified plumber in the United States. The airline pilot's professional responsibilities are confined to within the cockpit; his role and base location remain constant for a number of years and he can change his job at will. The cohesive forces which keep military aviators in the air are motivation for flying and a sense of dedication to the country's needs which are highly weighted at the initial Selection Board and later the fostering of *esprit de corps*. In civil aviation, airline *esprit de corps* also exists but more emphasis is laid on adequate remuneration to keep the aviator in the air.

It is against this background that we should look at the incidence of flying accidents and psychiatric wastage in the two groups. Figure 3 gives the flying accident wastage rates and, as might be expected, service flying carries a higher risk of fatal accident. This is especially so in the younger age group. The inverse ratio between accident rate and age in military aviation is nicely shown by ten years of experience in the Royal Air Force.

Figure 4 is a graph relating the number of fatal accidents (relative to aircrew strength) to age, for the 10-year period 1958 to 1967. The number of fatal accidents diminishes steadily with age, although this relationship does not hold when compared with hours flown.

Psychiatric wastage likewise is much higher in military flying, especially in the younger age groups. This reflects the more hazardous nature of military situation. The relationship between hours flown and psychiatric wastage in military flying is well shown in Figure 5. The psychiatric wastage is highest in the early stages of flying when the pupil pilot is first subjected to the hazards of aviation, but Figure 6 shows that both in military and civil flying there is a secondary peak on the psychiatric wastage age 40 to 49. In most of these later psychiatric casualties the precipitant of the psychiatric illness is not the flying *per se*, but is usually some domestic stress related to separation from family or, in the case of military aircrew, the desire to set up home after 20 years of living in Service quarters. Chronic, low intensity, domestic stress seems to lower the threshold for withstanding the strain of continuous flying and sometimes gives rise to the syndrome of phobic reaction to flying characterised by increasing the irrational anxiety about some aspect of flying which had previously been well tolerated.

The other causes of medical wastage are included in Figure 7. None of these causes approach the importance of cardiovascular disease, flying accidents and psychiatric wastage.

In summary, we confirm previous work showing that cardiovascular disease, flying accidents and psychiatric illness are the chief causes of medical wastage of aircrew. In civil aviation, cardiovascular disease (90% due to coronary artery disease) is the chief cause of wastage while in military flying, flying accidents and psychiatric wastage are expectedly higher.

LES MALAISES EN VOL DANS L'ARMÉE DE L'AIR FRANÇAISE: ÉTUDE ANALYTIQUE DE 1961 À 1968

P. PESQUIES, P. M. PINGANNAUD, J. NATHIE, et J. BORSARELLO

C.E.R.M.A. – 5bis, Avenue de la Porte de Sèvres, Paris 15, France

1. Introduction

De 1961 à 1968, l'Armée de l'Air Française a suivi une double évolution. Celle-ci a été marquée, sur le plan matériel, par la mise en service d'avions à hautes performances de la classe Mach II et le remplacement progressif des appareils à hélices par des réacteurs, principalement dans les Écoles de Formation, et, sur le plan logistique, par une nouvelle conception de la mission stratégique impartie à l'Armée de l'Air Française. Ces huit années ont donc représenté pour le personnel navigant une phase de transition et d'adaptation. Il est donc apparu intéressant d'analyser l'influence de ces modifications de la vie professionnelle des équipages sur ce chapitre de médecine aéronautique, toujours d'actualité, que constituent les malaises en vol.

L'étude des malaises en vol constatés pendant cette période a été menée à partir des comptes rendus d'enquêtes établis par les médecins de la Formation Aérienne en collaboration avec les Services Techniques locaux. Certaines enquêtes ont nécessité, en outre, une hospitalisation, en particulier dans le Service spécialisé de Médecine Aéronautique de l'Hôpital Dominique Larrey. Quelques malaises, enfin, ont dû faire l'objet d'une enquête approfondie.

2. Fréquence et répartition des malaises en vol

Le nombre total des malaises en vol, ayant fait l'objet d'une enquête médicale pendant ces huit dernières années, s'élève à 111, se répartissant en 98 cas observés chez des pilotes, 11 cas chez des navigateurs, et 2 cas chez des mécaniciens. Il est intéressant de comparer la répartition de ces malaises avec le nombre d'accidents aériens enregistrés et le nombre total d'heures de vol effectuées pendant la même période (Tableau I). L'étude de ce tableau conduit aux réflexions suivantes. Le rapport entre les malaises et le nombre d'accidents aériens, ainsi que le nombre total d'heures de vol effectuées est décroissant, mais sans qu'il soit possible d'attacher une signification à cette décroissance. On peut en outre, noter l'importance du pic en 1962. L'augmentation en valeur absolue et relative du nombre des malaises enregistrés cette année-là paraît être en rapport avec la période initiale d'adaptation du personnel. Il se peut que par la suite, ce phénomène ait perdu de son acuité.

3. Répartition suivent le type d'avions

Suivant les types d'avions utilisés dans l'Armée de l'Air, les malaises constatés se sont

TABLEAU I

Répartition des malaises en fonction du nombre total d'heures de vol

Années	1961	1962	1963	1964	1965	1966	1967	1968
Pourcentage du nombre total d'accidents	5.7	9.9	6.2	9	8	8.2	7.9	6.1
Taux pour 10 000 hr/vol	0.22	0.30	0.21	0.23	0.19	0.18	0.17	0.10

TABLEAU II

Classement des malaises suivant le type d'aéronef

Monoréacteurs combat			Biréacteurs combat		École			Transport et liaison	Hélicopt.
Subs.	Superson.		Subs.	Superson.	Début		Spéc.		
	Mach 1	Mach 2		Mach 2	Hélice	Réact.			
12	11	2	19 dt 10 navig.	0	6	10	34	16 dt 1 navig. + 2 méc.	1

ainsi répartis (Tableau II). Les données recueillies conduisent aux conclusions suivantes: (1) Le nombre des malaises en vol est particulièrement élevé en École de Spécialisation: il est moindre en École de Début. Cette discordance peut s'expliquer par les problèmes d'adaptation dus aux conditions nouvelles du travail aérien, plus difficile en École de Spécialisation qu'en Ecole Élémentaire.

(2) On observe un très faible pourcentage de malaises en vol chez les pilotes d'avions à hautes performances. Bien que ce phénomène puisse paraître surprenant dans la mesure où l'apparition d'un matériel nouveau est souvent génératrice de troubles d'adaptation, on est en droit de se demande si la rareté du nombre des malaises n'est pas en rapport avec la rigueur de la sélection médicale du personnel et sa grande motivation.

(3) Chez les navigateurs, tous les malaises en vol observés se sont produits sur des avions anciens et non sur du matériel à hautes performances, ce qui s'apparente au phénomène déjà constaté chez les pilotes. En règle générale, les malaises en vol apparaissent chez les jeunes navigateurs, lors de leur formation professionelle sur des avions de type conventionnel: les difficultés rencontrées sont la plupart du temps résolues avant leur passage sur avions modernes.

4. Répartition des malaises en vol chez les pilotes

L'analyse a porté sur la répartition des malaises en fonction de l'âge et de l'expérience aéronautique (Figures 1 et 2). On note que 70% des malaises observés ont eu lieu avant la trentième année. Ce phénomène s'explique par la conjonction de plusieurs facteurs

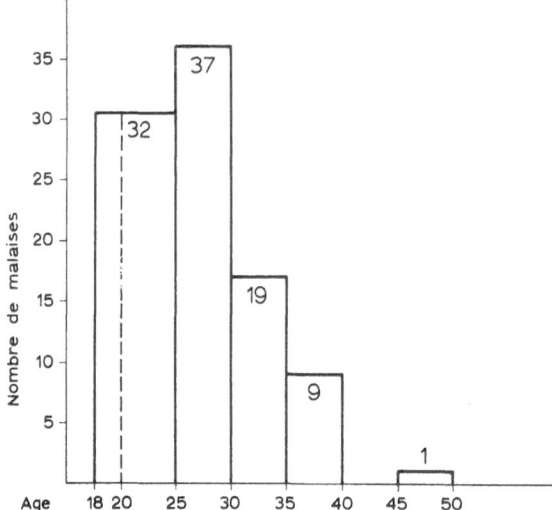

Fig. 1.   Répartition des malaises en vol en fonction de l'âge.

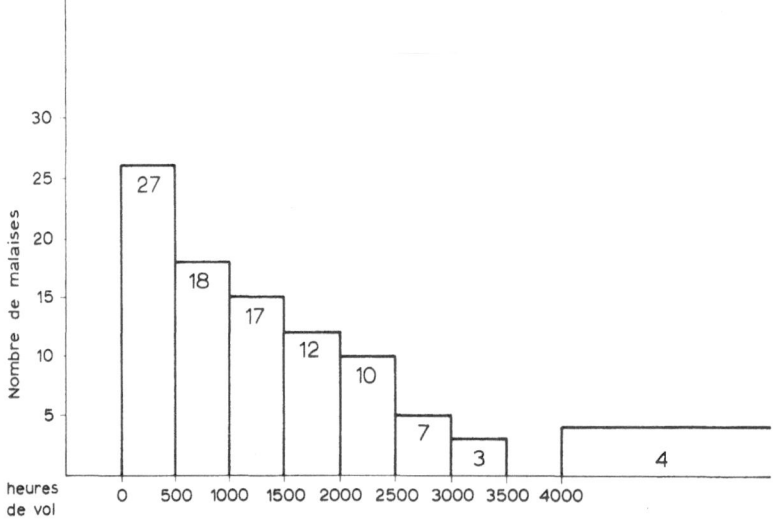

Fig. 2.   Malaises et expérience aéronautique.

qui sont: l'importance des difficultés d'adaptation en École, l'apparition de troubles liés à la désadaptation chez un personnel un peu plus âgé à l'occasion d'évènements divers (mariage, naissance des enfants, difficultés matérielles ou professionnelles etc.) et la découverte ou l'apparition beaucoup plus rare de certaines affections somatiques. Ces malaises frappent ainsi une population jeune qui correspond dans sa grande majorité à la population active chez le personnel navigant.

L'analyse de la répartition des malaises en vol en fonction de l'expérience aéronautique montre que la majorité des cas observés se situe avant le cap des 500 hr, ce qui correspond à la phase de formation des pilotes en École. Les malaises restants s'étendent sur un éventail plus large d'heures de vol, allant de 500 à 3500 hr, cette limite correspondant en général à la fin de la carrière aéronautique d'un grand nombre de pilotes militaires.

5. Étiologie des malaises en vol

Bien qu'il soit classique de distinguer dans la génèse des malaises en vol ce qui revient aux facteurs aéronautiques et aux facteurs humains, on a jugé préférable dans cette étude d'adopter une classification axée sur l'observation clinique des malaises observés. On a ainsi distingué:

(1) Les malaises en vol pour lesquels le diagnostic d'organicité est indéniable, ces malaises étant en relation avec des facteurs aéronautiques constatés lors de l'enquête ou avec une affection somatique précise et confirmée.

(2) Les malaises révélateurs d'emblée d'un état névrotigue dont le diagnostic a été fait après enquête en milieu spécialisé.

(3) Enfin, les malaises complexes, aux étiologies possibles multiples mais jamais vérifiées et dans lesquels, aux causes organiques, s'est associée une importante composante psychologique.

A. MALAISES EN VOL DE CAUSES ORGANIQUES

(1) *Malaises relevant d'une cause aéronautique:* Lors d'une enquête médicale, les facteurs aéronautiques (hypoxie, dépression, accélérations, etc.) sont souvent évoqués. En fait, c'est seulement pour 15 malaises sur 111 que l'intervention de ces facteurs a pu être dûment établie. Au premier rang se situe l'hypoxie, liée à un défaut de fonctionnement des équipements protecteurs. Parmi les causes plus rares, on relève l'intoxication oxycarbonée et la décompression rapide.

(2) *Malaises répondant à une cause médicale somatique:* Ils sont au nombre de 7 et leurs étiologies sont: 3 affections cardio-vasculaires, 1 accès fébrile chez un mécanicien d'équipage à l'état général déficient, 2 intoxications alimentaires et 1 insolation.

B. MALAISES EN VOL RÉVÉLATEURS D'UNE DÉFAILLANCE PSYCHOLOGIQUE

On en dénombre 26. Ils comprennent pour la plupart des névroses d'angoisse ou leurs nombreux équivalents somatiques, certaines névroses post-traumatiques (en particulier après un accident aérien) ou des états névrotiques réactionnels à des situations conflictuelles très pénibles pour le personnel.

C. MALAISES D'ÉTIOLOGIE COMPLEXE

Ce sont les plus fréquents, puisqu'on en dénombre 63. Dans ces cas, on considère comme probable qu'à une cause organique ou aéronautique réelle mais d'importance moyenne se surajoute une composante psychologique. Les facteurs aéronautiques ne seraient que les facteurs favorisants d'un état d'angoisse mal défini. Ce sont ces observations d'anoxie dite 'modérée' que l'enquête technique ne permet jamais de retrouver au niveau des équipements. Ce sont ces apparitions de voile noir ou même des pertes de conscience pour des accélérations relativement modérées et pour le diagnostic desquelles on envisage trop souvent la sommation des accélérations, de l'anoxie modérée et de l'hypoglycémie. Ce sont ces malaises que l'on attribue trop vite à la fatigue, à une banale affection saisonnière ou à l'hyperventilation.

Ainsi il ressort de cette enquête que sur les 111 malaises en vol observés de 1961 à 1968, 22 seulement avaient une origine purement organique, alors que les 89 autres étaient dûs en totalité ou en partie à un problème d'ordre psychologique.

6. Antécédents et évolution des malaises en vol

Sur les 98 malaises observés chez les pilotes, 29 ont fait l'objet au cours de l'enquête d'une hospitalisation pour bilan complémentaire. A l'issue de l'enquête, les décisions médico-aéronautiques furent: 8 propositions d'inaptitude définitive, 16 propositions d'inaptitude temporaire de durée variable. Dans 3 cas, cette inaptitude temporaire se transforma en une inaptitude définitive. 1 proposition de reclassement dans un emploi sédentaire, et 17 reclassements dans une autre spécialité aéronautique. Sur les 13 navigateurs et mécaniciens ayant fait l'objet d'une enquête pour malaises en vol, un seul fut déclaré inapte physique.

Chez les pilotes, l'importance des défaillances psychologiques comme cause principale ou secondaire des malaises en vol mérite d'être soulignée: elles représentent en effet 80% des cas. Devant une pareille étiologie, il est intéressant d'étudier les antécédents médico-aéronautiques de ces pilotes. Quarante-cinq d'entre eux, soit 50%, ont eu un ou plusieurs accidents avant l'apparition de leurs malaises en vol. Le laps de temps s'écoulant entre le dernier accident et le malaise varie entre quelques jours et près d'une année. L'accident est fréquemment un accident grave, surtout matériel. Il semble donc que les accidents aériens jouent un rôle important dans le déterminisme des malaises en vol d'origine psychologique. Sans pouvoir dire qu'ils les provoquent, il apparaît indéniable qu'ils peuvent cristalliser les difficultés rencontrées par les pilotes. De ces faits, doit se dégager la notion que le personnel accidenté devient un personnel fragilisé sur le plan psycho-affectif et qu'il convient de le surveiller étroitement.

Est-il possible ainsi d'établir un pronostic à long terme de ces malaises dus à la désadaptation ou à l'inadaptation à la pratique du vol? Sans pouvoir se permettre d'apprécier la prédisposition de ce personnel aux accidents aériens, on notera toutefois que sur les 83 pilotes ayant présenté des malaises en vol de cet ordre et n'ayant pas été éliminés, 20 eurent par la suite un accident aérien grave dans lequel le facteur humain joua un rôle déterminant: trois d'entre eux entraînèrent la mort du pilote. Les valeurs élevées de ces chiffres méritent de retenir l'attention.

7. Conclusions

L'analyse des malaises en vol établie à partir des 111 comptes rendus d'incidents aériens médicaux observés de 1961 à 1968 dans l'Armée de l'Air Française, a permis de confirmer encore l'importance des défaillances psychologiques dans l'étiologie de ces malaises. Le pourcentage élevé de ce type de défaillance par rapport à celles relevant d'un facteur aéronautique ou somatique résulte de la conjonction du progrès technique et de la qualité et de la rigueur de la sélection médicale : le premier a entraîné une diminution du rôle du facteur aéronautique, la seconde a réduit le nombre des affections organiques non détectées lors des expertises médicales.

Les antécédents d'accidents aériens paraissent jouer un rôle dans le déterminisme de ces malaises d'origine psychologique et il convient donc d'assurer une étroite surveillance, si possible dans un service spécialisé de Médecine Aéronautique, du personnel accidenté.

SELECTION OF AIRLINE TRANSPORT PILOTS
PSYCHIATRIC AND PSYCHOLOGICAL APPROACH

H. GARTMANN

Medical Service, Swissair, Zurich, Switzerland

Up to 1953 the number of well selected and fully trained military pilots applying for an airline transport pilot career was higher than the number of young pilot applicants needed by Swissair every year. During the past sixteen years, the situation has entirely changed.

From 1953 to 1968, the transport capacity of our airline has increased from 49 354 000 to 797 708 000 ton-kilometres, the number of employees from 2403 to 11 185, the number of pilots from 158 to 558, and the demand for new pilots from about 10 to approximately 40 to 50 every year. During this period, our Air Force did not show any appreciable growth, and due to continuous over-employment, many military pilots began to show more interest for jobs in private business rather than that of an airline transport pilot. Since 1954, this has necessitated our selecting more and more of our future pilots from groups of young applicants without any flying experience whatsoever, and so to train them right from the start.

Figure 1 shows the situation in 1968. Only 15, well qualified, military and experi-

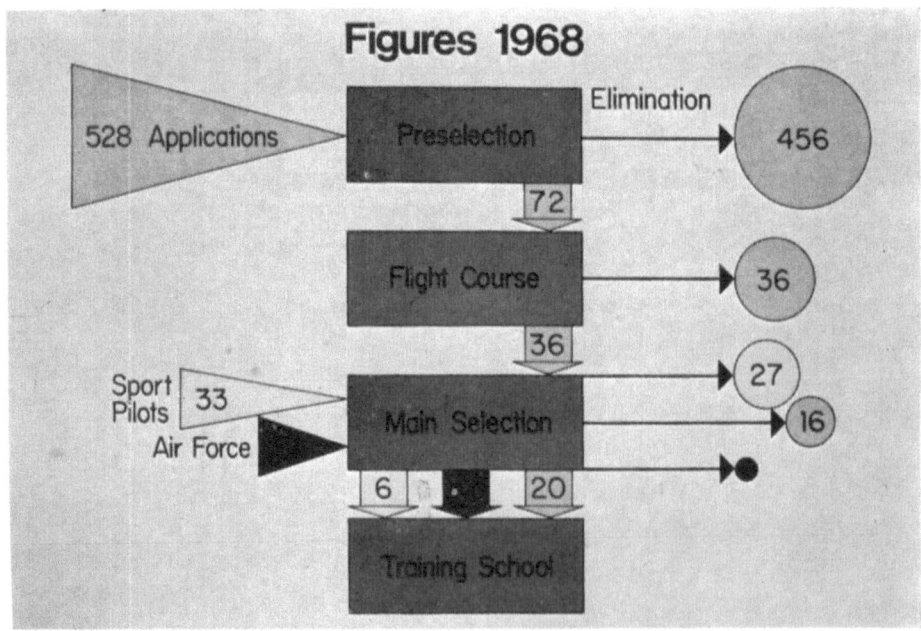

Fig. 1.   Results of Selection-1968.

D. E. Busby (ed.), Recent Advances in Aerospace Medicine, 106–112. All Rights Reserved.
Copyright © 1970 by D. Reidel Publishing Company, Dordrecht-Holland.

enced professional pilots applied; 14 of them were accepted. While only one candidate out of this group was eliminated, we had to eliminate 27 out of 33 applicants from the group of 'sport-pilots', as only 6 of them were considered suitable. A total of 528 young candidates without any flying experience were screened in a one day pre-selection program; 72 of them were considered suitable enough to be admitted to a two-week preliminary selection flying course. During this course, 36 were eliminated and dismissed. The remaining 36 were admitted to the main selection, lasting two days. Twenty of them were successful, and so were admitted to the flight school. Swissair assumes that the failure rate should not be higher than 12%. The average failure rate in the training courses 1959 to 1963 was 27%; in 1964 to 1968 it was only 13.5%.

Our Medical Service participates only in the main selection. The whole medical examination, including a psychiatric interview of 1 to $1\frac{1}{2}$ hours, takes about half a day. In the remaining $1\frac{1}{2}$ days the candidate is given:

(1) An interview by the chief pilot of the training school, directed especially to the professional side of the personality, and his flying and military experience.

(2) An interview by the head of the selection group of the training school, directed particularly towards depth motivation and also to the professional side, but with a slightly different approach to that of the chief pilot of the school.

(3) A Rorschach-test given by a separate examiner.

(4) A battery of paper and pencil tests (unless already applied in pre-selection).

(5) A particular pattern in the Link trainer (unless already applied in pre-selection).

(6) Psychomotor tests focused mainly on multiple attention under stress.

The results of all these examinations, the results of the pre-selection and the results of the two-weeks flying course, the credentials obtained by the Personnel Service and the report of a graphological expert are collected, discussed by the team of the Selection Service and integrated into an all-around personality picture, which is finally submitted to the Selection Board of Flight Operations Management.

Personally, this Medical Director has to participate in three different functions – first as the examining psychiatrist, then in the team session, and finally as a member of the Selection Board. This is complicated and time consuming, but it is the only way for him to participate in the pilot selection with both sufficient influence and sufficient flexibility at the same time.

Figure 2 shows the routine procedure; it is possible for the Medical Director to intervene on three different levels. If he has a clear medical veto (which is rather seldom), he is supposed to declare it immediately after his examination in order to save unnecessary work to other examiners. The result of this team work during 15 years can be summarized as follows:

(1) The integration of an all-around personality picture has proven to be more successful than a separate 'pass' or 'fail' decision at every 'gate'. Even the Medical Service takes a separate decision only in clear medical and psychiatric veto cases.

(2) Psychiatric examinations and psychological tests are not alternative to each other but essential complements. They open up quite different ways of approach to the candidate's personality.

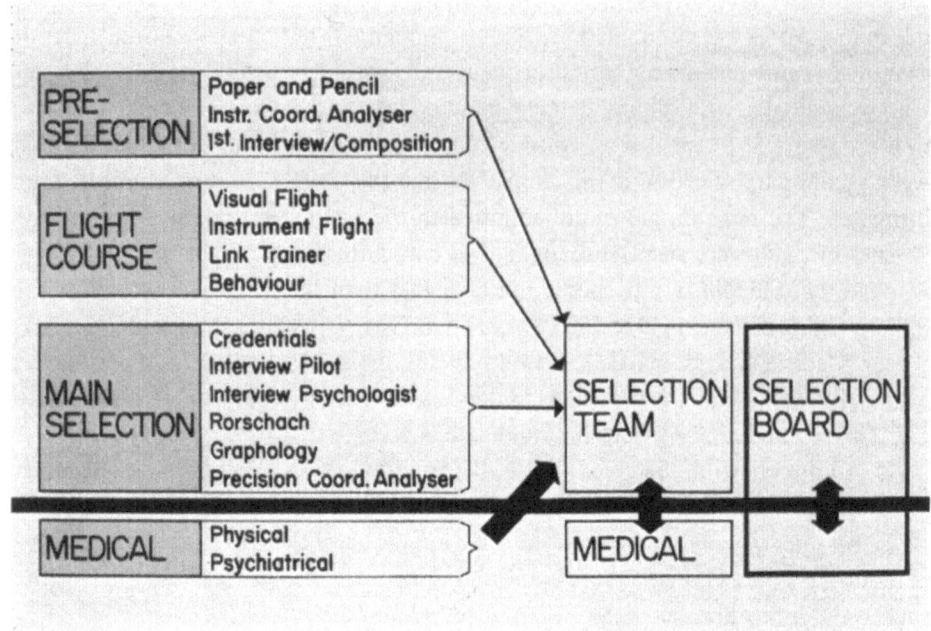

Fig. 2.   Routine procedures for Pilot-Selection.

(3) The extensive interviews are worthwhile because the structure of the personality is, in the long run, of equal importance to the strictly professional skill.

(4) If tests are applied at all, then there should be a sufficient number of them. Misjudgments are then less likely.

(5) For young applicants without proven flying skill, a preliminary flying course is of the greatest value if the instructors are pedagogically experienced and specially trained for selection tasks.

(6) Many examinations, especially those which cannot be mathematically calibrated (*e.g.* psychiatric and other interviews), should be applied as much as possible by the same examiners for all candidates.

All this is routine. If, however, during the main selection discrepancies between the results of different examiners arise, further clarification, rediscussion and additional examinations may become necessary. The Medical Service and the Selection Service can be very helpful to each other: certain otherwise inexplicable test results must and can be re-interpreted in the light of further psychiatric evaluation and *vice versa*.

This feed-back circuit for mutually relevant information may be illustrated by a few actual cases.

CASE NO. 1:

Medical pre-employment examination 1958 at age 29. Physical findings: vegetative lability, tendency to hypertony, tachycardia (figures follow later). Expert evidence of cardiologist: lowered S-T interval, borderline case; however, not yet pathological.

Psychiatric evaluation: good solid family background and personal history. Stable pleasant life situation, good contact, very well adjusted. Successful, but finally disappointed in his administrative profession; late but profound motivation for pilot's career.

Conclusion after medical and psychiatric examination: there were good reasons to presume that the high pulse rate and partially raised blood pressure were rather symptoms of a temporary personality reaction and of psychosomatic disorder than due to a fixed hypertensive disease. But the essential question was still left open: Is this the jammed aggressivity of a personality continuously overdemanded by his environment and by himself? Or is it the jammed activity of a clever personality able to fulfill much more than he has fulfilled until now?

A reconsideration of the results of all psychomotor tests answered this medical question at once. They unanimously proved so much technical skill, such a quiet, self-understanding and disciplined performance, tenacity and concentration that there was no doubt: this man had been, until now, rather under- than overstressed. He was accepted. Already during, and also after the so-called stress of the basic training, all figures of blood-pressure and pulse rate went back to normal and have remained so for ten years. The flying qualifications were always above average and the man is now a first-class pilot. Figure 3 shows the diagram of the blood-pressure (one minute after a slight exercise) and the pulse rate in the period from 1958 to 1968.

CASE NO. I

	BLOOD PRESSURE	PULS RATE
1958	160/105	96
1960	170/90	68
1962	145/85	88
1965	130/80	80
1968	130/80	80

Fig. 3.   Bloodpressure and pulserate (Case No. 1) 1958–1968.

CASE NO. 2:

Electronic engineer, age 20, examined as a pilot's candidate in 1950 in a selection system somewhat different from the one we are using now. In the physical examination, he was considered fit and also the results of psychiatric evaluation of his life history was quite acceptable: 'clever at school and during apprenticeship, intelligent, open-minded and frank'. Nevertheless, he was finally refused because his Rorschach-protocol was 'full of neologisms, funny abstractions, tremendous aggression'. This interpretation was verified by an excellent Rorschach-expert. The answers this candidate gave in the Rorschach-test were extraordinary indeed: Figure 4 shows the Rorschach-plate No. 3. He sees in the centre "two human structures destroying something" and further "this red thing behind them is a cunning thought. They play peace, but they are thinking of cunning aggression". Figure 5 shows Rorschach-plate No. 9: "Two figures in a fight with glittering irons. They look peaceful, but in their mind there is war. There is, however, a hope, a mutual hope, that the other one might not be fighting".

The candidate was seen again in 1952, when he was applying for a pilot's career again. In the interview he made an impression as healthy and reasonable as ever. He was shocked by the sudden

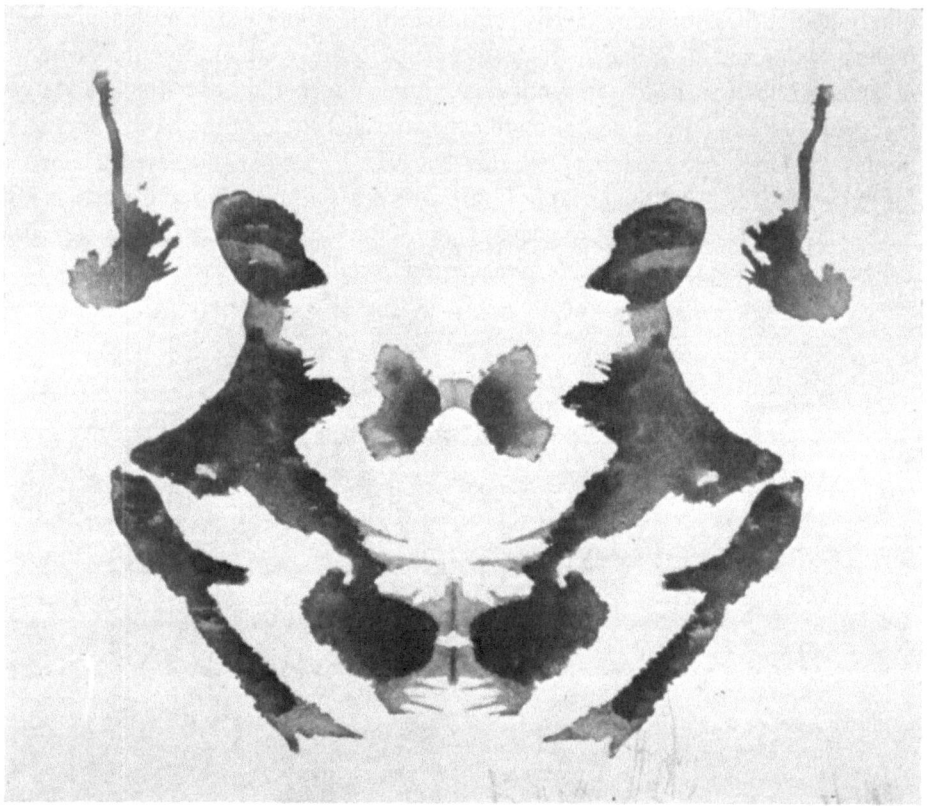

Fig. 4.   Rorschach-plate No. 3.

remark: "Your Rorschach is completely crazy but you are not. Please do not play the fool again". And then he told the examiner the whole story: Before applying as a pilot's candidate for the first time, he took advice from an older pilot as to what sort of answers in the Rorschach-test would make the best impression upon the examiner. His adviser's briefing was: "A pilot must be a fighter. The more of war and fights and tough aggressions you can interpret into these Rorschach-figures the better for you". Being rather reluctant in believing this story at once, he was asked: "You want to make me believe that you are such an actor that you can just play these funny answers without any inner necessity or urge?" "Of course, I have played", was his answer. "Alright then, let us check it. Let us presume you are not applying for a pilot's but for a clergyman's career, and I am a cardinal or something like that". His flexibility was surprising: not a single aggressive answer came this time; all the pictures seemed to be for him full of angels, chapels, churches and other holy things. When we look again at Rorschach-plate 3 on Figure 4 there are now "two priests swinging their incense, a praying figure with a light and red soul inside". Plate 9 in Figure 5 shows now "two praying monks".

After this re-examination it was clear that the problem raised by the Rorschach was not a pathological (possibly schizophrenic) abnormal aggression (as primarily believed), but rather a calculated cunningness of a very flexible personality. For reasons beyond our own control he was not admitted to a pilot's career, but he has been working very successfully now for more than ten years as a flight engineer. This case is not quoted to criticize the Rorschach-test: in continuous confrontation with the findings of the psychiatric evaluation of the life-history it can be an excellent test. This may be proven by Case No. 3.

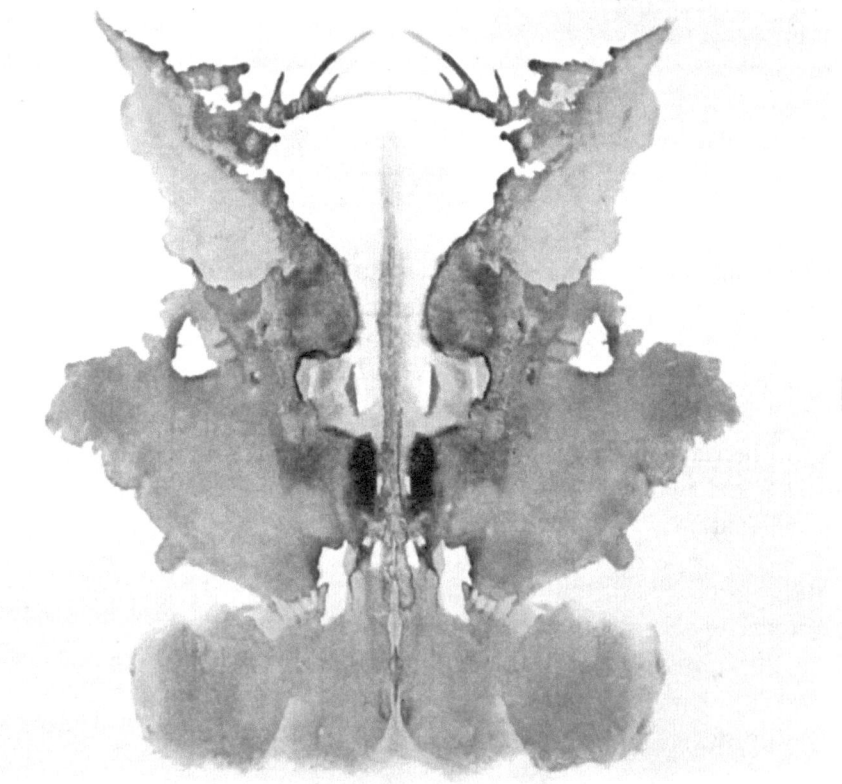

Fig. 5.   Rorschach-plate No. 9.

CASE NO. 3:

Engineer, age 23, acceptable results in most tests. Physically healthy, no serious symptoms in the psychiatric exploration, and apparently no hereditary disease in the family. But very frightened during the Rorschach-test and also some very strange answers. In plate 3 of the Rorschach (Figure 4) he can just see loose parts of a female body. Here a bosom, here an individual leg with this part of the knee considerably disturbing his view of the picture, a loose head here, but in spite of his intellectual capacity and vigilance he sees not a trace of a female figure as a whole. The reason for such a disintegration of the female image was not explainable. The candidate was summoned for another psychiatric examination. No really severe sexual problems at the present time could be found as an explanation for the disintegrated female body. However, after a prolonged investigation, it became clear that the personality of his mother was really as disintegrated as the female body seen by the candidate on Rorschach-plate 3. She had been temporarily in a mental hospital because of a psychosis. This trauma was only one side of his problem. Obviously, he had tried to dissimulate his heredity: altogether it was discovered later that there were more cases of rather abnormal personalities in his family. He was not accepted, not primarily because of the heredity, but rather because of the immaturity of his personality he proved in his behaviour and his dissimulation. This tendency to hide important things would not have been discovered without the Rorschach test.

CASE NO. 4:

Engineer, age 24; in the selection examination physically fit. Psychiatrically doubtful: reserved personality, little contact. Has worked through a severe conflict in his family intellectually but not emotionally. Very intelligent, full of brilliant irony, considerable tenacity. Also, to the Selection Service he seemed to be inhibited in his contact, but a reliable personality with good technical skill. There was some doubt as far as resistance against any continuous mental stress was concerned. The company finally agreed on a rather exceptional procedure: his not yet solved conflicts were discussed again with him. He agreed whole-heartedly with a psychoanalytically-oriented treatment by an experienced psychotherapist. This took him about one year. When he was interviewed again 1½ years later, he had gained a good deal of that 'corrective emotional experience', which is characteristic for every successful psychoanalytical approach. His private conflict was worked through to an extent that he was now fully disposing of all energy needed for a pilot's career. He was accepted to the flying school and succeeded there. He is now a co-pilot with average qualifications.

In conclusion, it was the purpose here to report fifteen years experience in pilot selection including its two important elements:

(1) The routine procedure which can be summarized under the slogan: 'Integration of an all-round personality picture out of as many and as different approaches as possible'.

(2) The handling of particular cases under the slogan: 'Discrepancies and unclarified findings as a mutual stimulus among the examiners to reconsider and re-examine the candidate again'.

À PROPOS DES RECOMMANDATIONS DE L'O.A.C.I. SUR LES NORMES AUDITIVES DU PERSONNEL NAVIGANT TECHNIQUE

J. PASQUET et J. LAVERNHE

Service Médical Air France, 1 Square Max Hymans, Paris 15e, France

Les conditions de travail des navigants ayant rapidement évolué depuis quelques années et notre expérience s'enrichissant, il est permis aujourd'hui de remettre en cause certaines notions précédemment acquises. En particulier, le syndrome de 'surdité des aviateurs' s'est, en aviation commerciale, profondément modifié. Il n'y a pas de formule audiométrique particulière du navigant si ce n'est celle dépendant, d'une part des conditions d'apprentissage ainsi que l'ont montré dans leurs études statistiques, Lafontaine *et al.* (1963) et, d'autre part, des anciennes conditions de vol traumatisantes pour l'oreille interne. Actuellement par contre, le niveau sonore dans les cockpits des jets est relativement faible. De plus les communications radio sont très améliorées grâce à la fidélité acoustique des hauts parleurs dont le réglage à la puissance de sortie est de bonne qualité. Quant aux accidents d'oreille moyenne, ils sont, sauf exception, sans séquelles en raison des faibles variations de pression et de la meilleure information des navigants qui entraîne un traitement précoce efficace comme l'a montré Hustin (1965).

Les dépassements des normes audiométriques constatés lors des examens révisionnels sont donc essentiellement en rapport avec le vieillissement, bien compensés par l'expérience acquise, alors que les agressions qui ont au départ constitué l'hypoacousie ont disparu ou se sont très atténuées. Ainsi nous constatons depuis huit ans qu'un nombre important de navigants se situe en dehors des normes requises pour le renouvellement de leur licence. Mais il nous semble exister là une situation discordante si on a pu estimer néanmoins qu'ils pouvaient continuer de voler.

Rappelons les recommandations du standard I de l'O.A.C.I. (1962). Pour les pilotes et radios navigants: "le candidat ne doit pas avoir une perte d'audition pour l'une ou l'autre des oreilles, supérieure à 25 décibels pour l'une quelconque des 3 fréquences 500, 1000 et 2000 cycles par seconde, ou à 40 décibels pour la fréquence 3000 cps".

Les normes de l'arrêté français de 1953 atténuent légèrement ces conditions pour le standard I: le candidat ne devant pas avoir une perte supérieure à 30 dB pour les fréquences 500, 1000, 2000 et à 40 dB pour la fréquence 3000 cps.

Dans l'enquête réalisée l'application de ces normes aurait conduit depuis 1961 à déclarer inapte 99 sujets, soit 8% de notre personnel navigant technique, se répartissant de la façon suivante: 59 pilotes, 14 radios navigants, et 26 mécaniciens navigants.

Or, tous ces navigants ayant fait la preuve d'une audition suffisante ont été déclarés aptes sur dérogation. En effet, dans tous les cas ont été effectués les examens capables de permettre outre un diagnostic étiologique et de localisation, une évaluation de la capacité auditive résiduelle par un bilan clinique avec examen otoscopique et examen de la perméabilité tubaire, une acoumétrie simple avec épreuves au diapason, une audiométrie liminaire tonale et supra-liminaire avec recherche de recrutement, et des tests en vol au cours desquels la compréhension des messages s'est effectuée normalement.

Mais cette situation qui paraît résulter de la relative sévérité des normes d'audiométrie tonale actuelle, risque d'être la source de difficultés ou de malentendus avec les navigants. Il est en effet psychologiquement inconfortable pour un navigant de voler sur dérogation, dérogation qu'il peut craindre de voir résilier à chaque contrôle. En outre, la stricte application des normes aurait conduit à déclarer ces navigants inaptes. Ils auraient alors été en droit de demander une indemnité spéciale au titre de l'imputabilité au service aérien, prévue par les réglements francais. Paradoxalement d'ailleurs, un navigant, sur son initiative, pourrait refuser de demander une dérogation pour bénéficier des avantages que lui confèrerait l'inaptitude.

Il nous semble donc souhaitable d'atténuer la sévérité des recommandations de l'O.A.C.I. qui pourrait être complétées comme suit: *"Lors des examens révisionnels d'aptitude, les navigants en fonction dont les seuils d'audition tonale se situent en dehors des normes recommandées feront l'objet d'un examen audiométrique vocal: l'intelligibilité devra atteindre 50% des éléments de langage à 40 décibels au-dessus du niveau de référence."*

L'introduction systématique de l'audiométrie vocal qui a l'avantage de contribuer au diagnostic des lésions acoustiques en recoupant les données de l'audiométrie tonale, permettrait d'évaluer le niveau de compréhension pratique, ce qu'il importe en définitive de mesurer pour établir le niveau d'invalidité. Bien entendu, cet examen n'exclue pas les très importants tests en vol.

En dehors des examens pratiqués par les autorités chargées de l'attribution d'une dérogation, nous avons nous-mêmes par ailleurs réalisé 18 examens audiométriques vocaux dont il nous paraît intéressant de rapporter les résultats en montrant les conséquences qu'aurait le nouveau texte proposé.

La plus mauvaise oreille étant prise comme référence pour le seuil d'intelligibilité de 50% en audiométrie vocale au casque dans le silence, les cas se répartissent comme donnés sur le Tableau I.

TABLEAU I

Décibels	10	15	20	25	30	35	40		45	50	55	60
Nombre de sujets	1	2	3	3	1	3	3		1	–	–	1

L'application à ces sujets du projet élaboré donnerait les résultats présentés sur le Tableau II.

L'adoption du texte proposé permettrait donc une atténuation notable de la sévérité des normes actuelles d'audiométrie tonale, les plus importants déficits restant

TABLEAU II

	Arrêté de 1953	Projet envisagé	Décision effective du C.M.A.C.
Aptitude (nombre de cas)	0	16	18
Inaptitude (nombre de cas)	18	2	0

de la compétence du Conseil Médical de l'Aviation Civile chargé de l'attribution des dérogations.

En conclusion, nous pensons que l'adoption du texte proposé aurait l'avantage de tenir compte du passé aéronautique et du vieillissement et de permettre une évaluation de la compréhension pratique qui, seule, entre en ligne de compte pour la sécurité aérienne. Enfin, en réduisant le nombre de sujets inaptes, il éviterait d'éventuelles demandes abusives d'indemnités pour imputabilité au service aérien.

Bibliographie

Hustin, A.: 1965, *Rev. Méd. Aéro.* **4**.

Lafontaine, E., Pialoux, P., et Lucas, A.: 1963, *Congrès International de Médecine Aéronautique et Spatiale*, Rome, Italy.

Standards Internationaux, Avril 1953, Annexe I de la Convention relative à l'Aviation Civile Internationale

A STUDY OF SIMULATED AIRLINE PILOT INCAPACITATION

Phase I – Obvious and Maximal Loss of Function

C. R. HARPER, G. J. KIDERA and J. F. CULLEN

Medical Department, United Air Lines, Denver, Colo., U.S.A.

1. Introduction

A sudden loss of ability to function in a pilot performing flight duties can be a dramatic topic. The possibility of its occurrence has been the subject of many discussions. It
has been the reason for many aviation industry rules and rigid governmental regula-
tions. The true incidence as it relates to accident causation is not reliable. A few
statistical reviews are published but the relatively poor 'state of the art' in reconstruct-
ing the events leading to an accident substantially negates any existing statistics or discussions regarding the subject and accident etiology.

The hypothetical dangers involved when related to a rapidly increasing population
of senior pilots commanding high performance jet aircraft could be significant. To the
authors' knowledge, studies of simulated inflight incapacitation are very limited.
In view of the many unknown factors regarding the subject, the United Air Lines
Medical Department initiated the present study. Two phases of study were planned:

Phase I – Gross sudden incapacitation simulating an abrupt functional loss such
as myocardial infarction or cerebrovascular accident.

Phase II – Involves the subtle or less obvious physiological deficit, such as a hypo-
glycemic reaction or psychomotor seizure. A situation where the pilot seems to be
functional to other crew members, but in essence is not performing.

Both phases of study are complete. Phase II results are still being evaluated. The
results of the obvious incapacitation are the purpose of this paper. Phase II results will
follow in a future presentation.

2. Method

A. PROTOCOL

Qualified line crews of the DC-8 and B-737 were utilized while performing flight tasks
in the respective aircraft simulator. To preclude subjective error regarding measurements and observations, sound movie photography was utilized to record the incapacitation and subsequent events. The aircraft attitude, airspeed, altitude and ILS
approach aid were duplicated and photographed in the radio-aids room or 'tower'.
The movies of these basic flight instruments were spliced and joined with the movie in
the simulator. This allows simultaneous viewing of pilot and simulator performance.
The cameras used in the study had a time limit of approximately twenty minutes.
The total number of 'incapacitations' was 45; 25 in the DC-8 simulator, and 20 in the
B-737. Three-man crews were studied in the DC-8 and 2-man crews in the B-737.

D. E. Busby (ed.), Recent Advances in Aerospace Medicine, 116–122. All Rights Reserved.
Copyright © 1970 by D. Reidel Publishing Company, Dordrecht-Holland.

The phase of flight distribution is shown in Table I for the DC-8. The DC-8 portion included one emergency descent with incapacitation during the descent and two episodes at about 50 ft above the ground right after aircraft rotation for take-off.

The phase of flight for the B-737 portion of the study is shown in Table II. Tables I and II also show the distribution of which pilot became 'unconscious' and who was

TABLE I

Pilot incapacitated and phase of flight (DC-8)

Captain incapacitated	12 Cases
First officer incapacitated	13 Cases
Pilot flying incapacitated	17 Cases
Pilot not flying incapacitated	8 Cases

Phase of flight distribution		Pilot incapacitated	
		Captain	First officer
Take-off	8	4	4
Approach	9	4	5
Missed approach	2	1	1
Climb	4	2	2
Descent	2	1	1

TABLE II

Pilot incapacitated and phase of flight (B-737)

Captain incapacitated	15 Cases
First officer incapacitated	5 Cases
Pilot flying incapacitated	14 Cases
Pilot not flying incapacitated	6 Cases

Phase of flight distribution		Pilot incapacitated	
		Captain	First officer
Take-off	8	6	2
Approach	10	8	2
Missed approach	2	1	1

TABLE III

Altitude of incapacitation

Altitudes (MSL)	Distribution	
	DC-8	B-737
Below 200 ft	4	12
200 ft–700 ft	8	8
700 ft–1700 ft	7	–
Above 1700 ft	6	–

flying at the time of 'incapacitation'. Due to observations in the DC-8 portion, which was completed first, all episodes in the B-737 were on take-off or approach, and all were performed at altitudes below 1500 ft. Table III points out the altitude of incapacitation.

B. CREW BRIEFING

During required proficiency checks, crews were requested to participate in the study at the time of their arrival for simulator (pre-flight) briefing. With the crew together, it was explained that one of the crew would become 'incapacitated' sometime during the 2-hour flight. The element of complete surprise could not be attained because of the strong possibility that the remaining crew members would ask for the simulator to be turned off and attempt to aid the 'unconscious' pilot. The exact time of the episode was unknown to the crew.

There was no explanation of how to handle the situation. Instructions were to

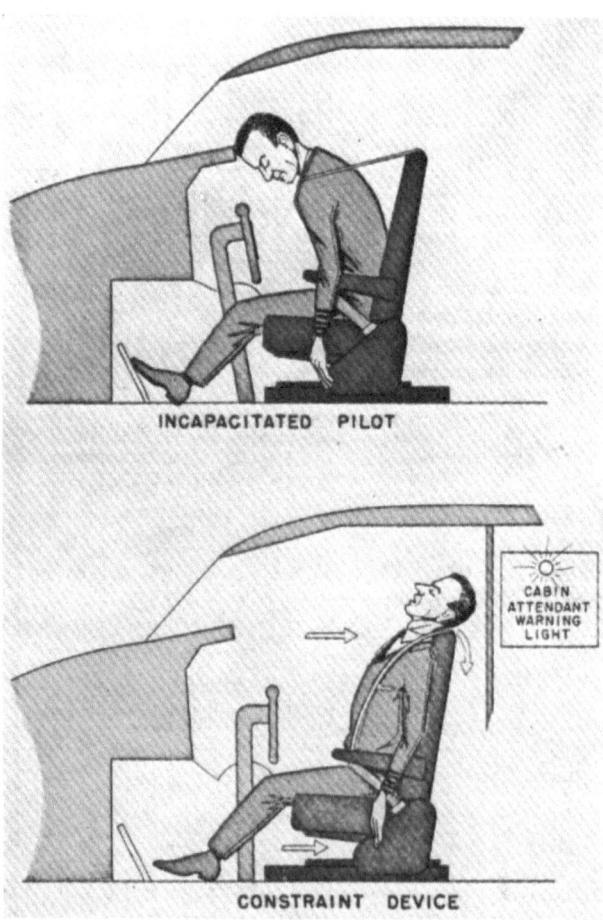

Fig. 1.   Experimental emergency pilot restraint device.

proceed as they would under actual flight conditions using their own judgement and planning.

The crew member to be affected was briefed separately and given a cue (fail flag appears on ILS) when to 'collapse'. As he collapsed he was to attempt to alter a control switch or throttle or produce pressure in roll or pitch to the control wheel. He was then to remain ineffective and silent until removed from his seat or until landing.

Persons outside the aircraft simulator were available as 'stewardesses' or 'passengers', if requested by the unaffected crew for aid.

The restraint effectiveness of the prevalent shoulder harness in use was evaluated. In one-half of the episodes, the shoulder harness was worn by the 'affected' pilot. The prevalent shoulder harness in use by United Air Lines is the inertia reel-lock type.

A new concept of emergency pilot restraint was given initial testing with the two man crew. This experimental device consists of a geared motorized unit (Figure 1) which, when activated, performs three tasks:

(1) Retracts a pilot back firmly in his seat (if he is wearing the shoulder harness).
(2) Pulls the seat to the full aft position.
(3) Alerts cabin attendants to come to the flight deck.

The activation switch will be guarded and one is accessible to either pilot. The optimal location is still under study.

C. METHOD OF EVALUATION

Each movie was evaluated by two flight instructors, a flight standards inspector, a flight surgeon and an aviation psychologist. The instructors and inspector were currently aircraft type-qualified for the DC-8 and B-737.

Each participating crew member was given a questionnaire to complete following the simulator session.

TABLE IV

Mean crew member experience

DC-8	Time in type	Jet time	Total time
Total Mean (hr) – All Pilots	2425.22	3020.9	8924.5
B-737	Time in type	Jet time	Total time
Total Mean (hr) – All Pilots	411.58	1485.14	4861.37

The experience levels of the crews participating in the study are shown in Table IV. Excluding time in type, the DC-8 crews were twice as experienced as the B-737 crews.

3. Results and Discussion

The large amount of data collected precludes a complete detailed review in this paper. The major observations, discussion and recommendations will be presented. The analysis is placed into two categories: the operational aspects, which examined the initial aircraft control and/or recovery as well as the command potential and degree of operational ability of the remaining pilot under the increased workload; and the medical human factors aspects, which examined when and what type of emergency aid was ordered and the overall effect, if any, of the 'startle reaction'. General observations of the above aspects are presented for a 3-man crew aircraft (DC-8) and 2-man crew (B-737) aircraft:

A. OPERATIONAL ASPECTS

(1) *3-man Crew (DC-8)* Forty-four percent of the incapacitations occurred on final approach or right after executing a missed approach. None descended below 150 ft above the ground before attaining a climb. Only one pilot (a captain) elected to continue to approach. In this case the co-pilot 'died' inside the middle marker at 200 ft. The remainder elected a 'go-around'.

Forty-two percent of the episodes took place during take-off or climb. The highest altitude was 2900 ft, the lowest at 70 ft (essentially at V_R). In 3 instances the pilot overshot the missed approach altitudes from 300 to 800 ft.

Evaluation of the films revealed the following concerning performance during these simulated emergencies:

	Good	Satis-factory	Fair	Poor
Initial A/C Takeover	54%	38%	4%	4%
Command Ability	33%	17%	38%	12%
Overall Performance	42%	22%	22%	16%

(2) *2-man Crew (B-737)* Sixty percent of the episodes occurred during a final or missed approach. One case descended to 50 ft above the ground before attaining a climb (one throttle idled by 'dying' captain unnoticed) and 5 cases continued the approach to landing.

Forty percent occurred on take-off or initial climb. Incapacitation altitudes varied from 50 to 150 ft. One pilot, as above, did not observe the 'dying' captain pull one throttle back to idle resulting in poor climb and airspeed and stall warning. In 4 cases the missed approach altitude was in error from 200 to 2000 ft.

The performance ratings during these simulated emergencies were:

	Good	Satis-factory	Fair	Poor
Initial A/C takeover	40%	50%	(0)	10%
Command ability	20%	35%	25%	20%
Overall performance	15%	50%	30%	5%

Considering the lower overall mean pilot experience, the 2-man crew performed favorably. This is pertinent when comparing the altitudes of 'incapacitation' in the B-737 versus the DC-8 (Table III). The reasons for this are conjecture. The stimulus and motivation of the remaining pilot to perform without immediate help from a third crew member should be considered. This factor may be relevant to the fact that 20% of the 2-man crew continued the approach to landing versus 4% of the 3-man crew. The reasons for a decision to continue final approach with a normal aircraft or execute a missed approach are both sound.

Although none of the 'aircraft' crashed, several reached relatively unsafe distances above the ground when the incident occurred during final approach. The lack of the ability to have the element of complete surprise should be considered here.

These emergency simulations showed the effectiveness of the inertia reel-lock type shoulder harness to be quite inadequate. The harness allows an unconscious body to fall from the sitting position to practically any portion of the control area, as if no shoulder harness were worn. This should be compared to the harness system that can also be hand-locked by switch.

On the other hand, the experimental pilot restraint device could be of considerable physical and psychological support to a remaining crew member. This would be particularly true during a critical phase of flight and/or an incapacitation of a violent nature, e.g. a grand mal seizure. Except for bodily removal from the seat, which can be performed by other people, the device can as effectively remove the pilot from the control area as could the third crew member (Second Officer).

B. MEDICAL/HUMAN FACTOR ASPECTS

The 2- and 3-man crews are discussed jointly, and comparisons made. The first aid attention given to the 'afflicted' crew member varied significantly in the two types of crews. Oxygen was offered by only 48% of the DC-8 crews versus 65% of B-737 remaining crew member. This is interesting considering the DC-8 had the extra crew member immediately available. The fact that B-737 crews have had more recent lectures on First Aid may explain this difference. Only 3 of all the pilots in command inquired concerning breathing and artificial respiration and only one requested that the pulse and presence of dilated pupil be checked. Only 2 pilots requested that 100% oxygen be used.

Sixty percent of the incapacitated pilots were ordered removed from the seat in the DC-8. Ten percent were removed in the B-737. The restraint device mentioned was made available in 35% of the cases. The crews who elected to leave the afflicted member in his seat ordered the shoulder harness put on in only 50% of the cases. Unfortunately, the inertia reel harness provided minimal, if any restraint protection. The real possibility of a tonic and/or clonic seizure during a terminal or hypoxic cerebral phase is of significance here. It seems apparent that the following are needed:

(1) A positive hand-lock type harness.
(2) Seat pulled to full aft position.
(3) The decision to always remove pilot from his seat.

(1) and (2) would allow an initially acceptable margin of safety concerning interference with the yoke and center pedestal (throttles) and allow a remaining crew member to observe any changes made by the affected pilot. This can be accomplished by the third crew member or by a restraining device as in Figure 1.

A universal decision to remove the pilot from his seat would allow a more thorough evaluation of the aircraft and give remaining crew a chance to think out the changes in responsibility and aircraft performance, *e.g.* nose wheel steering or high speed turnoff, check lists, *etc.*

The effect of the 'startle', or alarm reaction was impossible to measure in this study. It was, however, evident in varying degrees. For example, there was a request that cabin attendants notify passengers of a possible emergency evacuation. Moreover, a passenger was frequently placed in the Captain's seat, to later exchange seats with the First Officer. The concern to 'fly the airplane' first is, of course, vital. A tendency to over-react in this type of emergency was noticed in some cases. This is no doubt responsible for the complete disregard for the incapacitated pilot in so many cases after the aircraft was well under control.

4. Conclusions

Even though death or abrupt loss of function is statistically rare, the study indicates a future need for a recommended operational sequence of events for remaining crew members, and more emphasis on aid to the incapacitated pilot after the flight situation is well under control. The completion of these initial goals will be attempted by using selected portions of the study films in developing a training movie and written educational material. These will be used during initial and recurrent training periods.

PREVENTION OF FOOD-BORNE DISEASES IN CIVIL AVIATION

J. HOOGENDOORN and D. A. A. MOSSEL

Medical Department, KLM Royal Dutch Airlines, Amsterdam, The Netherlands

1. Introduction

This paper attempts to demonstrate the need for both continuous and increasing alertness with respect to food hygiene. The airlines already perform a considerable amount of preventive hygienic work. Nevertheless, a few months ago a serious outbreak of acute gastroenteritis occurred during a tour in the Orient. Twenty-three of a tour group of 42 passengers developed diarrhea, abdominal cramps and vomiting. One person died and 2 others had to be hospitalized. Epidemiological investigation incriminated part of a dinner (shrimp/crab salad) which was served during the flight between Bangkok and Hongkong on May 3, 1969. The mean incubation time for this food poisoning outbreak was 15 hr. The first symptoms were observed 5 hr after consumption of the suspected dish. No information could be obtained on the other passengers on the same flight who did not belong to the tour group, due to lack of information on where to contact them in Hongkong.

The size of such outbreaks of in-flight food poisonings will increase considerably after the introduction of the so-called 'jumbo' aircraft. The possibility of an incident of such magnitude must be a constant concern to the airlines.

2. Needs for Prevention

In spite of existing World Health Organization recommendations and utmost care in food preparation taken by many airlines, the potential risk for food contamination still seems to be great. An attempt has been made to estimate the overall chances of spreading food-borne infectious diseases in civil aviation to date by carrying out a world-wide survey of sanitary conditions prevailing in 25 airport catering establishments. The summary of this survey in Table I makes it obvious that numerous serious sanitary deficiencies still exist in a great number of these establishments.

TABLE I

Results of a world-wide check of 25 airport catering establishments

Toilets: 50% no hand basins
Toilets: 55% no soap or towels
Toilets: 55% no fly screens

Food preparation: 20% not separated from washing-up section
Food preparation: 45% no fly screens
Refrigeration: 30% inadequate

D. E. Busby (ed.), Recent Advances in Aerospace Medicine, 123–125. All Rights Reserved.
Copyright © 1970 *by D. Reidel Publishing Company, Dordrecht-Holland.*

When considering to intensify preventive measures, it should be recalled that the micro-organisms most frequently responsible for acute food poisoning are, in order of decreasing seriousness, *Shigella, Salmonella, Staphylococcus, Clostridium perfringens* and *Bacillus cereus*.

The ultimate reservoirs of many of these bacteria may be found in the digestive tract of healthy food-producing animals (especially *Salmonella*), as well as in human carriers (especially *Shigella*). The sources of contamination with *Clostridium perfringens* and *Bacillus cereus* are certain foods of animal and vegetable origin, respectively. In addition, flies, cockroaches and other insects play an important role in indirect fecal contamination. Contamination of food with *Staphylococcus aureus* stems from purulent skin lesions, or from the nose and throat.

When foods contaminated in one of these ways are stored in the temperature 'danger zone' of 45 °F (7 °C) to 140 °F (60 °C), bacteria multiply rapidly. Food initially contaminated with only a low number of pathogens can, within 6 hours, have sufficient numbers of bacteria and bacterial toxins to provoke acute symptoms and signs of illness, commencing from 3 to 30 hr after it is consumed.

Particularly hazardous are all foods which consist entirely or partly of milk and milk products, eggs, meat, poultry, fish and sea-food. In general, all foods with a high moisture- and protein content, must receive careful hygienic attention.

Finally, contamination of foods and beverages by protozoa or worm eggs must not be overlooked. Foods and beverages may act only as inert vectors.

3. Prevention

The practical measures of prevention can be summarized by what is called the '5-P' approach.

Purchasing: First class raw materials only. Contamination and deterioration of these raw materials must be prevented while stored. Storage separated from kitchen and prepared foods.

Premises: Excellent sanitary conditions. Food preparation area totally separated from all other parts of kitchen. Adequate storage and refrigeration rooms. Flies and vermin must be kept out by proper methods. All areas must be easily accessible for cleaning and inspection. Constant supervision, and frequent inspection by medical experts.

Personnel: No carrier of pathogenic organisms must work in a kitchen. Specialized pre-employment medical examinations and periodical re-examinations. Thorough indoctrination in the principles of personal hygiene and proper food handling. All personnel should report to the medical department after having been absent due to illness before resuming work. All physical complaints should be reported. The medical department should make bacteriological examinations of stools, naso-pharynx, *etc.*, whenever indicated.

Processing: all foods, unnecessary to say, must be processed under the most rigid hygienic circumstances. Storage of processed foods either below 40 °F (5 °C) or above

140 °F (60 °C). Bacteriological surveillance of prepared foods by simple but reliable methods.

Plane operations: it is potentially hazardous to serve food on board that has left the cooling stage (below +5 °C) more than 5 hours previously. Special attention should be paid to this time limit in case of a last-minute flight delay. Indoctrination of cabin personnel in the principles of proper food handling. Instructions to all crew members regarding the choice of safe restaurants abroad.

A rather simple procedure for catering establishment surveillance has been in use by KLM for many years. Specially trained inspectors provided with an extensive but simple check-list pay unexpected and unannounced visits to catering establishments abroad. During the course of the inspection, every item is checked and noted. After completion, the list is countersigned by the manager of the establishment.

The check-list gives the experts of the medical department a full insight in all aspects of the prevailing conditions in the kitchen concerned. If the check-list shows unsatisfactory conditions, measures are taken to remedy the deficiencies. When repeated inspections show no improvement, the contract with the caterer is be discontinued as soon as possible.

It is advisable that the inspectors are familiar with simple bacteriological methods for surface examinations of prepared foods. Medical departments should supervise the composition of menus, guaranteeing that dangerous foods, such as shell-fish, will will be excluded from meals.

4. Conclusions

The need for increasing sanitary supervision of food served by the airlines is stressed. The so-called 5-P approach compelling caterers to produce meals, snacks, etc., of better sanitary quality is recommended.

UNSCHEDULED LANDINGS FOR MEDICAL REASONS:
A FIVE-YEAR SURVEY OF THE EXPERIENCE AT
AMERICAN AIRLINES

V. SCHOCKEN and L. G. LEDERER

Medical Department, American Airlines, New York, U.S.A.

This report deals with the incidence and causes of unscheduled landings for medical reasons made by American Airlines planes during the 5-year period, 1964–1968. An unscheduled landing in this sense is a landing made optionally at the discretion of the crew in order to deplane a passenger who, because of some illness, infirmity or accident, should not continue on to the scheduled destination of the flight. This type of landing must not be confused with an emergency landing which is made when something occurs that threatens the airworthiness of the plane. The unscheduled landings are sometimes made on the initiative of the passenger. The passenger may ask for a landing and if he supports his request with sufficiently cogent reasons he may persuade the crew. At other times, the landing is made at the initiative of the crew. In such a case, one or more of the crew members who are attending to and observing an ill, infirm or stricken passenger decide that they can no longer cope with the situation or no longer take the responsibility for the welfare or life of the passenger.

However the decision originates, once the captain makes the decision for an unscheduled landing he is committed to a series of expensive and time-consuming steps. He must determine the location of the nearest airport at which he can land. That airport might be one normally served by his airline or it might be one that is strange to him and at which his company maintains no personnel or facilities. He must, in consultation with his dispatcher, decide whether his plane is above the permitted landing weight. If it is, he must jettison fuel – sometimes up to 20000 to 30000 lb. Arrangements must be made for medical personnel to receive the incapacitated passenger. If the stop is not on the airline's routes, then arrangements must be made for the use of another carrier's facilities, and so on. It is estimated that each unscheduled landing costs the company $2000 and usually delays a flight at least 1 hr. That hour must be multiplied by the number of passengers to arrive at the cost in man hours lost. The further loss of time caused by missed appointments and connections with other flights can only be guessed at. Therefore, an unscheduled landing is an important occurrence both from the point of view of the airline and of the travelling public.

The first aspect of unscheduled landings on which data was gathered is the incidence or rate of occurrence. It was found that over the 5-year period, 1964–1968, an average of 18 unscheduled landings per year were made. The figures for the individual years were: 1964, 14: 1965, 18; 1966, 17; 1967, 19; 1968, 22. The secular upward trend corresponds to the increase in air traffic during that period. In 1968, American Airlines boarded approximately 20 million passengers. Therefore the number of unscheduled

D. E. Busby (ed.), Recent Advances in Aerospace Medicine, 126–129. All Rights Reserved.
Copyright © 1970 by D. Reidel Publishing Company, Dordrecht-Holland.

landings represents an incidence of about 1 per million. Stated otherwise, of every million passengers who board an American Airlines plane, one will have to be deplaned in an unscheduled landing. This incidence is remarkably low and in most operations, inadvertencies that occur on a 'one in a million' basis are overlooked as acceptable risks. An analysis of the reasons for these unscheduled landings indicates, however, that even this occurrence rate is far from the irreducible minimum. As a rough estimate about half of the unscheduled landings made during the period of this study should have been avoided.

The information gathered on medical events preceding the unscheduled landing comes from the crew reports. In most cases a fairly detailed report was written by the stewardess and a briefer report submitted by the captain. In rare cases where a doctor happens to be on the plane, his opinion is sometimes obtained as to diagnosis and severity of the illness. For the most part, then, information concerning the illness of the passenger for whom the landing was made consists of the observations and impressions of one or more stewardesses and the captain. These impressions have been tabulated for the 90 unscheduled landings that took place during the period of this study. The principal manifestations listed in the order of frequency of occurrence are shown in Table I.

TABLE I

Reported reasons for unscheduled landings
American Airlines, 1964-68

Syncope	21 instances
Heart attack (real or suspected)	20 instances
Dyspnea (including asthma)	20 instances
Chest pain	13 instances
Convulsions or seizures	7 instances
Abdominal pain	7 instances
Hemorrhage (including epistaxis)	5 instances
Miscellaneous illness	5 instances
Injury aboard	2 instances
Diabetic	2 instances
Dead	2 instances
Drunk	1 instance

The number of occurrences for these signs and symptoms adds up to 105 for the 90 landings because where the reason was given as a multiple entity, such as 'chest pain and dyspnea', both are listed. The miscellaneous illness includes a passenger who simply demanded that the plane be landed because he was 'nervous' and a frank case of hyperventilation. There are also cases where no more information was given than that the passenger was 'extremely ill'.

The question of what effect the presence of medical personnel on the plane has on the likelihood of an unscheduled landing was raised. It was found that when a doctor who happened to be travelling on the plane responded to a call for assistance, he might be more conservative than the crew and militate for a landing, or he might reassure the crew and prevent a landing. In one case a doctor asked for a landing for an obvious case of hyperventilation; in others, doctors have attended passengers to the destination of the flight. However, when no doctor was on board and a registered nurse responded to the call for a doctor, then it was found that the nurse almost invariably recommended a landing.

The question of just how ill the stricken passenger was remains somewhat ambiguous. It is known that in at least 2 cases the evidence of mortal illness is incontrovertible. In other cases the landing was made on a false alarm. In several cases, the passenger for whom the landing was made declared himself fully recovered on touching *terra firma* and declined all medical attention. In one case, recovery on landing was so complete that when the plane was ready to take off again after the unscheduled landing the recently indisposed passenger insisted on re-boarding the plane to continue his flight.

In general, unscheduled landings fall into 3 categories or groups. In the first the landing is made because a passenger becomes ill or indisposed in a way that may be very distressing and frightening to him and to the crew, but his problem really does not represent a medical emergency. In this group are hyperventilation, intoxication, simple syncope, brief epileptic seizures, *etcetera*. The second category or group consists of landings necessitated by acute medical occurrences requiring medical care without delay. Included here are heart attacks, pulmonary emboli, acute cerebral vascular accidents, *etcetera*. The third category or group consists of landings made because of exacerbations of known illnesses or infirmities, such as asthma, angina pectoris, congestive heart failure, *etcetera*.

Efforts in attempting to minimize avoidable unscheduled landings are concentrated on reducing the occurrences in groups I and III. To help stewardesses cope with the passenger who becomes ill in a way which is neither emergent nor life threatening, lectures and demonstrations in first aid are given to them. An attempt has been made to indoctrinate them to recognize hyperventilation and treat it appropriately. The lecturers have tried to disabuse our stewardesses of the idea that the walk-around oxygen tank is a universal panacea. Specifically, it is impressed on them that in cases of syncope, lowering the head is more therapeutic than propping the passenger up with an oxygen mask. But our record of unscheduled landings for syncope suggests that this instruction has not been wholly successful.

Passengers who are involved in group III landings are those who were too ill to fly or who were not properly prepared for the flight. To help these people avoid trouble and complete their trips whenever at all possible, the Medical Department of American Airlines often contacts the passenger's doctor. If one of our ticket agents learns that a prospective passenger has some medical problem that might lead to complications in flight, the Medical Department is consulted. If necessary, the Company doctor contacts the passenger's doctor to get more information about the passenger's condition and to insure that all proper preparations and arrangements are made. The spirit of this type of communication with the prospective passenger and his doctor is not to deny anyone the convenience of air travel but to be sure that everyone who can safely fly, or who can be gotten into condition to fly will be able to do so. There has never been an unscheduled landing on American Airlines for a passenger who was checked in this way.

As larger equipment such as the Boeing 747 Jumbo jet is introduced, the cost and inconveniences associated with unscheduled landings will increase greatly. However, most unnecessary unscheduled landings could be eliminated by pursuing the following 4-point program:

(1) Continued indoctrination of the crews, especially the stewardesses, in handling indisposed passengers.

(2) Provision of a place on board where an ill passenger, especially if suffering from syncope, can recline.

(3) Close cooperation between sales personnel, the airline medical department and the personal doctors of passengers with medical problems.

(4) Avoidance of assaults on the passenger with immoderate quantities of food and alcohol.

U.S. AIRCRAFT HIJACKINGS –
EPIDEMIOLOGICAL CONSIDERATIONS

H. L. REIGHARD,

Office of Aviation Medicine, Federal Aviation Administration, Washington, D.C., U.S.A.

During the early part of 1969, the hijacking of American air carrier aircraft to Cuba increased in a manner suggesting an exponential rate of progression for this phenomenon (Figure 1). The rate had reached an average of 2 to 3 hijackings per week in early February, 1969, when positive efforts were initiated to stop this activity.

This study of the epidemiological aspects of aircraft hijacking began with the collection and recording of available information concerning hijacking events and the persons who had committed this crime. Its purpose was to describe the phenomenon and the involved persons in a way intended to lead eventually to preventive methods. The descriptive and analytical phases of the study involved the processing of data obtained from reports of investigations of the behavioral backgrounds of hijackers, aircrew reports regarding hijackers, data on airlines, aircraft and airports affected, and certain classified information. This information was provided from the great number of American hijacking attempts from 1961 to this time (Table I). The analytical effort was intended to provide refined information in at least the following areas:

(1) The nature of hijacking events.
(2) The characteristics of hijackers.
(3) The methods of operation used by hijackers.

TABLE I

Hijacking attempts in the United States from 1961 to 28 August, 1969

	Unsuccessful		Successful		
Year	General aviation	Air carrier	General aviation	Air carrier	Total
1961		. .		. . .	5
1962			.		1
1963	.				1
1964			.		1
1965		. . .		.	4
1966					0
1967			.		1
1968		. . . .	. . . . .	. . . .	22
1969		. . . . . .		. . . .	30
Total	1	15	8	41	65

D. E. Busby (ed.), Recent Advances in Aerospace Medicine, 130–134. All Rights Reserved.
Copyright © 1970 by D. Reidel Publishing Company, Dordrecht-Holland.

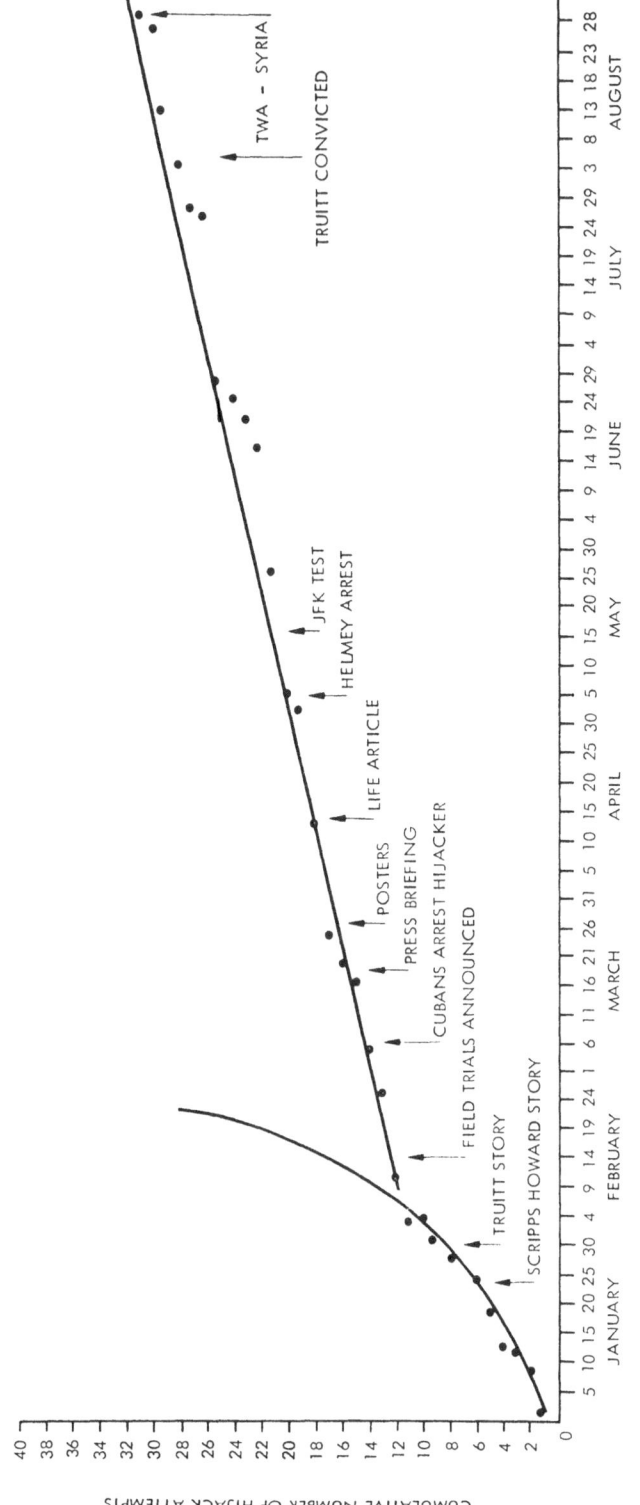

Fig. 1. Cumulative number of hijack attempts to Cuba.

(4) Motivations of hijackers.

(5) The nature of any changing trends in the phenomenon of hijacking in the United States.

The early data from American hijackings suggested the following possible motivations for hijackings which, in turn, tended to describe the type of person who commits this crime:

(1) Hijacking a planeload of passengers is an extremely dramatic way of defecting to a country whose political ideologies are significantly different from those of the country of origin of the flight.

(2) The hijackers expected to be received and honored as heroes in the country to which they fled.

(3) The hijacker was seeking to escape from his personal problems and past inadequacies, in a brief moment of power in a life of failure.

(4) Few of the hijackers were highly disturbed mentally but most had serious emotional problems.

(5) A common factor appeared to be the commission of a political demonstration in a manner chosen to embarrass the United States while at the same time escaping punishment and, hopefully, being rewarded for his efforts.

(6) Some hijackers were clearly using this means of escaping apprehension and punishment for past crimes.

Subsequent events and further analyses of the data proved that many of the assumptions of hijackers were erroneous. This was useful in later efforts to control the epidemic nature of the hijacking phenomenon.

Analysis also led to certain conclusions regarding the effect that certain environmental factors appeared to have on the rate at which hijackings occurred. This related especially to the type and quality of information which was made available in the public information media. In general it appeared that hijackings were more probable when the available information consisted of the following:

(1) Many hijackings were successful with no evidence of attempts to prevent or abort them.

(2) Airlines were consistently taking steps to ensure arrival in Cuba once a hijacker had announced his intention.

(3) Jokes about hijacking suggested it was a humorous interlude for those persons, such as crewmembers and passengers, who became involved.

(4) Hijackers were not returned from Cuba.

(5) Neither the government nor the airlines had any workable means of preventing hijacking.

(6) Naive and impractical suggestions made by members of the general public were highly publicized.

From these analyses, observations and other information obtained it was hypothesized that certain positive actions of the government and the airlines should have a beneficial effect. To this end, an action program was developed in an effort to modify the phenomenon. Since there appeared to be no single specific and certain cure for this condition, it was decided that multiple actions should be taken as suggested by the analytical results of the study.

First, it was quite apparent that there was a need to correct erroneous impressions which existed. In this connection, various methods were employed to disseminate information dealing with the following subject areas:

(1) Treatment of hijackers in Cuba. As information became available that hijackers were not treated as heroes on arrival in Cuba, this information was included in discussions with the news media and widely published. Hijackers themselves, speaking from Cuba, confirmed that they were jailed for varying periods of time and thereafter worked as agricultural laborers.

(2) Weapons detection system development. In the early days of the hijacking epidemic, it was widely publicized that efforts to detect weapons would be fruitless because of lack of ability to discriminate between concealed weapons and other similar objects. The improved state of development of weapons detection technology, for this specific application, has been publicized, most prominently in conjunction with field testing of the detection system at various large airports.

(3) Penalties for commission of criminal acts associated with flight. In the early days of the epidemic it was not generally known that the commission of a hijacking carried penalties similar to those for acts of piracy on the high seas – a minimum of 20 years in prison and maximum penalty of death. Being a capital crime there is no statute of limitations which would exonerate the hijacker after the passage of time. He may be prosecuted to the fullest extent of the law at any time he is apprehended and brought to trial.

Certain other acts related to flight, frequently committed in preparation for or in the course of hijacking, also carry severe criminal penalties. These include carrying a concealed deadly weapon, threatening any flight crew member or interference with the flight crew in the performance of their duties.

Eighteen persons have to date been convicted in the U.S. for acts associated with hijacking. This fact has been publicized.

(4) Search of passengers and baggage. Because of the evolvement of a legal environment in the United States in recent years which prescribes certain ill-defined but limiting conditions regarding the search of citizens and their possessions, there developed a general belief that searching of passengers for weapons could not be performed. The facts are that for many years all the major American airlines have had authority to refuse passage to anyone thought to be a hazard to a particular flight and, more specifically, authority to refuse passage to anyone who, upon request, refuses to permit a search of his person or possessions. Further, with the application of a detection screening system, such as has now been developed, in a manner which heightens the suspicion that a passenger may be carrying a concealed weapon, a search in an effort to discover a weapon has been found to be legally permissible. This set of circumstances permits one to move further toward the identification of would-be hijackers before they board aircraft.

The second part of the government's effort to modify the hijacking phenomenon involved efforts to develop a weapons detection system for this specific application. Such a system has been developed and extensively tested on passengers at several major airports in the United States. It consists of a behavioral profile of the known characteristics of past hijackers and a weapons screening device. The application of these two screening elements provides rather precise discrimination between ordinary passengers and those with the characteristics of known hijackers. If generally applied, more than 99% of all air passengers, in the United States, could be cleared from suspicion of being potential hijackers. Information regarding the development of this system has been disseminated to the news media.

Since the announcement of the government's plans to take positive actions intended to apprehend hijackers, there has been a noticeable modification of the hijacking phenomenon. As compared to the period during which the epidemic was at its peak, the phenomenon now differs in the following ways:

(1) The cumulative trend of hijacking events is now linear in nature as compared with the exponential progression through January 1969 (Figure 1).

(2) Hijackings previously affected only aircraft flying in the Eastern part of the United States. They now occur as well on flights originating elsewhere, including the West Coast.

(3) Hijackers are now much more likely to be Cubans (or Latins) as compared to the earlier period when many were mentally unstable or criminal white or black militant citizens of the United States.

A number of other United States Government efforts have been initiated to bring an end to the hijacking phenomenon. Among these have been attempts to have hijackers returned to the United States from Cuba, to obtain Cuban cooperation in returning hijacked aircraft promptly with its crew and passengers, to arouse the international community to the seriousness of this matter to the end that international agreements might be reached to punish or extradite hijackers, and to obtain the agreement of the Cuban government to receive Cuban refugees in the United States who desire to return to Cuba. The American government has so far been successful in obtaining agreement from the Government of Cuba to return the hijacked plane promptly with its crew and passengers. It has signed recently the Tokyo Convention, an international agreement which provides that a hijacked aircraft be promptly returned to the aircraft commander, and its passengers and crew be assisted in continuing their journey. Amendments to the Convention have been proposed, and are now under consideration by the International Civil Aviation Organization, which would provide that hijackers would either be punished by the receiving country or be extradited to the country of registry of the aircraft. The United States will continue in these efforts as well as those to detect would-be hijackers.

In summary, an epidemiological study of the hijackings in the United States has led to a better understanding of the nature of this phenomenon and has suggested specific steps which might be taken to modify it. Continuing analysis will be conducted to improve our understanding of this condition and to assess the effects of our efforts at modification.

EXPERIENCE WITH A PHYSIOLOGICALLY-BASED FORMULA FOR DETERMINING REST PERIODS ON LONG-DISTANCE AIR TRAVEL

L. E. BULEY

International Civil Aviation Organization, Montreal, Quebec, Canada

1. Background

Long-distance air travel by professional officers of the International Civil Aviation Organization (ICAO), most of whom are working outside their own countries, is extensive. It comprises principally travel by the Headquarters Secretariat, located in Montreal, and by personnel of the six Regional Offices and far-flung Technical Assistance Missions, on official assignments and on home leave. The rationale of providing for rest-periods during this travel, as related to its purpose, is:

(1) *Mission travel:* The prime consideration relates to the outward journey and is to ensure maximum effectiveness of the officer in executing his mission on arrival; of secondary importance is the efficiency of his resumption of work on return. His physical and mental well-being, although not of high priority *per se*, is clearly closely related to both the foregoing objectives.

(2) *Home Leave:* Promotion of the physical and mental well-being of the staff member (and of any dependents travelling with him), within the limits set by expenditure of time and money reasonable in the circumstances, is paramount. The secondary objective, the staff member's efficient resumption of duty on return, is largely synonymous with the primary objective.

(3) *Combined mission and leave travel:* A criterion of a well-planned itinerary is that it presents no significant incompatibility between the Organization's and the officer's interests.

Until January 1967, rest-periods during official air travel by ICAO staff had been predicated (as in other UN organizations) on rule-of-thumb 'allowable journey times', tabulated for various combinations of point of origin and destination. Arbitrary downward and upward adjustment of these times for non-medical reasons had apparently obscured the fact that (exigencies and expediency aside) the criterion of 'reasonableness' of rest-period durations is the physiological and psychological reaction of normally-healthy staff members to the itineraries involved. Recognition by ICAO's Staff Advisory Committee of this essentially medical rest-period rationale resulted in an attempt to develop a formula validly based on significant, broadly-quantifiable stress factors, and at the same time easily applicable by administrative personnel without exercise of judgment.

2. Selecting Usable Parameters of Stress

A passenger's physiological and psychological state following a normal long-haul

D. E. Busby (ed.), Recent Advances in Aerospace Medicine, 135–141. All Rights Reserved.

flight is principally influenced by factors which can be conveniently grouped as personal (age, state of health, individual tolerance), general operational (noise, vibration, low humidity, immobilization) and specific operational (flight duration and time of day, time-zone translocation in east-west-east travel and changes of climate and culture in north-south-north travel). The effects on passengers of factors in the first and second categories are not amenable to quantification, and the climatic and cultural variables in the third category are not directly accountable. Significant variables available for computation are therefore flight duration (which indirectly takes account of exposure to general operational stresses and in the North-South-North case, climatic changes), local times of departure and arrival, and time-zone translocation. It therefore appeared that the most likely practical determinant of rest-period duration(s) would be the sum of functions of flight duration and of number of time-zones traversed, weighted according to the psychophysiological unfavourability of local times of departure and arrival in such a way as to include an eastward/westward travel differential.

3. The Formula

As it has evolved the equation is:

$$\text{Rest period (in tenths of a day)} = \frac{\text{Flight duration (in hours)}}{2} + \frac{\text{Time-zones in excess}}{\text{of 4}} + \frac{\text{Departure time}}{\text{coefficient}} + \frac{\text{Arrival time}}{\text{coefficient}}$$

or, in symbolic form:

$$\text{R.P.} = \Delta T/2 + (Z - 4) + C_D + C_A.$$

Principal ground rules for application of the Formula are:

(1) The indicated rest period (R.P.) in tenths of a day is rounded upward to the next higher half day; however, R.P.'s summing to less than 1 day before rounding are not given unless an overnight flight on mission travel has been made.

(2) Departure and arrival times are in local time.

(3) A stopover exceeding 2 days (exclusive of an authorized rest period) constitutes termination of a journey, the onward flight being a new journey for rest-period purposes.

(4) The maximum rest-period allowable at any one place en route is 2 days.

A. FLIGHT DURATION TERM

Although this term was regarded as the cornerstone of the equation, it cannot be claimed that great subtlety was involved in its derivation. As a starting point, it was arbitrarily decided that the flight duration/rest-period ratio, in isolation, should be 1:1. This would have meant either an answer in twelfths of a day, or using a fractional flight duration denominator. On the premise that, in long-distance air travel generally, sleep loss is rather greater than perusal of airline schedules suggests, the ratio was liberalized to 1:1.2.

B. TIME-ZONE TRANSLOCATION TERM

As shown in Figure 1, the world's 24 time-zones are basically defined by meridians of longitude 15 deg apart, this being the angular distance traversed by the Earth each hour. The local standard time in any zone is therefore one hour later than that in the adjoining zone to its west and one hour earlier than in its eastern neighbour at any

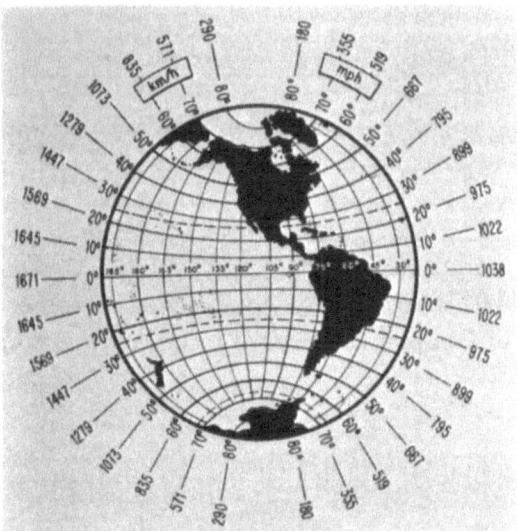

Fig. 1.   Ground speeds along parallels of latitude, in statute miles per hour, necessary to traverse 15 meridians (1 time zone) per hour.

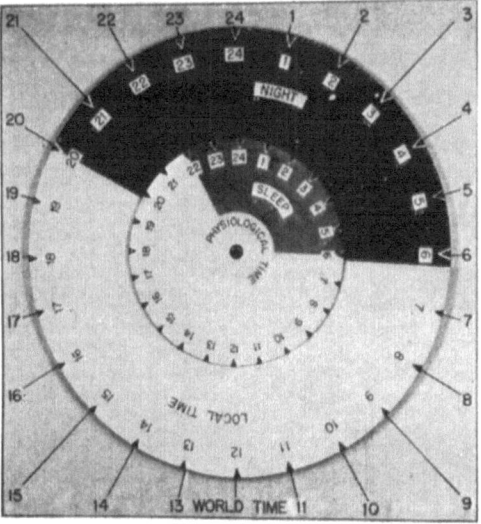

Fig. 2.   World Time (GMT)/Local Time/Physiological Time dial-board (after Strughold, 1952).

given world standard time (GMT). The Figure gives the groundspeeds, for various latitudes, necessary to 'pace the sun' in westward travel, or to 'compress time' by a factor of two in eastward travel. It is not for this paper to review the biological basis of human circadian rhythm or the physiological and biochemical manifestations of its disruption. Following Strughold's (1952) classic exposition, and particularly since the advent of large-scale turbojet transport a decade ago made circadian dysrhythmia a mass phenomena, these aspects have been ably researched and amply reported upon. This paper *is* concerned, however, with the likelihood of out-of-character behavior and inept decisions by those who allow themselves (or are allowed) inadequate time for physiological cycle adaptation before going about their high-level official tasks.

Since many intelligent people report difficulty in fully comprehending physiological cycle shift effects, no apology is made for inclusion of Figure 2 in which the three kinds of time involved are diagrammatically represented as elements of a simple rotary calculator. If these are moved differentially, any dynamic situation resulting from time-zone translocation can be illustrated. In Figure 3, the calculator is applied to return travel between a region of N. America 5 zones west of the Greenwich (0) zone and a region of Europe 1 zone east of it. In clockwise progression the juxta-

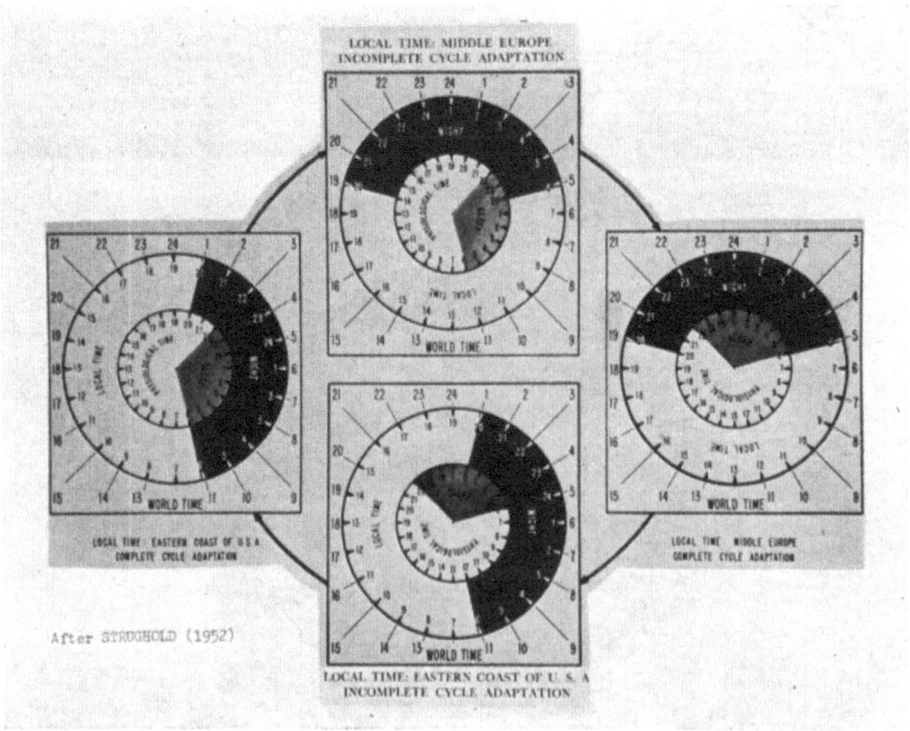

Fig. 3.   Application of World Time (GMT)/Local Time/Physiological Time dial-board
(after Strughold, 1952).

positions illustrate successive out-of-phase and adaptive conditions, but further information is needed to estimate the adaptation times.

It is pertinent to deciding what relative weight to assign to time-zone translocation in the Formula to know what order of behavioral and intellectual penalty out-of-phase conditions might carry, and for how long. Recent work by Klein *et al.* (1968) suggests that the peak variation in psychomotor performance due to this factor alone corresponds (in subjects in their 20's) to the maximal effect of about 0.1% blood alcohol and of an oral dosage of 500 mg of hexobarbital. Add to this the fact that the traveller is typically unaware of the extent of his behavioral impairment following rapid transit of 5 or more time zones. The choice of 4 zones as the threshold of significance for the purpose of the Formula was originally based on evidence that Geophysical Year and subsequent expeditions living under conditions of continuous summer daylight in northern latitudes could adjust to regimens of 21- or 28-hr 'days', but not to longer or shorter 'days'. The findings of much laboratory and civil aviation field research, subsequently available, suggest that this choice was somewhat conservative for young travellers, but not necessarily for the middle-aged who predominate among the ICAO staff concerned.

The relative importance given to the time-zone factor in the Formula, insofar as it

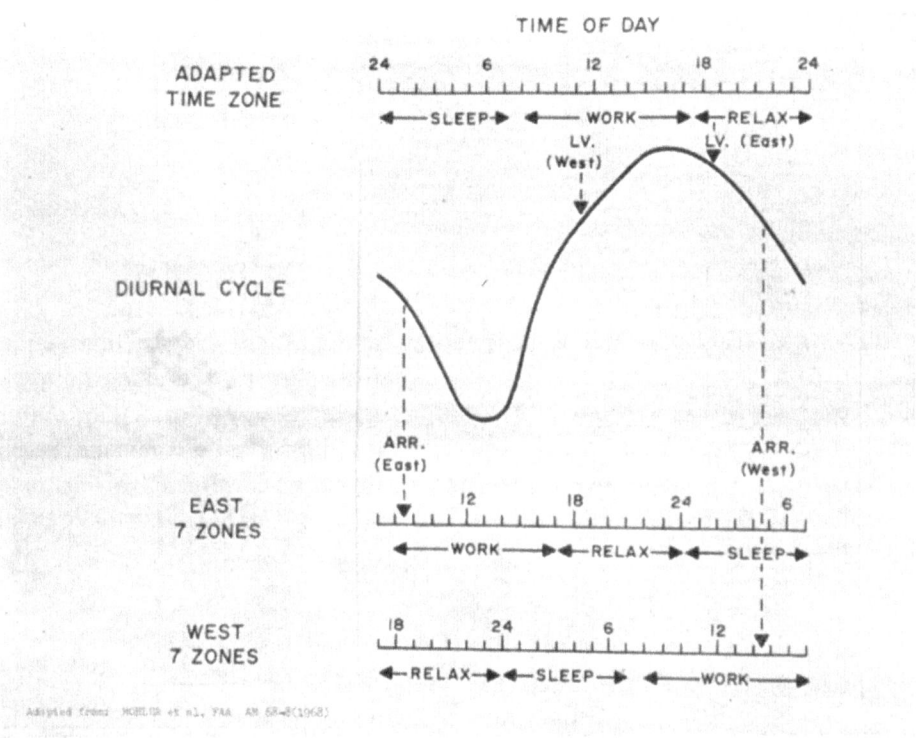

Fig. 4. Time-zone nomograph based on typical circadian curve, social pattern and places of departure and arrival (after Mohler *et al.*, 1968).

relates to persistence of functionally significant dysrhythmia, resulted from a value judgment based largely on the earlier work of Hauty and Adams (1966a, b, c) and the subjective investigations of Lavernhe *et al.* (1965). Subsequent work has not indicated a need to revise this judgment.

C. DEPARTURE AND ARRIVAL COEFFICIENTS

It was apparent that these should be predicated on the shape of a typical circadian curve for some performance or behavior index, and on the social pattern (in particular the community sleep period) of the places of departure and arrival. Figure 4 shows a time-zone nomograph based on these elements. A three-dimensional model was developed, with departure and arrival times forming the horizontal scales, and corresponding coefficients and local sleep periods as the vertical elements, with the objective of defining an 'equal-stress continuum'. This approach was defeated by interpretative difficulties and the overriding administrative desirability of coefficient values which were whole, relatively low numbers. The values finally selected are shown in Table I.

TABLE I

Departure and arrival time coefficients as
related to local times.

Period (local time)	Departure time coefficient	Arrival time coefficient
0800–1159	0	4
1200–1759	1	2
1800–2159	3	0
2200–0059	4	1
0100–0759	3	3

It will be noted that if the sums of the D and A coefficients for each local time period are plotted (at the period mid-points), a curve approximating the vertical mirror image of a typical diurnal performance curve (or approximating such a curve 12 hr out of phase) is produced. The curve peaks coincidentally with a typical community sleep period curve plotted on the same local time axis. This can be construed as giving some theoretical validity to the distributions and values chosen, although essentially these must always represent a compromise.

4. Application of the Formula

Before being placed in general use, the formula was tested for possible anomalous results by retrospective application to a large number of actual journeys made by ICAO personnel, and to hypothetical but typical journeys, using published airline schedules. Examples of results obtained are: Montreal-Lima, R.P. 1½ days; Montreal-

Sydney, via Vancouver, $2\frac{1}{2}$ days; Helsinki-Monrovia, $1\frac{1}{2}$ days; Montreal-Karachi, $2\frac{1}{2}$ days; London-Kathmandu, $1\frac{1}{2}$ days; Montreal-London, 1 day; London-Montreal, nil. Routine application of the formula to all official ICAO air travel over the past $2\frac{1}{2}$ years has been, in general, satisfactory in terms of efficiency and well-being of staff, and of administrative acceptability. It has minimized a long-standing source of contention between travelling staff and administrative staff, but has not completely achieved the objective of abolishing any need for 'interpretation' of the travel rules by the latter. The formula was presented to the UN Consultative Committee on Administrative Questions in 1967, but, partially due to ICAO's then small experience with it, it was not adopted as 'UN Common System' practice. At least two specialized agencies of UN other than ICAO have adopted it, however, and it is presently under consideration by the Federation of International Civil Servants Associations (FICSA). It is in use, in original or modified form, or is under consideration, by a number of governmental and industrial organizations including the U.S. State Department and U.S. Federal Aviation Administration, Canadian Forces Air Transport Command, Alcan Aluminium Ltd., Campbell Soup Co., and I.B.M. Corporation.

The validity of the Formula is reviewed from time to time in the light of new airline route structures and timetables and the possible effects of new equipment. Present indications are that the advent of supersonic airline travel will ease the time-zone translocation problem for flight crew, but will in general accentuate it for passengers, although reduction in flight durations will to some extent offset this in the overall post-flight fatigue picture. The weightings presently given to the various stress factors in the ICAO Formula will need radical reexamination in the context of SST operations.

References

Hauty, G. T. and Adams, T.: 1966a, *Aerospace Med.* **37**, 668.
Hauty, G. T. and Adams, T.: 1966b, *Aerospace Med.* **37**, 1027.
Hauty, G. T. and Adams, T.: 1966c, *Aerospace Med.* **37**, 1257.
Klein, K. D., Wegmann, H. M., and Bruner, H.: 1968, *Aerospace Med.* **39**, 512.
Lavernhe, J., Lafontaine, E., and Laplane, R.: 1965, in *Proceedings 36th Annual Scientific Meeting, Aerospace Medical Association*, New York, New York, U.S.A.
Mohler, S., Dille, J. R., and Gibbons, H. L.: 1968, AM68–8, Federal Aviation Administration, Washington, D.C.
Strughold, H.: 1952, *J. Aviat. Med.* **23**, 464.

HYPNOTICS AND JET-AGE TRAVEL

J. SNYDER

Hoffmann-La Roche Inc., Nutley, N.J., U.S.A.

1. Introduction

With the advent of trans-continental and trans-oceanic jet travel, problems of insomnia have been frequently observed in both flight crew and passengers (Siegel *et al.*,
1969; [1]). Difficulty in obtaining 'restful' sleep has resulted in the increasing use of
hypnotic drugs and other regimens aimed at correcting this problem. However, while
the use of drugs seems to aid in reducing sleep latency, the after effects are often worse
than the insomnia itself.

2. Characteristics of Sleep

Since the late 1950's, the subject of sleep has undergone intensive laboratory investigation. The original observation of Rapid Eye Movements (REM) by Aserinsky and
Kleitman has been confirmed in laboratories throughout the world, as has the concept that sleep is an active rather than passive state. More recently, sleep has been
divided into stages, i.e. I, II, III, IV and REM, scored by correlating electroencepha-
lographic (E.E.G.), electromyographic (E.M.G.) and electro-oculographic recordings
(Rechtschaffen and Kales, 1968). Briefly, these stages are characterized by the following parameters:

Stage 1 – a relatively low voltage, mixed frequency E.E.G., without rapid eye
movements (REM).

Stage 2 – 12 to 14 cps E.E.G., sleep spindles and K complexes on a background of
relatively low voltage, mixed frequency E.E.G. activity.

Stage 3 – moderate amounts of high amplitude, slow wave (delta) activity.

Stage 4 – large amounts (over 50% of the record) delta wave activity.

Stage REM – a relatively low voltage, mixed frequency E.E.G. in conjunction with
episodic REMs and low amplitude E.M.G.

In a normal sleep cycle the pattern would be as follows: awake, Stage 1, 2, 3, 4, 3, 2,
REM, 2, 3, etc. with Stage REM occurring approximately every 90 min throughout
the night. Some investigators prefer not to use these different stages, whose significance is not clearly understood, particularly Stage 4, but to speak of sleep as REM
or non-REM (NREM) (Dement, 1969).

It has been amply demonstrated that sleep patterns occur cyclically throughout the
night, and that of all the stages, REM remains most constant throughout life. It is the
slowest stage to adapt to phase shifts of circadian rhythm, taking up to 72 hr longer
than any of the NREM states (Weitzman, 1969). REM deprivation, whether by drug
or physical means has been shown to reduce reaction time, result in a 'hangover'
effect and with rebound, may cause extreme physiological and psychological stress

D. E. Busby (ed.), Recent Advances in Aerospace Medicine, 142–145. All Rights Reserved.
Copyright © 1970 by D. Reidel Publishing Company, Dordrecht-Holland.

(Berger and Oswald, 1962: Dement, 1960; Dement *et al.*, 1966; Derenzi and Faglini, 1966; Stern, 1969).

Crew members and passengers who cross multiple time zones are known to have difficulty in sleeping on schedule at layover stations, because of both circadian disruptions and psychological factors [1]. While advice is commonly given to go to sleep at a normal time, this is usually neither practical nor possible. This delay in sleep onset, of itself, brings on a slight REM deprivation, when added to the circadian shift and REM suppressant activities of most active hypnotics, it can become a serious problem for the subject. Ideally, in order to alleviate this situation, flights should be scheduled so as not to interfere with normal sleep time. Since this is not economically feasible at the present time, it was thought that an alternative, the use of hypnotics, should be assessed.

3. Use of Hypnotic Drugs

Several hypnotic compounds studied elsewhere for their physiological properties have been categorized into two groups – REM suppressants and NREM suppressants (Kales *et al.*, 1969a, b). Unfortunately, most hypnotics suppress Stage REM; when their use is discontinued, a withdrawal 'rebound' is usually seen (Kales *et al.*, 1969b). This suppression and rebound phenomenon is frequently associated with nightmares and dependency lasting for extended periods of time (Oswald, 1969; Oswald and Priest, 1965). One must remember that suppression and rebound of Stage REM places physiological stress on the organism that is not ordinarily present. The goal in the use of hypnotics must be to provide sleep which is natural – restful, not stressful.

4. Study of Hypnotic Drugs

Eight hypnotics have been tested under sleep laboratory conditions by this investigator. The results of this study are summarized in Tables I and II. It is noted that only two

TABLE I

Stage REM alterations following drug administration and withdrawal. Eight-night studies.

| | % Stage REM on study nights (Ni) | | | | | |
| | Baseline | | Drug | | Withdrawal | |
	Ni 3	Ni 4	Ni 5	Ni 6	Ni 7	Ni 8
Group A						
glutethimide 500 mg ($N = 5$)	27.0	14.3	16.2	18.0	31.4	30.7
methyprylon 300 mg ($N = 7$)	25.3	18.4	18.9	25.3	31.5	31.6
secobarbital 100 mg ($N = 2$)	20.2	15.3	19.8	19.0	21.1	21.2
methaqualone 300 mg ($N = 5$)	23.4	18.8	23.4	21.6	27.6	22.4
pentobarbital 100 mg ($N = 4$)	21.7	18.3	21.1	20.9	26.4	25.6
Group B						
chloral hydrate 1000 mg ($N = 5$)	23.0	21.7	23.7	22.4	23.3	24.8
RO 5-6901 30 mg ($N = 8$)	22.5	21.5	18.0	19.1	21.9	22.3

TABLE II

Sleep latency

Drugs							
Sleep latency (min)	Flura- zepam 30 mg N = 8	Chloral Hydrate 1000 mg N = 5 or 3	Metha- qualone 300 mg N = 5	Glute- thimide 500 mg N = 4	Methy- prylon 300 mg N = 7	Seco- barbital 100 mg N = 2	Pento- barbital 100 mg N = 4
B	39.4	38.5[a]	20.8	16.8	20.3[b]	13.7	38.8
D	30.5	25.4	32.2	18.9	21.2	11.8	30.8
W	22.8	25.4	34.5	29.1	30.5	13.5	19.8

[a] 3 only used for baseline.
[b] 2 figures not available.

hypnotics, chloral hydrate and flurazepam, did not suppress Stage REM, and that these drugs and secobarbital did not produce rebound on withdrawal. Only one hypnotic, flurazepam, proved effective in reducing sleep latency. In a more recent study during which a hypnotic drug was administered for 14 consecutive nights, flurazepam did not alter Stage REM and remained effective over the entire period, chloral hydrate did not alter Stage REM. Glutethimide suppressed Stage REM. Both chloral hydrate and glutethimide decreased sleep latency for 3 nights; however, there was then a gradual return of sleep latency to baseline or above before the eleventh drug night.

5. Conclusions

Trans- or intercontinental jet travel interferes with normal circadian and sleep-wake patterns, causing problems of insomnia. These problems are compounded by the use of Stage REM suppressant drugs which result in impaired ability to function at peak level and possibly increase the danger of drug dependence. Data have been presented here evaluating these hypnotics for REM suppression and efficacy.

These studies indicate that in order to minimize the effects of normal sleep patterns and provide the most desirable rest, flurazepam (30 mg dose) and chloral hydrate (1000 mg dose) are the most logical choices of the hypnotic drugs studied here.

References

Aeromedical Applications Division, Federal Aviation Agency, Washington, D.C. (personal communication): 1969.

Berger, R. and Oswald, J.: 1962, *J. Ment. Sci.* **108**, 457.

Dement, W.: 1960, *Science* **131**, 1705.

Dement, W.: 1969, *Sleep and Dreaming Symposium*, E. R. Squibb Co.

Dement, W., Greenberg, S., and Klein, R.: 1966, *J. Psychiat. Res.* **4**, 141.

De Renzi, E. and Faglini, P.: 1966, *Arch. Psicol. Neurol.* **27**, 552.

Kales, A., Kales, J., Scharf, M. *et al.*: 1969a, presented at *7th International Congress of E.E.G. and Clinical Neurophysiology*, San Diego, Calif., U.S.A.

Kales, A., Malstrom, E., Scharf, M., and Rubin, R.: 1969b, in *Sleep Physiology and Pathology* (ed. by A. Kales), J. P. Lippincott, Philadelphia, pp. 331–343.

Oswald, I.: 1969, in *Sleep Physiology and Pathology* (ed. by A. Kales), J. P. Lippincott, Philadelphia, pp. 317–330.

Oswald, I. and Priest, R.: 1965, *Brit. Med. J.* **2**, 1093.

Rechtschaffen, A. and Kales, A.: 1968, *A Manual of Standardized Terminology, Techniques and Scoring System for Sleep Stages of Human Subjects*, U.S. Department of Health, Education and Welfare, Bethesda, Md., U.S.A.

Siegel, P., Gerathewohl, S., and Mohler, S.: 1969, *Science* **164**, 1249.

Stern, W.: 1969, presented at *Meeting of the Association for the Psychophysiological Study of Sleep (APSS)*, Boston, Mass., U.S.A.

Stroebel, C.: 1969, personal communication.

Weitzman, E.: 1969, presented at *Second International Symposium on Experimental and Clinical Chronobiology*, Florence, Italy.

PSYCHOTHÉRAPIES ET CHIMIOTHÉRAPIES EN MÉDECINE AÉRONAUTIQUE

C. J. BLANC et R. J. DIGO

Service Médical d'Air France, 1, Square Max Hymans, Paris 15e, France

1. Introduction

L'importance croîssante des états dépressifs et névrotiques dans toutes les collectivités constitue l'une des caractéristiques essentielles de la médecine moderne. Cette étude est basée sur les données de 2300 consultations psychiatriques portant sur 1500 sujets, pratiquées au cours de ces six dernières années parmi le personnel d'une grande compagnie aérienne française. Elle comporte trois groupes de sujets: personnel au sol, personnel navigant commercial et personnel navigant technique.

Parmi les sujets appartement au personnel au sol la neuropsychiatrie vient au premier rang parmi les facteurs d'absentéisme (37% des cas). Chez les navigants les taux de morbidité psychiatrique sont élevés, chez les hôtesses (environ 20%), importants chez les stewards (environ 10%) et minimes mais non négligeables chez les navigants techniques. Il nous est difficile de fournir pour ce dernier groupe des chiffres précis, un nombre relativement élevé de sujets échappant à la consultation psychiatrique.

Les états dépressifs et névrotiques constituent dans nos trois groupes de sujets les syndromes les plus largement représentés (40 à 80% des sujets examinés). Les progrès thérapeutiques acquis en psychiatrie depuis une quinzaine d'années nous permettent dans la plupart des cas d'apporter une aide efficace à nos patients.

(1) La psychopharmacologie avec les antidépresseurs (ou thymoanaleptiques); les anxiolytiques (ou tranquillisants) et les antipsychotiques (ou neuroleptiques) permet d'abréger considérablement la durée des épisodes psychiatriques chez le personnel au sol. Elle s'avère particulièrement efficace dans la thérapeutique des dépressions.

(2) Les psychothérapies connaissent également un développement considérable depuis une quinzaine d'années. La chimiothérapie rend perméables à un abord psychologique certains sujets autrefois réfractaires à la psychothérapie. Les études psychopathologiques d'inspiration psychanalytique ou phénoménologique, ont permis d'approfondir notre connaissance des mécanismes psychogénétiques dans les dépressions névrotiques et les névroses. Chimiothérapie et psychothérapie ne doivent pas être opposées. La plupart des traitements psychiatriques sont aujourd'hui des thérapeutiques conjointes utilisant simultanément les actions restructurantes des médicaments et le pouvoir cathartique et thérapeutique de la parole.

(3) Les antidépresseurs ne doivent être utilisés qu'exceptionnellement chez les navigants techniques et réservés exclusivement aux cas graves. La prescription de ces produits entraîne toujours des inaptitudes au vol de longue durée. La préférence doit

D. E. Busby (ed.), Recent Advances in Aerospace Medicine, 146–149. All Rights Reserved.
Copyright © 1970 by D. Reidel Publishing Company, Dordrecht-Holland.

être donnée ici à la psychothérapie associée à une pharmacologie mineure tranquillisante ou hypnotique.

(4) La psychanalyse freudienne classique (cure type) nous paraît contre-indiquée chez les navigants techniques en activité. Cette thérapeutique de longue durée entraîne en effet des modifications structurales de la personnalité et à certains stades des phénomènes de régression qui peuvent compromettre l'aptitude au vol. Nous lui préférons des psychothérapies en 'face à face' fondées sur des techniques plus 'flexibles'.

2. Modalités pratiques d'utilisation

Le traitement des dépressions névrotiques et des névroses comporte pratiquement toujours l'utilisation conjointe d'une psychothérapie et d'une cure pharmacologique. Plusieurs principes essentiels doivent être respectés au cours de ces traitements.

La cure pharmacologique comporte de façon constante une association de plusieurs produits ayant des actions sélectives différentes. On utilise en effet simultanément:

(1) Un antidépresseur qui 'relève' l'état thymique. Les produits les plus couramment utilisés appartiennent soit au groupe de l'Imipramine et de ses dérivés, soit au groupe des I.M.A.O.

(2) Un tranquillisant qui neutralise ou 'tamponne' les effets anxiogènes de l'antidépresseur.

(3) Un neuroleptique administré à petites doses le soir (lévomépromazine) et associé le plus souvent à un barbiturique. Ces produits régularisent les désordres hypniques constants dans les dépressions névrotiques et les névroses et en général accentués par les antidépresseurs.

Les doses de produits doivent être modulées au cours de la cure afin de réduire au minimum les effets secondaires et les phénomènes d'intolérance dont l'intensité est imprévisible au départ. Ces réactions dépendent en effet de la structure psychopathologique et de la personnalité antérieure. On commence en général par des doses faibles ou modérées que l'on augmente progressivement.

La psychothérapie est un élément essentiel du traitement. Il s'agit le plus souvent d'une psychothérapie de catharsis, de soutien et de reconstruction de la personnalité. Dans le cadre de la relation malade-médecin elle exploite les modifications structurales de la personnalité induites par les médicaments (relèvement de l'état thymique, réduction de l'angoisse, neutralisation des symptômes obsessionnels ou phobiques).

L'amélioration de l'état thymique s'observe en général après un délai de réponse thérapeutique de l'ordre d'une quinzaine de jours. Dans les cas moyens la disparition des symptômes majeurs est obtenue au bout d'un mois de traitement.

Il est toujours nécessaire de poursuivre le traitement chimique plusieurs semaines après la guérison clinique objective, la réduction des doses de médicaments doit être très progressive. Il est souvent nécessaire de maintenir de petites doses de barbituriques et de neuroleptiques le soir au coucher six à huit semaines après l'interruption des antidépresseurs.

3. Les méthodes psychothérapiques

Les psychothérapies en profondeur de type psychanalyse freudienne classique sont à déconseiller chez les sujets appartenant au personnel navigant technique. Ces traitements peuvent entraîner à certains stades de la cure des phénomènes de régression affective avec modification de l'équilibre psychodynamique de la personnalité et par voie de conséquence, incidenses sur l'aptitude technique du sujet au vol. Leurs bénéfices ne répondent le plus souvent ni à nos besoins ni à ceux de nos malades car ils ne se manifestent qu'après plusieurs années de traitement alors que nous avons affaire le plus souvent à des situations conflictuelles aiguës nécessitant une intervention restauratrice urgente.

Les entretiens psychothérapiques en 'face à face' à la fréquence d'une séance par semaine, se sont montrés dans notre pratique les plus rapidement efficaces. Il s'agit de psychothérapies de courte durée (quelques semaines, quelques mois) à visée cathartique et restauratrice. Elles utilisent la technique dite de 'flexibilité' préconisée par Alexander et French. Elles ne visent pas à modifier les structures profondes archaïques de la personnalité mais au contraire elles tendent à restaurer les formes d'équilibre antérieur à l'évènement traumatisant ou au conflit actuel.

Dans le contexte de la relation malade-médecin elles permettent d'obtenir assez rapidement des résultats positifs:

(1) Sédation de l'angoisse par l'effet cathartique de la confession face à un interlocuteur compréhensif, bienveillant mais neutre.

(2) Lutte contre les phénomènes de régression affective et les comportements auto-punitifs inconscients qui en résultent. On doit interdire au patient toute décision engageant de façon irréversible sa vie privée pendant la période aiguë de souffrance névrotique ou dépressive.

(3) La prise de conscience par le sujet de certains mécanismes auto-punitifs inconscients à travers la verbalisation de ses problèmes grâce à quelques conseils directifs. Ces conseils pratiques ont le plus souvent pour objet l'aménagement tactique d'une configuration strategique figée. Il faut rétablir le contact du patient avec les dures réalités de son existence.

Ces psychothérapies brèves en 'face à face' peuvent être associées à un traitement tranquillisant et hypnotique à doses modérées pendant la période d'inaptitude au vol. Chez les pilotes et mécaniciens navigants la reprise d'activité est généralement possible après un arrêt de travail de quatre à six semaines. Le traitement psychothérapique peut souvent être poursuivi avec des séances beaucoup plus espacées après la reprise d'activité.

La mise en pratique de ces psychothérapies se heurte souvent à des difficultés:

(1) Réticences et préjugés des patients vis-à-vis du pouvoir thérapeutique de la parole et du dialogue.

(2) Peur d'une maladie organique assez facilement neutralisée par un bilan médical complet dont le caractère négatif favorise la prise de conscience de l'importance des facteurs psychogénétiques.

(3) Enfin et surtout crainte d'une violation du secret professionel. C'est la raison pour laquelle un grand nombre de nos sujets a été orienté vers des collègues exerçant en pratique privée.

4. Discussion et conclusions

Chez le personnel au sol la thérapeutique des dépressions et des névroses ne pose pas de problème particulier. Il n'est pas toujours indispensable d'interrompre l'activité professionnelle. Dans tous les cas le recours à la psychopharmacologie permet d'abréger considérablement la durée de la période d'incapacité.

Chez les pilotes et les mécaniciens navigants l'utilisation des antidépresseurs doit être limitée aux cas heureusement exceptionnels de dépressions graves. La prescription d'un comprimé unique d'Imipramine entraîne de facto une inaptitude au vol d'une durée minimum de cent jours. Le sujet cliniquement guéri après un mois de traitement comprend mal l'inactivité forcée qui lui est imposée. Il peut en résulter une réactivation de l'angoisse et de la dépression centrée sur la crainte d'une perte définitive de licence. La nocivité d'un repos forcé dans les états anxieux, névrotiques ou dépressifs est bien connue de tous les psychiatres. D'où l'importance des traitements psychothérapiques dans les dépressions et les réactions névrotiques d'origine conflictuelle chez nos navigants. La psychopharmacologie antidépressive se présente chez eux comme une arme thérapeutique à effet 'boomerang'.

Chez les hôtesses et les stewards il nous semble possible d'envisager dans certains cas précis une attitude plus flexible. L'aptitude au vol devrait pouvoir être accordée après guérison clinique chez des sujets qui poursuivent un traitement tranquillisant et neuroleptique d'entretien à doses faibles, administrées exclusivement le soir au coucher. Sur ce point les consignes de la Federal Aviation Administration mériteraient peut-être d'être reconsidérées et assouplies au cours des prochaines années.

LA PART DE LA RADIOLOGIE DANS L'ENQUÊTE MÉDICALE APRÈS ÉJECTION DES PILOTES MILITAIRES D'AVIONS À RÉACTION

R. P. DELAHAYE, G. GUEFFIER, H. SERIS, et R. AUFFRET

Hôpital Dominique Larrey, 78 – Versailles, France, et Laboratoire de Médecine Aérospatiale du Centre d'Essais en Vol, 91 – Brétigny-sur-Orge, France

1. Introduction

L'éjection constitue la principale possibilité de sauvetage des avions de haute performance. Avec les perfectionnements actuels (système zéro seconde en particulier), elle offre un pourcentage important de succès.

Les travaux sur l'éjection des pilotes militaires d'avions à réaction sont très nombreux, mais peu d'auteurs ont précisé la part et la valeur de la radiologie. Nous étudierons successivement dans ce travail:
· les lésions observées par la radiologie après éjection,
· l'étude radiographique du rachis du pilote assis sur un siège éjectable,
· l'examen radiographique post-mortem.

2. La radiographie après éjection

L'examen clinique est dans tous les cas indispensable mais seule la radiologie apporte des arguments irréfutables sur les mécanismes des lésions non seulement squelettiques mais aussi viscérales et la relation de cause à effet des lésions observées après l'éjection. Les radiographies contribuent donc à la prévention des accidents et possèdent un intérêt évident et fondamental dans le bilan d'aptitude. Elles sont des documents médico-légaux.

La technique radiologique doit etre rigoureuse, clichés standards, clichés localisés, tomographies, épreuves radiodynamiques.

La radiologie rachidienne permet le diagnostic exact des lésions traumatiques en précisant le nombre, la localisation et le type de fractures. Celles avec intégrité du mur postérieur sont les plus fréquentes, la moitié des fractures siègent à la charnière dorso-lombaire. Elles révèlent surtout l'aspect non spécifique du tassement cunéiforme antérieur.

Les rayons X facilitent l'étude de la détermination du mécanisme d'apparition de la lésion. Les fractures survenant lors de la propulsion du siège (éjection proprement dite) siègent généralement au niveau de la colonne dorsale moyenne, (D6-D7-D8). Elles résultent de deux facteurs. (1) L'accélération appliquée au siège varie selon le type de siège de 16 à 18 g pendant 0.18 à 0.20 sec à 0.20 à 0.21 pendant 0.08 à 0.10 sec. (2) La position défectueuse du pilote en hyperflexion ainsi que l'ont démontré des radiographies sur siège éjectable. Les fractures de l'arrivée au sol sont créées par une compression verticale sur une colonne en discrète flexion (bras de levier dorsal) et se localisant à la charnière dorso-lombaire.

Le diagnostic de ces fractures, même cliniquement muettes a toujours été affirmé par les radiographies rachidiennes obligatoires après tout accident aérien. L'importance et la primauté du risque rachidien ont imposé cet examen radiologique. Mais, il faut noter que tout organe ou partie du squelette traumatisé peut être intéressé par le traumatisme et la radiologie jouera également la un rôle fondamental.

La radiologie oriente la thérapeutique et permet de poser avec précision le pronostic.

TABLEAU I

Résultats observés dans l'Armée de l'Air Française
(octobre 1951 à juin 1969 inclus)

Nombre total d'éjections	Éjections manquées (décès)	Éjections réussies
295	71	224
100 %	24 %	76 %

TABLEAU II

Résultats des éjections en fonction de l'altitude

Altitude	Nombre d'éjections	Décès	Blessés graves	Blessés légers	Indemnes
Supérieure à 3000 pieds	183	17	25	31	110
De 1000 à 3000 pieds	53	13	2	8	30
Inférieure à 1000 pieds	47	34	3	5	5
Inconnue	12	7	1	1	3
Total	295	71	31	45	148

TABLEAU III

Résultats des éjections en fonction de la vitesse propre

Vitesse	Nombre d'éjections	Décès	Blessés graves	Blessés légers	Indemnes
Supérieure à 500 nœuds	24	12	5	4	3
De 100 à 500 nœuds	211	33	23	30	125
Inférieure à 100 nœuds	10	4	1	1	4
Inconnue	50	22	2	10	16
Total	295	71	31	45	148

Un tassement simple avec intégrité du mur postérieur sera traité par la kinésithérapie.

Éjections manquées et réussies dans l'Armée de l'Air Française sont présentées dans le Tableau I. Les conditions d'utilisation du siège éjectable (altitude, vitesse de l'avion) ont une influence majeure sur la réussité du sauvetage (Tableaux II et III).

En cas d'éjection à altitude basse, le pourcentage des décès est très important. Une forte proportion d'accidents graves est particulièrement observée dans les éjections non automatiques. Les résultats se sont nettement améliorés avec l'automaticité des différentes séquences. La plupart des éjections se sont produits à des vitesses propres comprises entre 100 et 500 nœuds. Au-dessus de 500 nœuds, le pourcentage de mortalité atteint 50. La vitesse constitue un facteur aggravant.

On observe des lésions bénignes et des lésions graves (entraînant des incapacités). Les pilotes présentant des ecchymoses dues aux sangles ou aux chocs à l'aterrissage qui entraîne aussi des érosions cutanées ou des plaies. Parfois, on note des entorses tibio-tarsiennes ou plus rarement des entorses du genou. Certaines intéressent le rachis: d'autre les membres, le thorax, le crâne. La radiologie joue là un grand rôle dans le bilan de ces traumatismes.

Les fractures vertébrales (Tableaux IV et V) surviennent chez 26 pilotes soit 11.6%

TABLEAU IV

La répartition des lésions vertébrales

Siège	Nombre
D5	1
D6	2
D7	5
D8	6
D9	1
D10	3
D11	1
D12	5
L1	11
L2	2
L4	1
	38 (26 pilotes)

TABLEAU V

Les lésions vertébrales multiples

Siège	Nombre
D6–L2	1
D7–D8	2
D7–L1	1
D8–L1	1
D7–D8–D9–D10–D11	1
D12–L1	1
D12–L1–L2	1

des éjections réussies. Ces lésions siègent surtout au niveau de la charnière dorso-lombaire (16 cas). Le plus souvent isolées (18 cas), elles sont parfois multiples (8 cas). La grande fréquence de localisation à la charnière dorso-lombaire s'explique par la manœuvre de ces fractures à l'arrivée au sol (fracture du parachutiste). Dans l'étude des pilotes ayant des fractures multiples il faut retenir le plus souvent l'association de deux facteurs: (1) la mauvaise position au départ du siège, et (2) l'arrivée au sol dans de très mauvaises conditions (vent violent, sol accidenté).

TABLEAU VI

Fractures non-vertébrales

	Nombre
Omoplate	2
Épaule – Clavicule	2
Humérus	10
Radius	5
Cubitus	6
Luxation du coude	1
Bassin	1
Fémur	9
Tibia	8
Péroné	7
Pied	2
Luxation ouverte du genou	2
Côtes	7
Sternum	4
Crâne (voute – base)	5
Face	3

Assez fréquentes, les fractures non-vertébrales intéressent surtout les membres (24 pilotes). Assez souvent, elles sont multiples (Tableau VI). Elles s'associent parfois à des fractures du rachis.

3. La radiographie du rachis en position assise: son intérêt dans la compréhension physiopathogénique des fractures rachidiennes de l'éjection

Dans le service d'Électro-radiologie de l'Hôpital d'Instruction des Armées Dominique Larrey, nous avons étudié l'aspect radiologique du sujet assis sur siège éjectable. La mise en place s'est effectuée sur siège type Martin-Baker MK 4, avec un équipement composé d'une combinaison de vol, d'un casque et d'un inhalateur, en utilisant successivement la commande haute, puis la commande basse.

Les études des modifications de la statique rachidienne en position assise ont bien montré que, lorsque l'homme passe de la station debout à la position assise, l'ensellure lombaire tend à s'éffacer et le cyphose dorsale physiologique se réduit. En général il n'existe pas de changement de la courbure cervicale. Nos constations vont dans le même sens, en faisant ressortir l'influence de l'état antérieur du rachis, de l'inclinaison du siège et du degré 'd'enfoncement' du sujet dans le siège.

Les radiographies de profil pratiquées au cours des enquêtes après éjection, objectivent des fractures vertébrales attribuées à l'accélération imprimée au siège. Ces atteintes rachidiennes se localisent électivement en D5, D6 et D7, ce sont des fractures par compression verticale du rachis discrètement fléchi (Mécanisme I de Watson-Jones). Cette localisation ne s'observe que si la force est appliquée dans l'axe de poussée au niveau du centre de courbure du rachis dorsal et si les vertèbres sont bien alignées. Donc, la position du rachis du sujet assis sur le siège éjectable est un facteur important avant celui de l'accélération.

Nos examens en salle de radiodiagnostic montrent que sur un sujet correctement assis, l'axe de poussée du siège passe au niveau de centre de courbure du rachis dorsal, c'est-à-dire selon flexion en D5, D6, D7 et parfois D8. Ceci explique cette localisation haute des fractures de l'éjection constatée lors des enquêtes. Par contre chez des cyphotiques, la courbure pathologique ne s'efface pas en position assise et l'axe de poussée intéresse alors toujours plusieurs vertèbres de la colonne dorsale moyenne.

D'où l'intérêt d'éliminer les cyphotiques et les scoliotiques importants. Les radiographies pratiquées montrent qu'il n'existe pas de nette modification de l'aspect du rachis en fonction du système de commande d'éjection utilisé.

Le réglage en hauteur du siège est à considérer car la position basse rétablit l'ensellure lombaire et accroit la cyphose dorsale. Le port des casques influe aussi sur la statique rachidienne, certains tendent à fléchir la région D4–D5–D6, action qui ne fait qu'accentuer la position basse du siège. Donc le casque ne doit pas être trop volumineux.

La radiographie en position assise permet de mieux comprendre l'importance de la position du pilote, fonction notamment de la position du siège, des équipements et de l'état antérieur du rachis. On a précisé plusieurs facteurs défavorables à l'éjection: les contours défectueux de certains dossiers de siège, la flexion de la tête en avant, la mauvaise adaptation des sangles et la mauvaise adaptation du coussin.

4. La radiographie post mortem après éjection

Peu d'éjections supersoniques ou transsoniques ont été publiées. Certaines n'ont pas été rapportées, et parfois on ne peut déterminer la vitesse réelle lors de l'éjection.

Une éjection survenue récemment dans l'Armée de l'Air Française à Mach 1.20, nous a permis d'objectiver le rôle de la radiographie dans les enquêtes *post mortem* après éjection.

A. CIRCONSTANCES DE L'ACCIDENT

Le Sergent G., pilote de chasse, âgé de 26 ans, a effectué 680 heures de vol dont 110 sur le type de l'appareil accidenté Mirage IIIE. Au cours d'un retournement de combat, à partir d'une configuration de vol à 30000 pieds, le pilote met son avion en piqué à 70° environ pour une raison indéterminée. Vers une altitude de 15000 pieds, jugeant, compte tenu de sa vitesse (Mach 1.20, 700 nœuds) qu'il n'avait plus la possibilité d'effectuer une ressource, le pilote a pris la décision de s'éjecter. Mis à feu au moyen de la poignée haute, le siège s'est séparé de l'avion à une altitude estimée de 9000 pieds et à une vitesse corrigée de 690 nœuds.

Ces données correspondent, compte tenu de l'altitude à une pression dynamique légèrement supérieure à 1000 millibars. A la suite des essais, on admet que la trainée d'un siège peut être assimilée à une surface plane d'un mètre carré. La force subie par l'ensemble siège-pilote à la sortie de l'avion a été dans ce cas de l'ordre de 10 tonnes.

Les séquences automatiques de l'éjection s'étant effectuées normalement, le parachute-pilote s'est déployé à une altitude approximative de 3500 pieds. La descente se termine dans un petit étang à 500 mètres de l'impact-avion. Le pilote a été retrouvé décédé, flottant à la surface. La jambe gauche arrachée est retrouvée à 300 mètres de l'étang.

B. DESCRIPTION DES LÉSIONS

L'examen externe du pilote montre des lésions de la face (fractures du nez, ecchymoses périorbitaires bilatérales), des fractures des deux humérus, un abdomen ouvert avec éviscération partielle du bassin, un arrachement du membre inférieur gauche au niveau de l'articulation sacro-iliaque, et des fractures des deux fémurs dont une ouverte à droite.

Nous avons pensé que des examens radiologiques pratiqués avant l'autopsie, permettraient d'obtenir des documents complétant les données anatomo-pathologiques. Leur description fera l'objet d'un paragraphe particulier.

L'autopsie nous a révélé en particulier au niveau des poumons des marbrures importantes avec hémorragies en surface, un aspect emphysémateux, œdémateux. A la coupe les lobes sont crépitants, rosés, spumeux et œdémateux. Nous avons noté un infarcissement des lobes supérieur et inférieur de chaque poumon. L'examen histologique a conclu à des lésions d'œdème pulmonaire sur un fond d'alvéolites catarrhales et hémorragiques au stade aigu. L'examen du péritoine, de l'épiploon, des intestins, du mésentère, de la rate, de la vessie, de la prostate et du pénis n'ont pu être pratiqués, car ces organes ont disparu à l'éviscération. Les examens histologiques du cerveau et de la mœlle épinière, ne mettent pas en évidence de lésions pathologiques.

Le rapport entre la vitesse du son et celle de l'avion, n'est pas le paramètre le plus important à considérer. Le facteur essentiel est la valeur de la pression dynamique, car il détermine l'importance des forces agissant directement sur le pilote, donc l'amplitude de la décélération qu'il subit.

Dans l'accident que nous citons les valeurs numériques ont été établies à partir des enrégistrements du contrôle régional, du témoignage d'un pilote, témoin de la première partie de la trajectoire et de calculs effectués sur ordinateur en utilisant les paramètres de base. La trajectoire a été reconstituée sur simulateur Mirage IIE.

C. RADIOGRAPHIES POST MORTEM

L'examen radiologique pratiqué à l'Hôpital A. Baur a mis en évidence les lésions suivantes:

(a) une fracture multifragmentaire du tiers moyen de l'humérus droit:

(b) une fracture du col chirurgical de l'humérus gauche avec luxation de la tête humérale;

(c) une fracture transversale sans déplacement du corps des deux omoplates;

(d) une luxation sterno-claviculaire gauche;

(e) une fracture de D6 (tassement latéral gauche);

(f) une fracture-luxation du sacrum avec disjonction des deux articulations sacro-iliaques (rotation de 90° du sacrum) et disjonction de la symphyse pubienne,

(g) une fracture symétrique du tiers moyen des deux fémurs;

(h) une fracture de la styloïde du 5ème métatarsien gauche;

La radiographie pulmonaire montre des opacités arrondies ou ovalaires à contours flous et estompés, prédominant essentiellement au niveau des bases.

D. PHYSIOPATHOGÉNIE DES LÉSIONS CONSTATÉES RADIOLOGIQUEMENT

Les calculs effectués ont permis de fixer les conditions de l'éjection: altitude à 15000 pieds; vitesse à 1.20 Mach, vitesse corrigée à 690 KTS. L'enquête à établi que le serrage des sangles du harnais était insuffisant, ce fait joint à l'angle de piqué et à la saturation maximale de la servocommande expliquent la fracture de D6, au départ du siège (20 g pendant 0.20 sec).

Les autres lésions surviennent à peu près simultanément et sont dues au souffle. L'évaluation des efforts subis par les membres inférieurs conduit à une estimation d'une force de 855 kgs, ce qui explique les fractures des fémurs et l'arrachement de la jambe gauche, a l'exception de la fracture vertébrale, provoquée par la mauvaise position du pilote, toutes les autres lésions sont le fait de la pression dynamique.

E. INTÉRÊT GÉNÉRAL DE LA RADIOGRAPHIE POST-MORTEM APRÈS ÉJECTION

La traumatologie des pilotes tués lors d'éjections est très complexe. Aux vitesses subsoniques, il n'apparaît pas de lésions traumatiques importantes lors de l'éjection proprement dite, sauf si le largage de la verrière est déficient.

Dans la plupart des cas, les éjections non réussies se sont produites à basse altitude ou à très grande vitesse. On observe de fréquentes fractures ouvertes ou fermées des membres s'associant à de grandes dislocations articulaires. Les côtes sont multi-fracturées, le crâne et le rachis également. Les viscères sont lésés; foie et rate éclatés, le poumon embroché ou porteur de lésions de 'blast'. Dans tous ces cas, l'examen radiographique systématique contribue à établir avec précision le mécanisme pathogénique des lésions observées.

5. Conclusions

La radiologie joue donc un rôle important dans l'enquête après éjection de pilotes d'avions à réaction. Elle permet le diagnostic exact des lésions. Elle apporte des renseignements d'ordre physiopathogénique et contribue ainsi à la prévention des lésions. Elle oriente la thérapeutique éventuelle et le pronostic. Avec H. Mangin, nous insisterons aussi en concluant sur l'importance d'un examen radiologique systématique du rachis en particulier.

A l'admission dans le personnel navigant, pour éliminer les lésions graves incompatibles avec la profession, mais aussi dans le but de constituer un dossier de référence d'intérêt diagnostic et médico-légal.

THE CENTRIFUGE AS A THERAPEUTIC DEVICE

R. PELLIGRA, S. STEIN, J. MARKHAM, P. LIPPE, J. NOYES,
J. DICKSON and K. SKRETTINGLAND

Ames Research Center, National Aeronautics and Space Administration, Moffett Field, Calif., U.S.A.

1. Introduction

The role played by the centrifuge in man's epic journey from Kitty Hawk to the moon has overshadowed its humble beginnings as a crude therapeutic device.

As early as 1795, Erasmus Darwin, an imaginative physician of his day, speculated as to the possible use of centrifugation to induce sleep, reduce heart activity, and suppress fever (White, 1964). The centrifuge was, in fact, used throughout nineteenth-century Europe for the treatment of the mentally ill. By the turn of the century, it was generally accepted that the acceleration forces of gravity and centrifugation exerted identical effects upon man's body. Application of this concept (later formulated as the 'Equivalence Principle' by Einstein) to the problems being generated by the recently invented airplane completely altered the future course of centrifuge research and technology. The centrifuge became the ideal, indeed, the only, practical and safe means of studying man's response to prolonged exposure to increased acceleration environments. This function was reinforced by rapid developments in aircraft design stimulated by two World Wars and the advent of the Space Age.

In recent years, the suggestion that centrifugation be used to prevent or alleviate the effects of weightlessness on the cardiovascular and musculoskeletal systems of man in space has renewed interest in its potential as a form of treatment for other clinical conditions. One such application in which centrifugation was used as an alternative to neurosurgery in the treatment of an elderly assault victim is reported below.

2. Case Report

Although complete details of this case will appear in a future report in the neurosurgical literature, it is felt that the following clinical aspects are of immediate interest to the aerospace medical community and are indispensable to a full appreciation of the technique employed.

A. PAST HISTORY

In October 1968, J. B., a 63-year old male of Mexican extraction sustained bullet injuries of the abdomen and head when he attempted to prevent holdup of the restaurant in which he was employed as a cook.

He was brought to the hospital in a conscious state and underwent emergency surgical debridement and repair of the abdominal and head wounds. Fragments of the .22 caliber bullet and splinters of bone were removed from the left frontal lobe along the missile tract. Because of the absence of abnormal neurological findings, no attempt was made to retrieve a fragment measuring approximately 10mm × 6mm × 4mm which had found its way into the ventricular system of the brain and was floating freely in the left lateral ventricle. The fragment could be demonstrated on X-ray to migrate from the occipital horn to the frontal horn of the left lateral ventricle by placing the patient's head in the brow-up or brow-down position (Figures 1, 2). His postoperative course was uneventful, and he was discharged from the hospital after 13 days with no apparent neurological deficit or other serious complaints. Physical examination on discharge revealed a well-developed, obese, elderly male who appeared younger than his stated years. Vital signs were normal. The abdominal and scalp incisions were healing well with no evidence of infection. The remainder of the physical and neurological examination was unremarkable.

Past History: The patient has enjoyed good general health all his life. In 1955, at age 50 years, he underwent transurethral resection for benign prostatic hypertrophy and in 1964, responded to medical treatment for a peptic ulcer which was documented by X-ray studies. He was discovered to have diabetes mellitus during his October hospitalization and his blood sugar and glycosuria have been easily controlled with diet and tolbutamide therapy. Although he has had no complaints referable to the cardiovascular system, ECG taken October 1968 showed general T wave flattening and small QII, III, AVF suggestive of an old posterior wall myocardial infarction.

Subsequent Course: Routine follow-up X-rays of the skull during an outpatient visit one month after surgery revealed that the bullet fragment that had been allowed to remain in the left lateral ventricle was now located in the third ventricle (Figure 2).

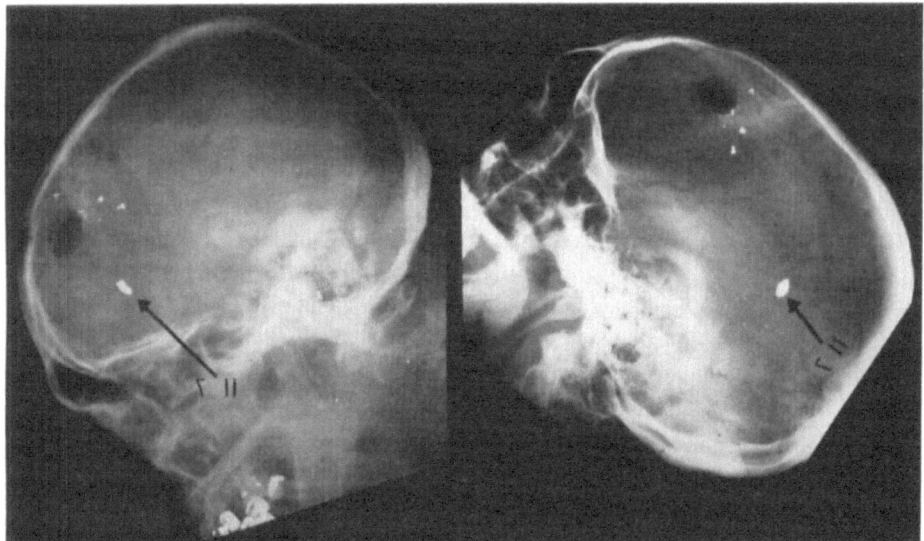

Fig. 1. Lateral X-rays of the skull taken in brow-down (left) and brow-up (right) positions demonstrate excursion of the bullet fragment from the frontal horn to the occipital horn of the left lateral ventricle.

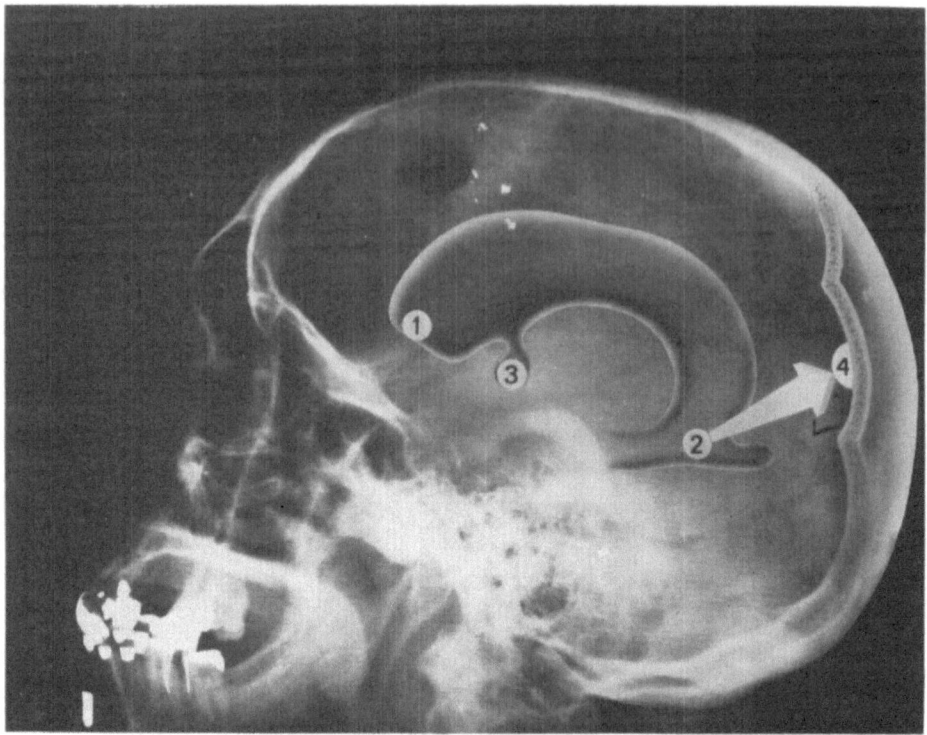

Fig. 2.   Indicates position of bullet fragment in: (1) the frontal horn of the left lateral ventricle, (2) the occipital horn of the left lateral ventricle, and (3) the third ventricle. The arrow indicates the anticipated migratory path of the fragment in an increased acceleration environment from its location at (2) to a point in the posterior parietal lobe just beneath the calvarium (4).

Except for occasional mild dizziness and slight blurring of vision, the patient had experienced no neurological symptoms during this period. He was brought to the X-ray department where, under fluoroscopic control, the bullet fragment was directed from the third ventricle to the left lateral ventricle by manually applying small impacts to the patient's head in various positions. In order to prevent the fragment from once again returning to the third ventricle and possibly obstructing the flow of cerebrospinal fluid, the patient was admitted to the hospital and restricted to bed rest in the left lateral decubitus position.

B. CENTRIFUGE TREATMENT

Preliminary studies by one of us (S.S.) utilizing gelatin molds of a consistency comparable to that of human brain tissue indicated that acceleration levels of 4 to 6g should be sufficient to cause the bullet fragment to penetrate the wall of the left lateral ventricle. It was felt that brief exposure in a centrifuge to forces of this magnitude, although unprecedented in a man of this age and cardiovascular status, would nevertheless involve less risk than surgical removal.

In order to avoid injury to critical areas of the brain, the fragment migrating under the influence of centrifugal force must be directed from its position in the left lateral ventricle, posteriorly, laterally, and superiorly along a direct path extending to a point in the posterior parietal lobe just beneath the inner surface of the calvarium (Figures 2, 3). Future management would depend on the extent of travel of the fragment along this path. If it came to rest at or near the terminal position just beneath the cranial bone, it would be readily accessible by simple craniectomy. If movement was minimal, but sufficient to penetrate the ependymal lining of the ventricle, it was hoped that glial reaction would hold it in place, thereby relieving the threat of migration within the ventricular system.

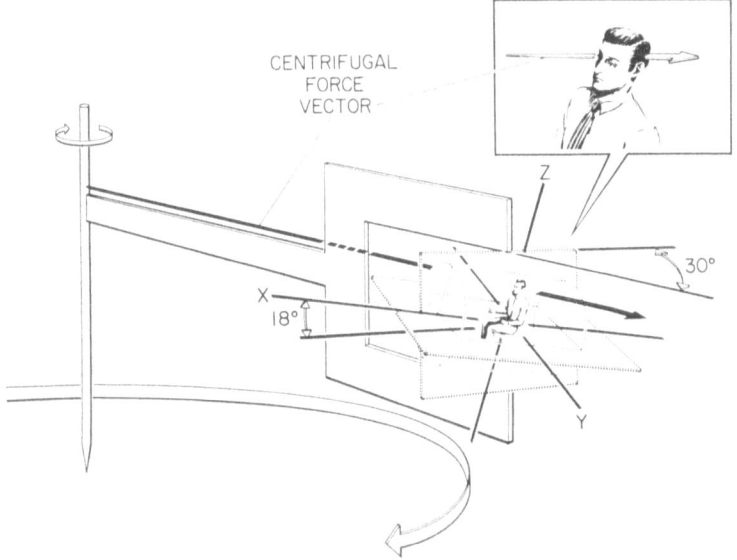

Fig. 3.   Position of the patient in the Ames Five-Degree-of-Freedom Centrifuge. At 6g, the accelerations acting along the patients G_x, G_y, and G_z axis were, respectively, $+5.1$ g, $+2.6$ g, and -0.9 g.

Consultation with our engineering staff revealed that with the Ames Five-Degree-of-Freedom Centrifuge operating at 4g, the force vector required to direct the fragment toward the desired position would be obtained by positioning the patient toward the center of rotation, pitched up 20.5°, and yawed 30° to the left. For 6g, the pitch angle would be 18°, the yaw angle 30° (Figure 3), and the accelerations acting along the patient's G_x, G_y, and G_z axis would be 5.1 g, 2.6 g, and -0.9 g, respectively (Figure 4).

Two of the investigators, experienced in centrifugation (K.S. and R.P.), rode the centrifuge with the cab in this unorthodox position without apparent ill effects.

The patient was exposed initially to 4 g for 30 sec. He experienced no nausea, dizziness, pain, or other subjective ill effects, and electrocardiogram, except for the occurrence of two premature atrial contractions, remained unchanged. Blood pressure and pulse rate responded normally. Polaroid X-rays taken immediately after centrifugation indicated that the fragment was still floating freely in the left lateral ventricle (Figure 1). The cab was then adjusted to a pitch-up angle of 18° and a yaw-left angle of 30° (Figure 3), and he was exposed to the following acceleration profile (Figure 4): 0.39 g/sec onset rate to peak 5 g maintained for 20 sec, then increased at 0.33 g/sec to 6 g for 3 sec. Initial offset rate was 0.8 g/sec and total exposure time approximately 58 sec. The rationale for the abrupt change in acceleration from 5 g to 6 g was to attempt to facilitate penetration of the ependymal lining. Again, the patient tolerated the exposure exceedingly well. He offered no subjective complaints. Electrocardiogram demonstrated approximately ten premature extrasystoles with coupling of one pair (Figure 5). Because of difficulties in identifying *P* waves, it cannot be determined if the

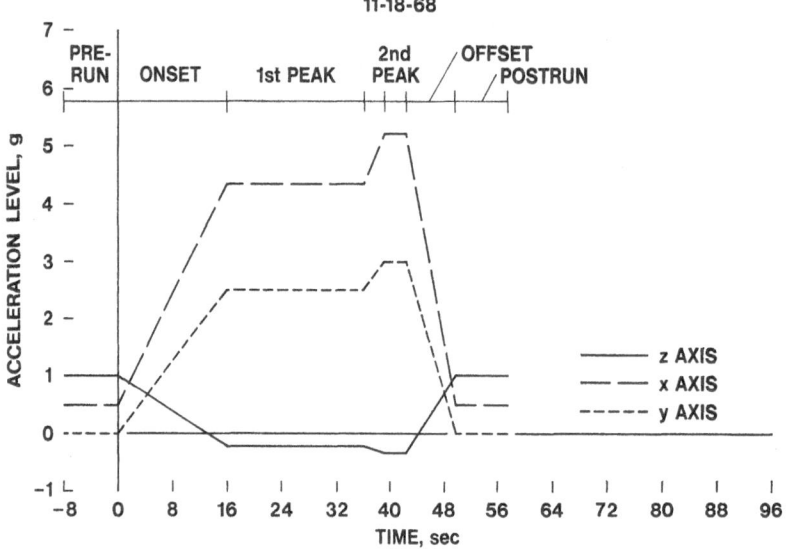

Fig. 4.   Acceleration profile, second run.

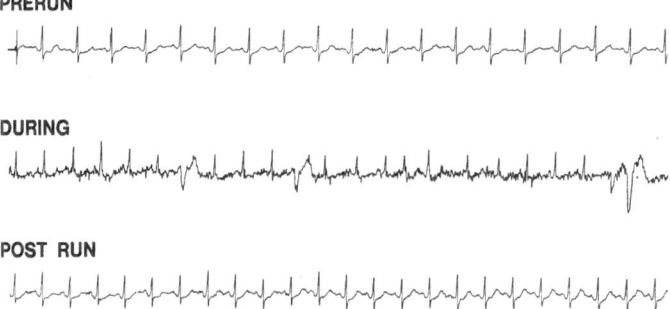

Fig. 5.   Electrocardiogram, October 18, 1968. Upper tracing – immediately prior to exposure to 6g acceleration profile (Figure 4). Middle tracing, during exposure (see text). Bottom tracing, immediately after exposure.

premature contractions were ventricular of multifocal origin, or unifocal premature ventricular contractions and premature atrial contractions with aberrant conduction (Figure 5). X-rays taken in the supine position indicated that the bullet fragment was still in approximately the same location in the left ventricle and that if penetration of the wall had occurred at all, it was certainly minimal. No further manipulation of the head to determine mobility of the fragment in the ventricle was attempted, and the patient was returned to the hospital. On the following day, an electrocardiogram showed diffuse minor T wave changes which reverted in several days. Blood enzyme levels were normal except for one transient of serum glutamic oxaloacetic transaminase (SGOT) to 70 units (normal 10 to 45 units). The patient continued to have no complaints referable to his cardiovascular system. After 10 days of bed rest, repeat skull X-rays revealed that the bullet fragment did not change its position with movements of the head. It was no longer floating freely in the ventricle. It appeared to be embedded in the posterolateral wall of the left lateral ventricle.

In an attempt to gain some insight into the mechanical events which had occurred intracerebrally, a fresh human brain autopsy specimen with a bullet fragment im-

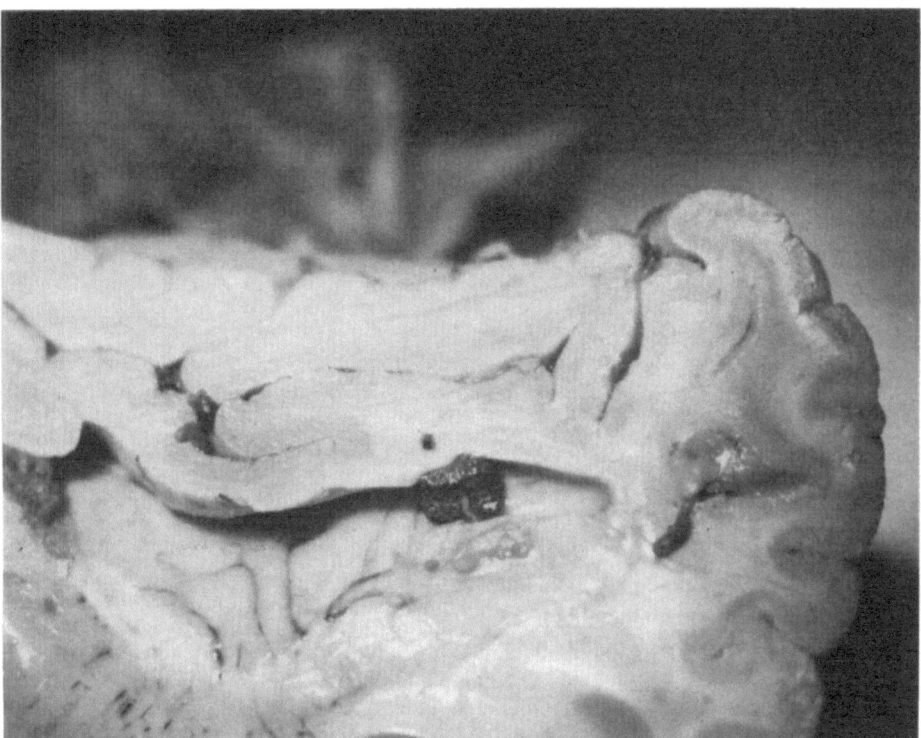

Fig. 6. Sagittal section of human brain autopsy specimen with bullet implanted in the frontal lobe of left lateral ventricle following exposure to the same acceleration profile as the patient (Fig. 4). *Note:* The bullet fragment has migrated posteriorly under the influence of centrifugal force and appears to be wedged in the posterior horn of the left lateral ventricle.

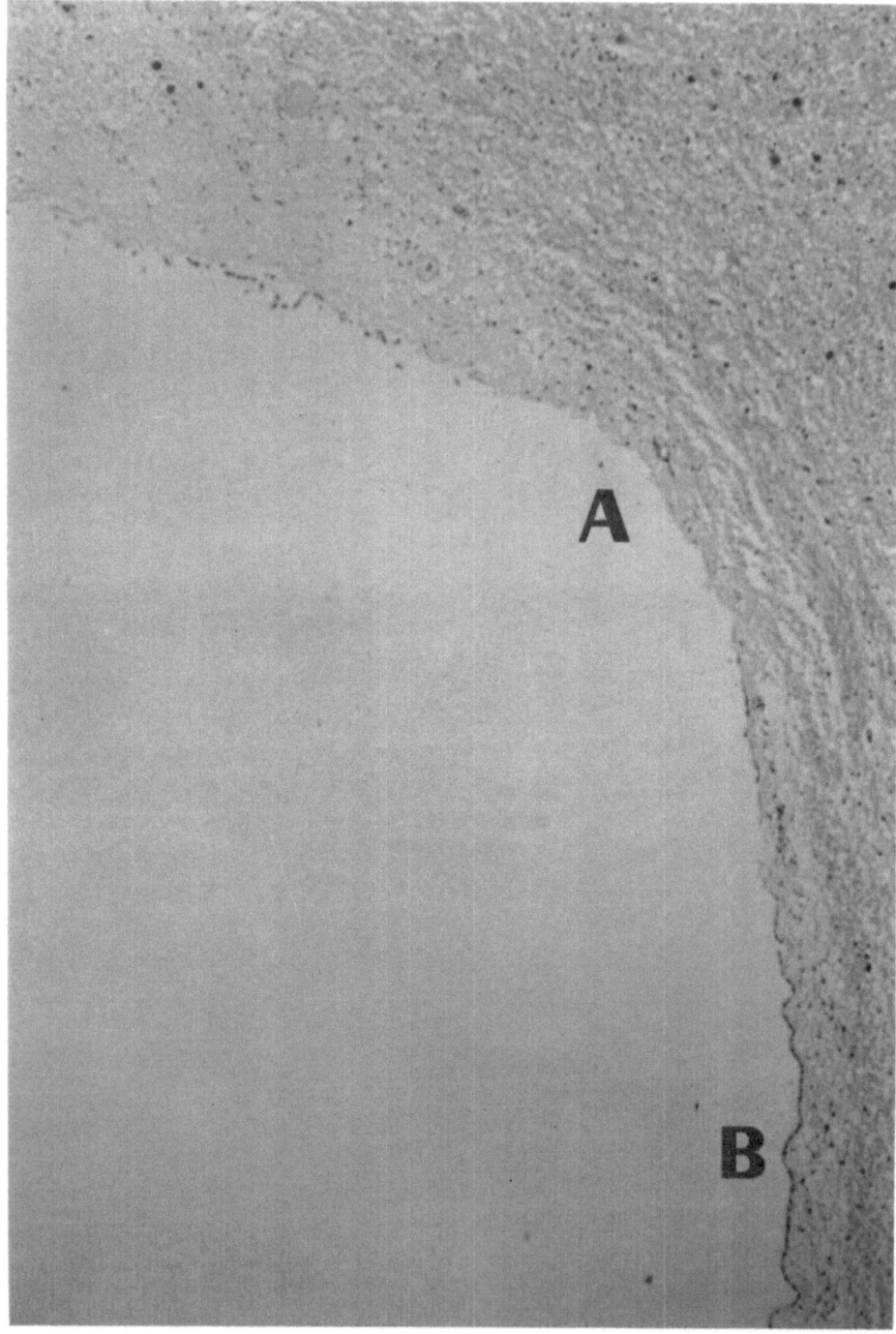

Fig. 7.   Microscopic section (H & E Stain) of the ependymal lining of the posterior horn of left
lateral ventricle of the human brain autopsy specimen exposed to the same conditions as the patient
Figs. 4, 6). *Note:* There is mechanical disruption of the ependymal lining (A) beneath the bullet
fragment and normal lining (B) in adjacent areas.

planted in the left lateral ventricle was exposed to the same acceleration profiles as the patient (Figure 4). On gross examination, the ependymal lining appeared to be indented by the bullet fragment which was wedged in the posterior horn of the left lateral ventricle (Figure 6). Microscopic examination showed mechanical disruption of the ependymal lining underlying the bullet fragment (Figure 7A), and no involvement of the adjacent areas (Figure 7B). Fully aware of the shortcomings of this model as representative of the events occurring in the intact human, it was presumed, nevertheless, that the bullet in the patient's brain was being held in place by the combined effects of wedging in the posterior horn and glial reaction due to disruption of the ependymal lining. The patient was discharged from the hospital in December 1968. He was permitted to carry on normal activities of daily living, but was cautioned to avoid situations which might accidentally involve abrupt jarring of the body or head.

Pneumoencephalograms (Figure 8), and serial tomograms (Figure 9), taken in

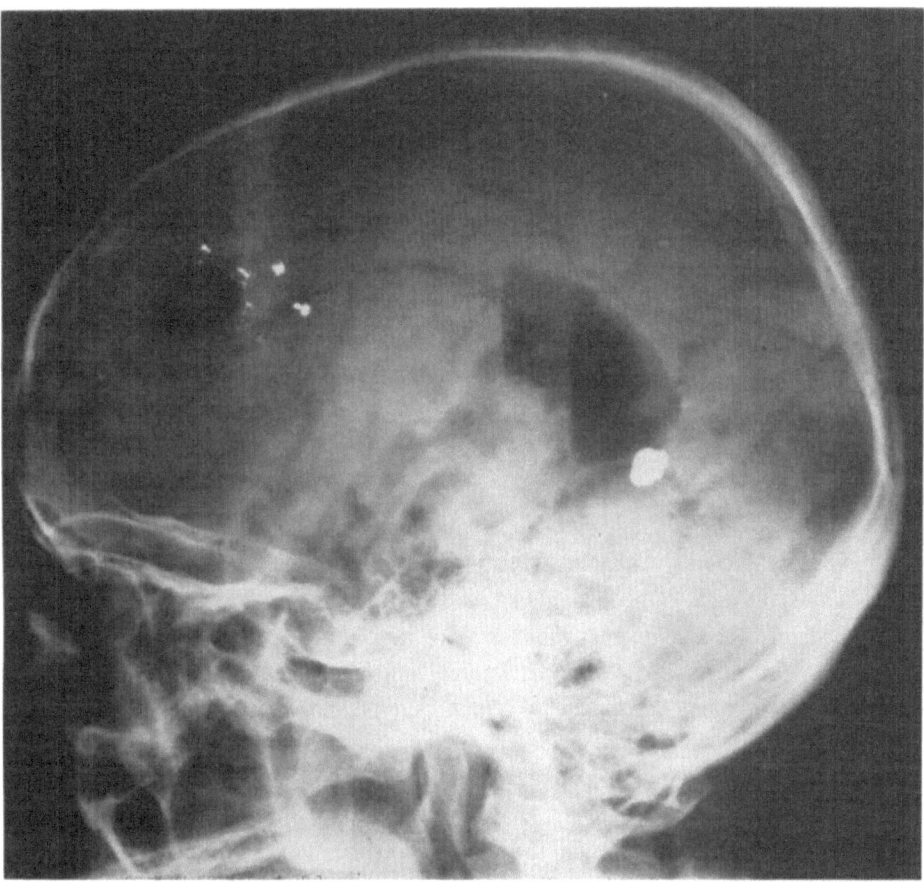

Fig. 8. Pneumoencephalogram: demonstrates air in ventricular system outlining both lateral ventricles. The bullet fragment is located at the postero-lateral wall of the left lateral ventricle.

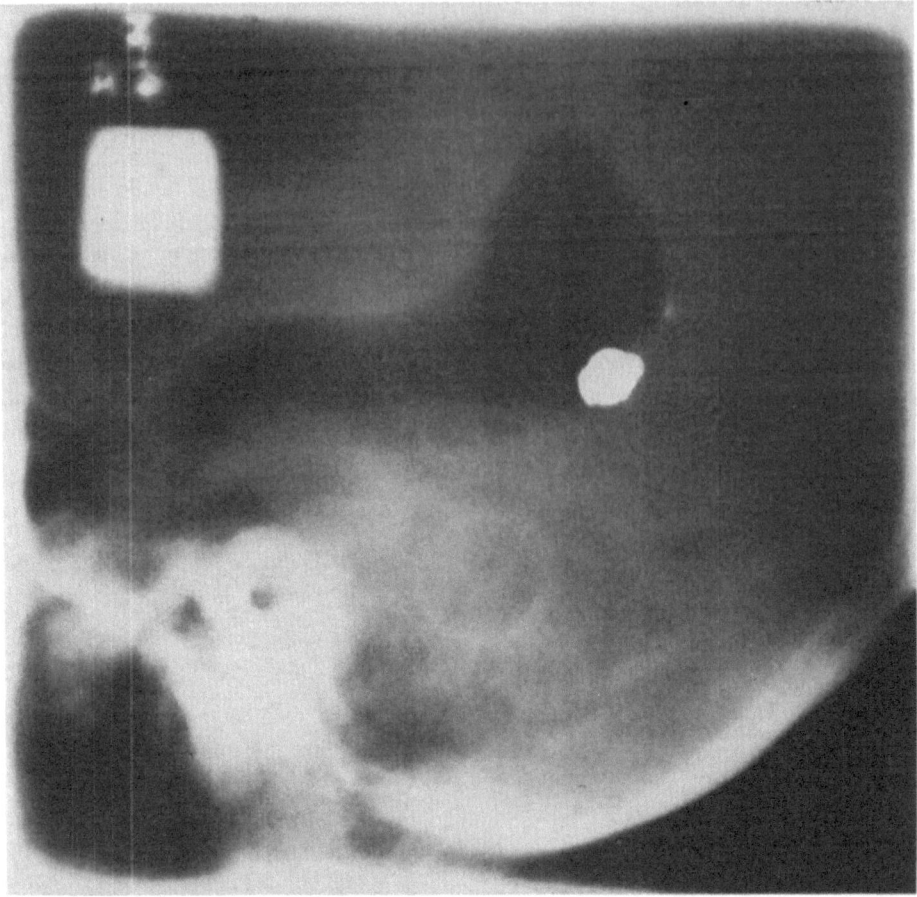

Fig. 9. Tomogram: at the level of the bullet fragment demonstrates that approximately 30 to 40 percent of the body of the fragment is embedded in the wall of the left lateral ventricle and the remainder is protruding into the ventricular cavity.

June 1969, six months after centrifugation, show approximately 30 to 40% of the body of the fragment imbedded in the wall of the left ventricle and the remainder protruding into the cavity. It is interesting to note that the patient has a minimally developed posterior horn in the left lateral ventricle, a not uncommon congenital anomaly. The patient continues to remain symptom-free and enjoys a normally active life.

3. Discussion and Conclusions

A bullet fragment floating freely in the ventricular system of the brain of a 63-year old male assault victim was moved to a fixed, safe position by briefly exposing him to an increased acceleration environment in the NASA Ames Research Center's Five-Degree-of-Freedom Centrifuge. The patient has returned to normal activity and, six months following the procedure, has no apparent neurological deficit or serious complaints. It is felt that this case demonstrates that:

(1) The centrifuge can, in select circumstances, be used as a safe, effective, therapeutic modality. This patient experienced little discomfort and no pain during the brief period of centrifugation and was spared the hazards of anesthesia, major neurosurgery, and postsurgical complications. Although asymptomatic free-floating foreign bodies in the ventricle following trauma are rare, retained intracranial fragments in other parts of the brain are not uncommon. Moreover, they usually occur in younger patients such as soldiers and assault victims who are considerably better medical risks than our patient. It may be possible by brief exposure to a centrifugal force field to move fragments that are deeply embedded in the brain to more accessible locations towards the periphery of the brain.

Only two other reports appear in the modern literature where centrifuge is used for the treatment of a patient. As part of a pain threshold study, Ham and coworkers, in 1943, attempted to relieve the symptoms of migraine headache by centrifuging otherwise healthy young male military personnel. In 1966, Neault and coworkers utilizing the Mayo Clinic Centrifuge, were partially successful in replacing a traumatically-detached retina in an 18-year old football player by exposing him to 2 to 2.7 g for a total of 2 hr in five sessions.

No attempt will be made here to catalogue the possible clinical uses of centrifugation. However, on the basis of the finding here, there appear to be select clinical situations in which it is desirable to displace an object which is denser than surrounding tissue, as for example a foreign body, gallstone, or ureteral calculus, the use of centrifugation should be considered.

(2) At least in this patient, advanced age and the presence of fairly advanced cardiovascular disease did not adversely affect tolerance to prolonged acceleration levels of 4, 5, and 6 g. This is, as far as can be ascertained, the first report of a man of this age and cardiovascular status being exposed to these conditions in a centrifuge. The implications of this finding for future manned space flight are significant. If elderly scientists are able to safely tolerate the acceleration forces of rocket liftoff, it will be possible for them to participate first-hand in experiments being conducted in Earth-orbiting, Moon-, or Mars-based scientific laboratories. The same might apply to commercial space flights or, exercising the imagination, to patients being sent to Earth-orbiting hospitals to be treated or to recuperate in a weightless environment. Furthermore, normal space flight attitudes do not involve exposure to significant acceleration levels along the $\pm G_y$ axis which we feel may have accounted for the transient cardiac ischemia observed in our patient on the day following centrifugation. Studies in live monkeys are currently being undertaken to determine whether the cardiac stresses in the patient could have been diminished by directing the acceleration force along the pure $\pm G_x$ axis of his body and positioning only his head such that the force would move the bullet fragment in the desired direction.

(3) Lastly, this case appears to demonstrate once again that aerospace technology can be applied usefully to solving mundane problems. There have been many examples

of the contributions of space technology to clinical medicine in recent years: biomedical monitoring, hyperbaric oxygen therapy, fiber-optics, lasers, to mention a few. Still, the current climate of lay opinion reflects a feeling that technology, cold and impersonal, exists for its own sake and is oblivious to the needs of mankind; that at least some of the energies being spent to further expand technology should be redirected towards effectively utilizing current knowledge. Whatever one's feelings are in this matter, it is undoubtedly true that hidden within the vast resources of aerospace know-how, are solutions to many common clinical problems. Aerospace physicians in general, and the members of the aeromedical field in particular, are in an ideal position to tap these resources for the benefit of mankind.

References

Gilles, J. A. (ed.): 1965, *A Textbook of Aviation Physiology,* Pergamon Press, New York.
Ham, G. C.: 1943, *War Med.,* pp. 30–56.
Neault, R. W., Martins, T. G., Code, C. F., and Nolaw, C. A.: 1966, *Proc. Mayo Clin.* **41**, 145.
White, W. J.: 1964, *A History of the Centrifuge in Aerospace,* Douglas Aircraft Company, Santa Monica, Calif., U.S.A.

SELECTIVE g-FORCE APPLICATION
IN THE TREATMENT OF RETINAL DETACHMENT

J. TEN DOESSCHATE, R. HOPPENBROUWERS and M. P. LANSBERG

National Aeromedical Center, Soesterberg, The Netherlands

1. Introduction

The treatment of retinal detachments is by no means a solved problem. Considerable effort is being given to find new and more reliable methods to bring about a good repositioning of the retina. However, the results are not always equal to the hopeful expectations when these methods are introduced.

One recent example of these (1962) unsuccessful attempts was the use of liquid silicone, advocated by Cibis (1962). The applied silicone caused destructive lesions of the retina and a situation in the anterior chamber that might be described as an 'inverse hypopyon'.

A completely new approach to treating the retinal detachment came from Neault and Martens (1966). Their idea was to make use of higher than normal gravity that would act as an improved driving force upon the retina. To this end the human centrifuge seemed to offer the best possibility to create the desired force environment. The case presented by Neault and Martens concerned a healthy 18-yr old high-school athlete with a greater than 280 deg traumatic superior disinsertion folded downwards, so that it covered both inferior quadrants except at the extreme periphery. The treatment consisted of a centrifuge ride at the end of the long centrifuge arm for a period of 2 hr, 15 min with a resultant force of 2.7 g. The treatment met with some success, and so inspired these investigators to try this method on the centrifuge shown in Figure 1.

2. Technique

It was recognized the construction of this centrifuge was not ideally suited for this kind of treatment, as there is no possibility of placing the subject easily in any desired position. This centrifuge has a free-swinging gondola, the subject being seated in the center facing forwards. Since the g-force acts along the Z-axis and always downwards, it would be applicable only in cases of inferior retinal detachments.

Interest was focused, however, on all types of retinal detachments, most especially on those where a headward or near-headward acceleration would be required *i.e.*, in cases of superior detachments. It was reasoned that in such instances, the centrifuge might constitute a g-force configuration that would theoretically be ideal. Conversely, without a centrifuge and just relying on normal gravity, nothing can be done in those cases as this would mean putting the patients on their heads. This was reason for considering the potential benefits that could be derived from a well chosen, centrifugal force environment. 'Well chosen' meant that the body and, more specifically, the

D. E. Busby (ed.), Recent Advances in Aerospace Medicine, 169–173. All Rights Reserved.
Copyright © 1970 by D. Reidel Publishing Company, Dordrecht-Holland.

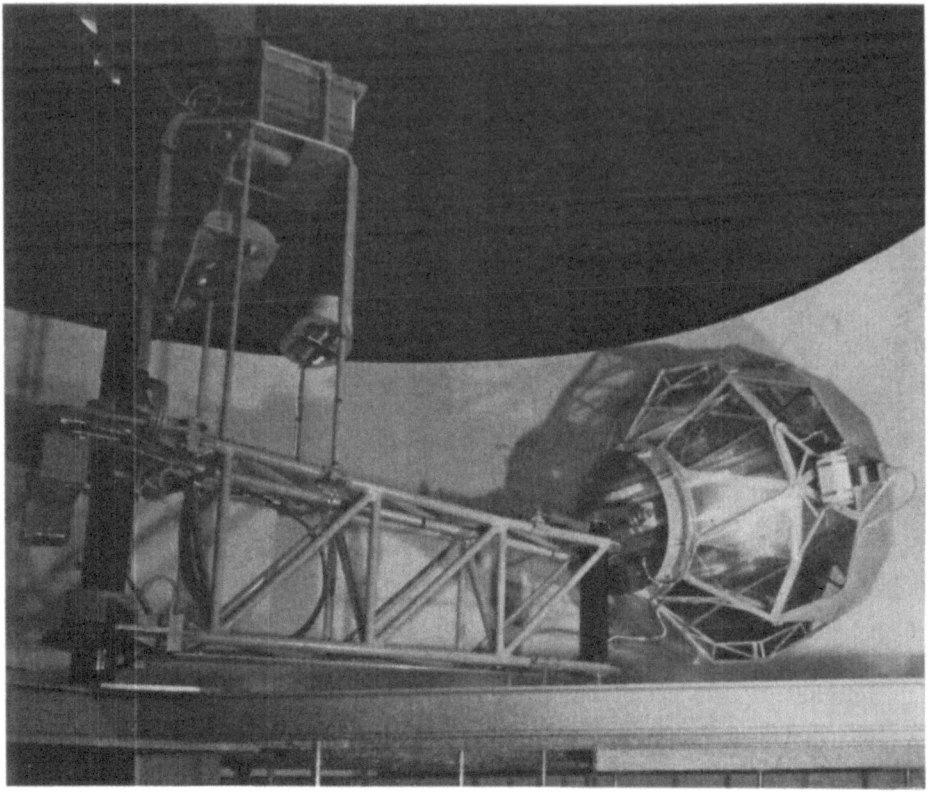

Fig. 1. The centrifuge of the National Aeromedical Center, while in operation.

circulatory system, should not be overstressed whereas, conversely, the retina should receive the peak load.

In order to achieve such a selective, differential loading, the patient should be positioned on the centrifuge so that the g-load on the circulation is minimized, and the g-load on the retina is optimized. This can be accomplished by placing the subject near to, or even over the axis. Both magnitude and direction of the resultant force at heart level will then differ substantially from those at head level. Under such conditions, the g-force which can be obtained at heart level is almost perpendicular to the long body axis, and at the eye level nearly parallel to it and of greater magnitude.

A fully centralized position with the subject placed over the axis is by no means necessary. With a little more eccentric position, the principle of selective loading is still available. The centrifuge in the Institute of Professor Meyer Schwickerath in Essen is an example of this. A disadvantage of the short or very short radius is the high angular velocity involved. The well-known $\omega^2 r$ formula governs this relation. A consequence of the high angular velocity lies in the vestibular stimuli it may generate. To prevent any unpleasant untoward effects from this standpoint the subject should be instructed to keep his head steady during rotation.

A second point of consideration is the pressure build-up in the cerebrospinal fluid and in the intracranial blood vessels. If one was not dealing with a complicated mechanical system like the human body but with a fluid filled disk, then the pressure at the outside would be $\frac{1}{2}\varrho\omega^2 r^2$; if, again one was dealing with a fluid filled ring, then the pressure at the outside would be $\frac{1}{2}\varrho\omega^2(r_E - r_I)^2$ where r_E is the external radius, and r_I is the internal radius.

Pressure relations within the human body are as indicated much more complicated (Weiss *et al.*, 1954a, b).

3. Case Reports

In July, 1966, the first clinical trial was performed with the centrifuge. The treatment

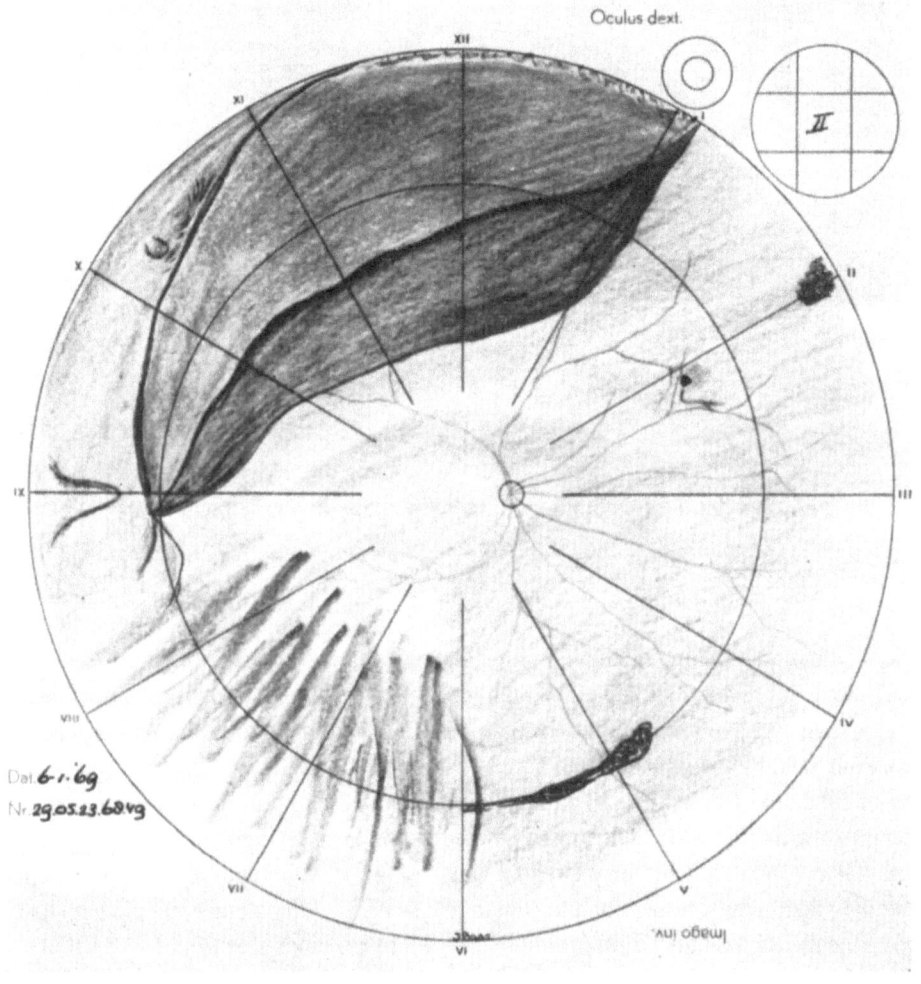

Fig. 2.   Right eye before centrifugation.

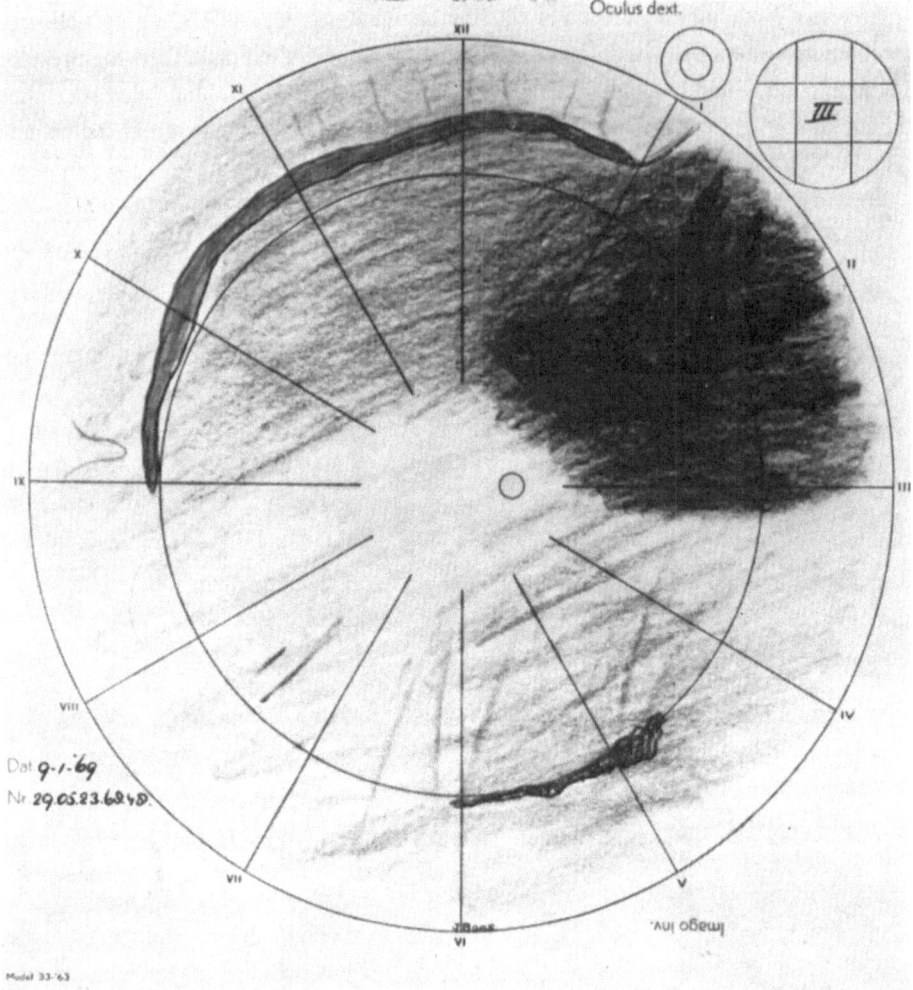

Fig. 3.   Right eye after centrifugation.

consisted of two runs in which a 2*g* value at eye level was maintained for 7 min. The result was not overwhelming, although some improvement occurred. Since then, 7 more patients have been submitted to centrifugation with *g*-profiles nearly similar to that exerted in the first case. Good results were obtained in only 2 patients. A resettling of the retina was achieved and the eye was ready for operation. However, then a new problem arose which is illustrated by the following case report.

A 40-yr old man who underwent a cataract extraction without complications 4 weeks previously, was admitted to the hospital with a retinal detachment in the right eye. A large tear was found extending from the 9 to 1 o'clock position. In addition, a minor hole was present at the 2 o'clock position. The retina was folded downwards in such a manner as to appear as a disinsertion. After centrifugation, the retina was moved to the choroid and it became clear that the tear was some distance away from the ora. The reapposition was so good that immediate surgery seemed indicated in order to prevent the retina from becoming elevated again. However, prompt action was regretted, for during surgery, the retina moved away and a second trial on the centrifuge to reappose the retina failed completely. It is felt now that some time should elapse between the moment of reapposition and surgical fixation.

The other case that responded very well to the centrifugal force was a young man who was blind in one eye. He then was struck by a water jet on the good eye and a very serious detachment ensued with the macula obscured by the folded-down retina. This was the second patient of this series. After successful centrifugation, surgery was performed with a good result.

4. Conclusions

In reviewing this series of 8 cases, the application of centrifugal force to a detached retina appears to have some virtue in special instances, but there is certainly no reason for exaggerated optimism. Perhaps these results would have been better if the $2g$-value had been exceeded. If a proper position is chosen, higher g-loads are very well tolerated. Other aspects which need further investigation are the selection of the cases that are suitable for this kind of treatment and the time lapse allowable after the detachment has occurred. A further point concerns the optimum interval between centrifugation and surgery.

The second case reported above was the only completely successful one. This might seem a discouraging result. However, when one realizes that that patient would have been blind if it were nor for the centrifuge, the conclusion should rather be that further efforts to find improvements in indication and technique are fully justified.

References

Cibis, P. A.: 1962, *Arch. Ophthal.* **68**, 590.
Neault, R. W. and Martens, T. G.: 1966, *Proc. Mayo Clin.* **41**, 145.
Weiss, H. S., Edelberg, R., Charland, P. V., and Rosenbaum, J. I.: 1954a, *J. Aviat. Med.* **25**, 5.
Weiss, H. S., Edelberg, R., Charland, P. V., and Rosenbaum, J. I.: 1954b, WADC-TR-53-139, Part 2, Wright Air Development Center, Wright-Patterson Air Force Base, Ohio, U.S.A.

SECTION III

MAN IN HIS GASEOUS ENVIRONMENT

DECOMPRESSION SICKNESS IN AVIATION

J. ERNSTING

R.A.F. Institute of Aviation Medicine, Farnborough, Hants., U.K.

1. Introduction

Although the clinical syndrome of decompression sickness was recognized in divers and compressed air workers as 'caisson disease' some 120 years ago, the first clear description of decompression sickness arising in men exposed to sub-atmospheric pressure was not made until 1930. Bert (1878), whose extensive studies of the effects of changes of environmental pressure upon animals, including man, form the basis of our knowledge of this subject, postulated that caisson disease was due to the evolution of bubbles of gas in body tissues and fluids. Surprisingly, however, he did not foresee the possibility of bubble formation on exposure to altitude. This possibility was considered in the early years of the present century by several investigators, including Boycott and Haldane (1908) and Henderson (1917), but no experimental evidence was forthcoming to support it.

It is fitting to recall at this Congress that it was a native of Holland, Dr. Jongbloed, who first recognized and described decompression sickness in men exposed to low environmental pressure. He presented his findings to the Fifth International Congress of Aerial Navigation at The Hague 39 years ago. He had exposed himself and his colleagues in a decompression chamber to a pressure of 124 mm Hg (equivalent to an altitude of 42 650 ft) where they had experienced repeatedly pain in limb joints. Jongbloed (1930) concluded that the pains experienced at high altitude were analogous to those found in men after rapid decompression from a high atmospheric pressure. During the following few years, there were a series of conflicting reports with regard to the occurrence of caisson disease at altitude but, by the end of the third decade, it was generally acknowledged (Armstrong and Borum, 1938; Boothby and Lovelace, 1938; Matthews, 1939) that symptoms of decompression sickness occurred in subjects exposed to high altitude. The great military importance of high altitude flight in unpressurized aircraft between 1939 and 1945 led to very extensive research programs. During and immediately after World War II, very large numbers of aircrew were exposed in flight for periods of up to several hours to altitudes above 25 000 ft. This resulted in a considerable number of cases of decompression sickness. With the subsequent widespread adoption of pressurization of the cabins of military aircraft, the numbers of aircrew routinely exposed to high altitudes fell markedly.

Certain groups of individuals are still exposed to altitudes at which decompression sickness can occur. Many Air Forces today employ jet trainer aircraft in which the cabin is not pressurized. The cabin altitudes of older aircraft with a low cabin pressure differential frequently exceed 25 000 ft. The possibility of exposure to very low pressures due to a failure of cabin pressurization is always present in aircraft flying at high altitude. Many military aircrew are routinely exposed to such altitudes during training in the use of their personal equipment in decompression chambers. With the advent of manned space flight, experimental subjects have been exposed to conditions in which decompression sickness may occur. A recent source of cases of altitude decompression sickness is the indulgence in underwater activities before flight which, if the depth and duration of the dive are sufficient, can reduce the altitude at which decompression sickness may occur to as low as 5000 to 8000 ft, the cabin altitude of many civil transport aircraft.

The purposes of this paper are to describe the clinical picture of decompression sickness arising as a result of exposure to altitude, to discuss briefly the physiological mechanisms underlying this syndrome and to summarize the current treatment of the condition. The experience and practice of the Royal Air Force, as detailed in the thesis on Sub-atmospheric Decompression Sickness in Man by Fryer (1967), has been used in the preparation of this paper.

2. Clinical Features

Since the clinical picture of altitude decompression sickness is so variable, this condition is usually defined in negative terms as denoting those symptoms and signs associated with reduction of environmental pressure, but not due to expansion of trapped or enclosed gas and not primarily due to hypoxia. Classically, the symptoms and signs which can occur in a subject suffering from decompression sickness at altitude include limb pains ('the bends'), respiratory disturbances ('the chokes'), skin manifestations, various disturbances of the central nervous system and cardio-vascular collapse. These disturbances are almost always corrected by recompression to ground level. Rarely, however, recovery may not occur immediately after descent, or the symptoms and signs may increase in severity after return to ground level post-decompression collapse).

(A. LIMB PAINS ('THE BENDS')

The most common severe symptom of altitude decompression sickness (Table I) is a

TABLE I

Relative incidence of symptoms of altitude decompression sickness
(modified from Fryer, 1967)

Symptoms	Incidence (%)	
	280000 ft for 2 hr	37000 ft for 2 hr
Bends	73.9	56.5
Chokes	4.5	6.5
Skin disturbances	7.0	1.6
Visual disturbances	2.0	4.8
C.N.S. disorder	1.0	0
Collapse	9.0	25.8
Miscellaneous	2.5	4.8

deep-seated pain ('bend') in or near a limb joint. This pain, which generally starts as a mild discomfort, almost always increases in severity with time. It is virtually always relieved by descent. If, however, the altitude is maintained, further disturbances, of which vasovagal syncope is the most common, supervene. The commonest site for the bends is the knee, followed in descending order of frequency by the shoulder, elbow, wrist or hand, and ankle or foot. The hip is affected only very rarely. Movement of the affected part usually increases the intensity of the pain, whilst local pressure by means of a pneumatic cuff or immersion of the limb in a fluid may well cause the pain to disappear.

B. RESPIRATORY DISTURBANCES ('THE CHOKES')

Respiratory disturbances, which are a serious manifestation of decompression sickness, occur much less frequently than do limb pains (Table I). The initial symptom is virtually always a feeling of constriction around the lower chest with a sense of tightness in the epigastrium. An attempt to take a deep breath causes an inspiratory 'catch', which limits inspiration. Soreness develops beneath the sternum. The subject frequently feels generally unwell and, as the condition develops, any attempt to take a deep breath causes coughing, which frequently becomes paroxysmal. If the altitude is maintained, the chokes almost variably progress to collapse.

C. SKIN MANIFESTATIONS

Itching, tingling and formication frequently occur at altitude. These symptoms are usually transient and of little significance. Much less common is mottling of the skin which, when it occurs over the chest, is generally associated with the chokes Gross vascular stasis may occur in the skin in association with post-decompression collapse.

D. NEUROLOGICAL AND VISUAL DISTURBANCES

Serious neurological disturbances, such as weakness or paralysis of limbs, occur very infrequently at altitude. Only one case of persistent paralysis has been reported (Höök, 1958). Numbness is also an unusual symptom. The most frequent neurological disturbances are blurring of vision, scotomata, fortification spectra and hemianopia. These often accompany other symptoms, such as headache, which often occurs in those with a past history of migraine.

E. COLLAPSE

A small but significant proportion of cases of decompression sickness present with a general feeling of malaise, anxiety and diminished consciousness (Table I). This syndrome may occur either without other manifestations of decompression sickness (primary collapse) or in association with the bends, the chokes or central nervous system disorder (secondary collapse). Typically, the individual becomes restless, pale and his hands and face are cold and clammy with sweat. At this stage he generally feels hot and cold alternatively. It is followed by impairment of consciousness. The radial pulse is virtually absent and there is usually a bradycardia. Finally, the subject loses consciousness and he may or may not jactitate. Descent is usually followed by a rapid recovery.

F. POST-DECOMPRESSION COLLAPSE

As has already been emphasized, the vast majority of individuals with decompression sickness recover either immediately or very shortly after descent to ground level. In a few instances, however, the symptoms may persist after return to ground level and, in a small number of cases, the symptoms and signs may become worse after descent. Those cases in which symptoms persist or become worse after return to ground level are described as having post-decompression collapse. The best available estimate of the incidence of post-decompression collapse is that given by Adler (1950), who calculated that 1 million man-flights to altitudes greater than 30000 ft (in decompression chambers) had resulted in 400 cases of collapse persisting or arising after return to ground level; 150 of these cases were serious. It is extremely rare for post-decompression collapse to follow an exposure to altitude in which no symptoms of decompression sickness occurred. (Adler, 1950; Fryer, 1967). Collapse after descent to ground level can be preceded by any of the manifestations of decompression sickness at altitude, although it is very unusual for collapse to follow an exposure in which the only symptom is the bends.

The clinical picture of post-decompression collapse is variable. There may be an interval between the descent to ground level and the appearance of symptoms of up to several hours duration. Typically, the patient becomes anxious, develops a frontal headache, and feels sick. He has facial pallor and cold, sweaty extremities. There is nearly always peripheral cyanosis. General or focal signs of neurological involvement, such as weakness of the limbs, apraxia, scotomata and convulsions, may occur. Mottling of the skin across the chest and shoulders is commonly very marked. The arterial blood pressure is generally well maintained until late in the development of the illness. Finally, in the worst cases, coma supervenes. Recovery can, however, occur at any stage, although in the past it has been very rare once coma has supervened. To date there have been 17 deaths due to decompression sickness reported in the world literature (Fryer, 1967). A very consistent, early finding in all cases of severe post-decompression collapse is an increase in the blood hematocrit. There is often also a polymorphonuclear leucocytosis, and the patient may have a high fever.

3. Incidence

There is considerable evidence for an altitude threshold for decompression sickness at 18000 ft. Above this threshold, the incidence of decompression sickness in a standard population depends primarily upon the altitude, the duration of the exposure and the degree of physical activity (Table II). Thus, for a 2-hour exposure, the incidence of symptoms of decompression sickness in seated subjects increases from 3.2% at 28000 feet to 75% at 35000 feet (Figure 1). The corresponding incidences of forced descents

TABLE II

Proportion of subjects requiring descent during various types of decompression tests (Fryer and Roxburgh, 1965)

Exposure	Failure rate (%)
35000 ft for 4 hr	45.0
37000 ft for 2 hr	21.0
40000 ft for 1 hr	20.0
37000 ft for 1 hr	13.0
35000 ft for 1 hr	8.0
25000 ft for 1 hr and 37000 ft for 1 hr	6.0
28000 ft for 2 hr on two occasions	1.65

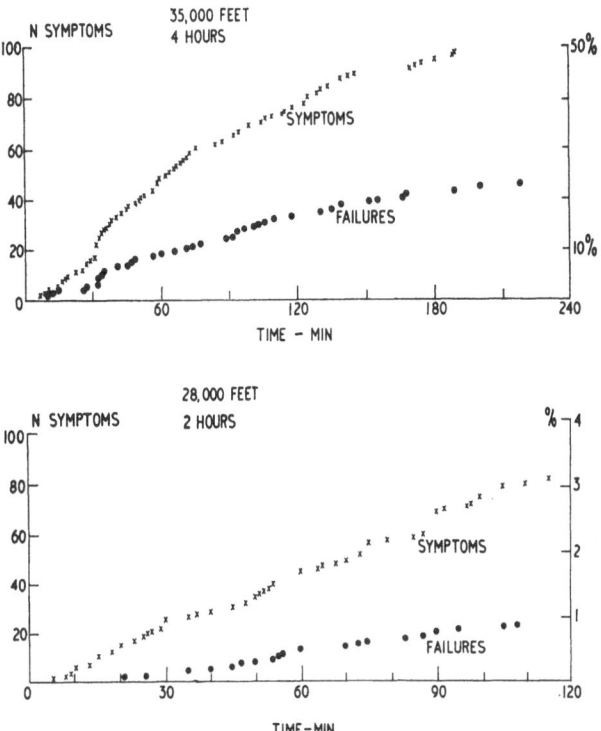

Fig. 1. Time course of development of symptoms and of incidence of forced descents in normal seated subjects exposed to simulated altitudes of 35 000 ft for 4 hr (upper figure) and 28 000 ft for 2 hr (lower figure) (Fryer, 1967).

are 1.6% and 20%. The rate of ascent within the practical aviation range of 100 ft/min to 200000 ft/min has an insignificant effect upon the subsequent development of decompression sickness. On ascent to a given altitude there is generally an interval of 5 to 10 min duration before any symptoms of decompression sickness arise. Thereafter, the occurrence of cases with time has a sigmoid distribution. The ultimate total incidence of cases varies with the conditions of the exposure. Exercise has a

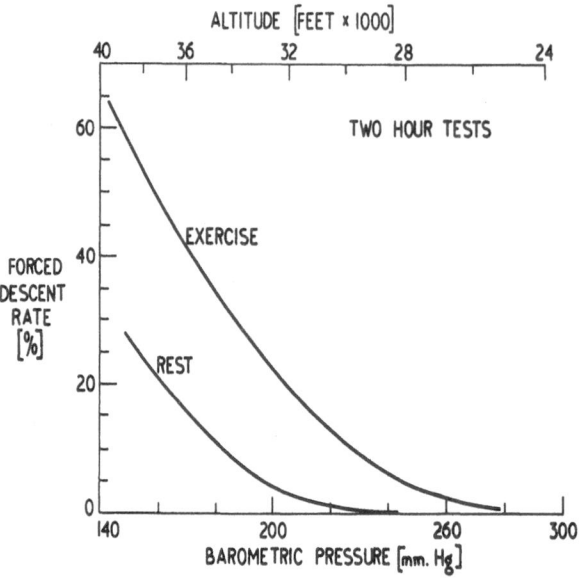

Fig. 2.   Effect of heavy exercise upon the relationship between the incidence of cases of decompression sickness requiring forced descent and altitude for exposures of 2 hr duration (Fryer, 1967).

marked effect (Figure 2). It raises the incidence of symptoms at a given altitude and lowers the altitude at which symptoms appear (Fulton, 1951). Hard exercise is roughly equivalent to an increase in the altitude of the exposure of 5000 feet.

A. FACTORS AFFECTING INDIVIDUAL SUSCEPTIBILITY

There has been some doubt in the past as to whether or not certain individuals were truly more susceptible than others to altitude decompression sickness, or whether or not the occurrence of decompression sickness in a population was a random process. Fryer (1967) has shown, by the analysis of the responses of over 2500 men to a standard test which consisted of exposure to 28 000 ft for 2 hr on two separate occasions, that there is a true individual susceptibility to this condition. In this series an individual who developed mild or moderate symptoms during the first exposure was 10 times more likely to develop symptoms during the second test than his colleagues who did not have symptoms on the first exposure.

The susceptibility to decompression sickness increased markedly with age, there being a nine-fold increase in the liability to experience symptoms during a 2 hour exposure to 28 000 ft between the ages of 17 to 20 years and 27 to 29 years. Obesity is known to increase the susceptibility to decompression sickness, but a reduction of the weight of an obese individual who has experienced serious symptoms of decompression sickness does not generally reduce his susceptibility to the condition.

A previous exposure to altitude increases the likelihood of an individual developing decompression sickness if the interval between the exposures is less than 12 hr. This increase in susceptibility occurs whether or not symptoms of decompression sickness are present during the initial exposure. The effect of a prior exposure to an environmental pressure greater than 1 atm has already been mentioned. For example, a sponge diver who had spent 30 min at a depth of 120 ft in the sea complained of pain in his chest and became grey, dyspneic and collapsed during a flight in an airliner the next day at a cabin altitude of 5000 ft. Recompression in a chamber resulted in a rapid and complete recovery (Preston, quoted by Fryer, 1967).

4. Etiology

There is little doubt that the basic mechanism responsible for the production of altitude decompression sickness is the supersaturation of the tissues with nitrogen, since this syndrome does not occur if nitrogen is removed from the body by breathing 100% oxygen before ascent to altitude. Nitrogen supersaturation occurs in a tissue on decompression to altitude because the rate of removal of the nitrogen dissolved in it to the lungs, and thence the environment, by the circulating blood is slower than the rate of fall of the absolute pressure in the tissue produced by the ascent to altitude. It is believed that the occurrence of decompression sickness is associated with the formation of bubbles of gas, the main constituent of which is nitrogen, in specific tissues of the body. Although there is considerable indirect evidence in support of this hypothesis, the unequivocal demonstration that bubbles are formed in the tissues under conditions in which altitude decompression sickness occurs in man is lacking.

Physical considerations suggest that the driving pressure for bubble formation in a fluid is the difference between the tension of the gas dissolved in the fluid and the hydrostatic pressure (Harvey, 1944). Thus, the greater the degree of supersaturation the greater is the tendency for bubble formation. The rise of local nitrogen tension, and hence the magnitude of the driving pressure which occurs with a given decompression will depend upon the gas solubility, the rate of diffusion of the gas in the tissue, and the local blood flow. The driving pressure would be expected to be larger in a tissue which contains a large proportion of lipid with its high solubility for nitrogen and a low blood flow. Bubbles will not form in a fluid, however, even when the driving pressure is large, unless suitable nuclei are present. These consist of microscopic masses of gases attached to irregularities on the walls of a cavity or small particles in suspension. The distribution of such gas nuclei may account in part for the sites at which the disturbances underlying decompression sickness occur. It is probable also that bubbles have to be of a certain size before the deformation pressure which they produce in the tissue is sufficient to cause symptoms or a disturbance of function (Nims, 1951). Thus, for example, bends are most likely due to the formation of extravascular bubbles in the ligaments and muscles surrounding a joint. A pain which closely resembles that of the bends can be produced by the local injection of small quantities of physiological saline into the muscles and ligaments around a joint.

The etiology of serious decompression sickness, in particular post-decompression collapse, is uncertain. There have been intensive studies of the clinical courses and pathology of the 17 fatal cases (Haymaker, 1957; Fryer, 1967). No common, underlying disease was present in these cases, although virtually all the individuals were over

30 years of age and overweight. The duration and altitude of the exposure which eventually led to death were often such that no symptoms of decompression sickness would have been expected (for example 22 min at 22000 ft; 28 min at 30000 ft). In every case, severe symptoms of decompression sickness occurred during the period at altitude. Clinical deterioration was virtually always associated with hemoconcentration, polymorpholeucocytosis and fever. There was intense peripheral vasoconstriction, and neurological signs were variable and often slight. Death generally occurred between 5 and 18 hr. Amongst the main pathological findings, effusions in serous cavities, congested and edematous lungs, fatty changes in the liver and accelerated renal tubular autolysis were found in virtually every case. Fat emboli were often present in small numbers in the lungs, and less commonly in the systemic vascular bed. A patent foramen ovale was found in 5 of the 9 cases in which the heart was examined critically (approximately 20% of normal individuals have a patent foramen ovale).

The basic mechanism responsible for death in this condition would appear to be loss of fluid from the circulating blood due to a widespread increase of capillary permeability, leading eventually to circulatory failure. This increased capillary permeability may be produced by a generalized dissemination of bubbles throughout the systemic circulatory tree (Fryer, 1967). It is suggested that the bubbles arise in fat, pass into the venous side of the circulation and produce a large scale pulmonary gaseous embolism, with transpulmonary passage of gas by way of capillaries and shunts. However, there is no detailed experimental evidence to support this hypothesis.

5. Treatment

The primary treatment of decompression sickness arising at altitude is recompression to ground level as rapidly as possible. When a case occurs in flight, it may not be possible to descend rapidly for operational reasons. In this circumstance, descent should be carried out to as low an altitude as possible and, if the chokes or collapse occur, the individual should, where possible, be placed flat and given 100% oxygen to breathe. As pointed out above, the vast majority of cases of decompression sickness recover completely on return to ground level. In order to ensure that post-decompression collapse is detected at the earliest possible moment, every case of decompression sickness, other than uncomplicated bends, should be observed for at least 4 hr after descent. Cases in which symptoms are not relieved by descent should be observed closely for symptoms and signs of impending collapse. The most valuable investigation is the serial measurement of the hematocrit. A high initial reading (greater than 54%), or a significant increase in the hematocrit over 30 min is indicative of serious decompression sickness.

Until about 10 years ago, the treatment of severe decompression sickness was based upon measures designed to combat the reduction of the blood volume and to maintain the oxygen supply to the tissues. However, the most obvious way of reducing the effect of bubbles in tissues and body fluids is to decrease their volume by overcompression. Although this method of treatment had been used for many years in the therapy of caisson disease, it was not until 9 years ago that Donnell and Norton (1960) reported the use of this technique in the treatment of a serious case of altitude decompression sickness. A 39-year old aviator developed weakness of his left arm and mild chokes. Within 5 hr of descent to ground level, he was moribund. One and a half hours later he was compressed to 6 ata, where there was a dramatic improvement in his condition; he eventually recovered. By 1964, Goodman (1964) was able to collect 14 cases of altitude decompression sickness which had been treated by compression to pressures between 2 and 6 ata. The value of over-pressure therapy in the treatment of this condition is now established beyond doubt (Workman, 1968).

Initially, severe cases of altitude decompression sickness were treated by compression to 6 ata followed by slow decompression to 1 ata over a period of 10 to 45 hr. In some cases (Cannon and Gould, 1964), compression was carried out only to the pressure at which symptoms were relieved. More recently Goodman (1964) showed that the combination of relatively mild compression and the administration of 100% oxygen could be used successfully for the treatment of severe altitude decompression sickness. The rationale of this procedure is that compression to 3 ata produces a considerable decrease in the size of bubbles whilst breathing 100% oxygen at this pressure produces a very large partial pressure gradient for nitrogen, driving this gas from the bubbles into the tissue fluids, and thence to the alveolar gas. The advantage of this technique is that it reduces to a minimum the risk of converting a case of altitude decompression sickness to one of compressed air decompression sickness, by reducing the time for which air is breathed at pressures greater than 1 ata. It also improves tissue oxygenation.

It is believed that the present treatment of choice for post decompression collapse is compression to 3 ata with intermittent oxygen breathing. The patient, breathing 100% oxygen, is compressed rapidly to 3 ata. If this procedure produces a marked improvement in his condition within 10 min, then the exposure to 3 ata is maintained for a further 30 to 60 min with short periods of air-breathing to reduce the possibility of oxygen toxicity. If the improvement is maintained, ascent to the surface is carried out slowly with the intermittent administration of oxygen. On the other hand, if there is not a marked improvement after 10 min oxygen-breathing at 3 ata, or if deterioration occurs at any time during the treatment, oxygen-breathing is discontinued and the patient is compressed immediately to 6 ata. The subsequent decompression depends upon the clinical state of the patient and is carried out according to standard diving therapeutic tables. It may be necessary to carry out supportive therapy during the overpressure treatment (for example, to administer fluids intravenously to restore the circulating blood volume). The need for this form of treatment is decided on clinical signs and the results of serial measurement of the hematocrit and blood electrolyte concentrations.

6. Prevention

The primary method of avoiding the occurrence of decompression sickness in the crew and passengers of aircraft is to limit the reduction of environmental pressure to

which they are exposed during flight. In military aircraft, in which the probability of
rapid decompression with its possible harmful effects had to be taken into account, it
was decided at the end of World War II that a maximum cabin altitude of 25 000 ft
represented an acceptable compromise between the need to reduce the frequency of
hypoxia incidents and decompression sickness on the one hand, and to avoid un-
acceptably high cabin differential pressures on the other. However subsequent experience showed that cabin altitudes of this order resulted in a significant number of cases
of decompression sickness, whilst the fears of rapid decompression and its harmful
effects had been over-emphasized. Although a maximum cabin altitude of 18 000 ft
would remove completely the possibility of decompression sickness occurring in
flight, other considerations, such as the weight of the pressure cabin, result in the
present compromise of a maximum cabin altitude of 22 000 ft (Ernsting, 1963).

The need to avoid an exposure to pressures greater than 1 ata and the consequent
increase in the amount of nitrogen in the tissues before flight even at cabin altitudes
as low at 5000 to 8000 ft have led to special instructions for aircrew, both military and
civil. These prohibit underwater swimming and diving for 24 hr before a flight.

During and immediately after World War II, the selection of relatively unsuscepti-
ble individuals by testing in a decompression chamber was used widely to prevent
decompression sickness in aviation. Such testing is uncommon today. However, in
certain circumstances, such as the use of unpressurized training aircraft at high altitudes, selection tests are still used to eliminate those aircrew who have a high susceptibility to decompression sickness. Experience has shown that the most successful
approach to the design of such tests is to simulate, in a decompression chamber,
exposure to the most severe cabin altitude/time profile to which the aircrew will be
exposed during flight. In order to reduce the occurrence of serious cases of decompression sickness in selection testing to an absolute minimum, it is essential that the
tests are carried out by experienced medical officers and that full facilities including
a 6 ata compression chamber are immediately available for the treatment of any case
of decompression sickness which may arise.

Finally, the removal of the nitrogen which is normally dissolved in the tissues and
fluids of the body by breathing 100% oxygen for an adequate period of time before
exposure to reduced pressure will prevent the occurrence of decompression sickness.
This method of prevention is widely used in the training of aircrew in the use of
personal oxygen equipment and pressure clothing. It is present policy for aircrew
who are undergoing such training in decompression chambers to breath 100% oxygen
for a period of 30 to 60 min (depending upon the nature of the subsequent exposure)
before they are exposed to altitudes in excess of 25 000 ft. Preoxygenation can also
be used to protect experimental subjects who are to be exposed to high altitudes in
decompression chambers and aircrew flying to high altitudes in unpressurized aircraft.

References

Adler, H. F.: 1950, U.S. Air Force Sch. Aviat. Med., Randolph AFB, Texas, U.S.A.

Armstrong, H. G. and Borum, F. S.: 1938, Eng. Sect. Memo Rept. Q-54-59, U.S. Army Air Corps, Wright Field, Ohio, U.S.A.

Bert, P.: 1878, *La Pression barométrique; Recherches et Physiologie Expérimentale*. Masson, Paris, p. 1168.

Boothby, W. M. and Lovelace, W. R. II: 1938, *J. Aviat Med.* **9**, 172.

Boycott, A. E. and Haldane, J. S.: 1908, *J. Physiol. (London)* **37**, 355.

Cannon, P. and Gould, T. R.: 1964, *Brit. Med. J.* **i**, 278.

Donnell, A. M. Jr. and Norton, C. P.: 1960, *Aerospace Med.* **31**, 1004.

Ernsting, J.: 1963, *Aerospace Med.* **34**, 991.

Fryer, D. I.: 1967, *Subatmospheric Decompression Sickness in Man*, Doctoral Thesis, University of London, London, U.K.

Fryer, D. I. and Roxburgh, H. L.: 1965, in *A Textbook of Aviation Physiology* (ed. by J. A. Gillies), Pergamon, Oxford.

Fulton, J. F.: 1951, in *Decompression Sickness* (ed. by J. F. Fulton), Saunders, Philadelphia, p. 437.

Goodman, M. W.: 1964, *Aerospace Med.* **35**, 1204.

Harvey, E. N.: 1944, *Harvey Lectures* **40**, 41.

Haymaker, W. E.: 1957, *Handb. Spez. Path. Anat. Histol.* **13(i)**, 1600.

Henderson, Y.: 1917, *Aviation* **2**, 145.

Höök, O.: 1958, *J. Aviat. Med.* **29**, 540.

Jongbloed, J.: 1930, *5me Congr. Int. Navig. Aérienne (The Hague)* **2**, 1418.

Mathews, B. H. C.: 1939, FPRC Rept. 60 and 70, Flying Pers. Res. Comm., Air Ministry, London, U.K.

Nims, L. F.: 1951, in *Decompression Sickness* (ed. by J. F. Fulton), Saunders, Philadephia, p. 192.

Workman, R. D.: 1968, *Aerospace Med.* **39**, 1076.

DECOMPRESSION SICKNESS AND THE CARDIOVASCULAR SYSTEM

N. G. MEIJNE

Dept. of Surgery, Wilhelmina Hospital, Amsterdam, The Netherlands

1. Introduction

With the reduction of barometric pressure, gases that are present in the body tend to expand in accordance with Boyle's law. Nitrogen physically dissolved in the blood and tissue fluid may become supersaturated with respect to the ambient nitrogen pressure. Current thinking and investigation implicate the evolution of bubbles of inert gas in the supersaturated extravascular and intravascular fluid compartments of the body as the primary cause of decompression sickness. This phenomenon occurs in tunnel and caisson workers, divers, flying personnel, and high and low pressure-chamber workers.

At first look, the incidence of decompression sickness in aviation seems to be rather low. However, the literature has reported a great number of cases of decompression sickness occurring in flight and in decompression chamber operations; several cases have been fatal. It is considered possible that several unexplained airplane crashes may have been caused by decompression sickness.

The cardiovascular system is the most vital body system in the production of decompression sickness, for it must remove a certain amount of inert gas from body tissues when the ambient pressure is lowered. Thus the incidence of decompression sickness can be expected to be higher in individuals who have poor cardiovascular system function and in instances where the total amount of inert gas to be removed from the body is high. Also, environmental factors such as rate of ascent, exposure time and temperature are known to influence this incidence.

Signs and symptoms of decompression sickness are caused by intravascular and extravascular bubble formation. Once bubbles form in tissues, a vicious cycle leading to further bubble growth may occur, for these bubbles can diminish perfusion, and so the rate of inert gas removal from the tissue. When intravascular bubbles begin to develop, they increase in diameter by coalescing. These bubbles, which form initially in veins, may pass from the venous to the arterial side of the circulation through arteriovenous shunts, to produce serious ischemia in several organs of the body. Finally, decrease of the arterial blood pressure favors bubble formation in arterial blood vessels.

This paper discusses various pathophysiological aspects of decompression sickness, centering interest in particular on the role of the cardiovascular system in the production of this phenomenon.

2. Pathogenesis of Decompression Sickness

Bubbles result when the body tissues are subjected to reduction in pressure at a rate

D. E. Busby (ed.), Recent Advances in Aerospace Medicine, 188–197. All Rights Reserved.
Copyright © 1970 by D. Reidel Publishing Company, Dordrecht-Holland.

faster than the body can eliminate inert gas, so the tissues become supersaturated with this gas. This theory is widely held and is supported by much experimental and pathological evidence. There seems to be no obvious reason to look for a different pathogenesis of decompression sickness in flying personnel as compared to those who work under increased atmospheric pressure.

Upon ascent, gas bubbles are formed in the fat depots, creating a generalized feeling of discomfort. As ascent is continued, the bubbles grow in size. A disruption of tissues may occur, with bubbles entering the blood stream along with globules of fat from the site of disruption. The lungs initially filter out many of these bubbles and fat emboli. Pulmonary hypertension may then result from blockage and irritative spasm of pulmonary blood vessels by these emboli. Then, changes in intracardiac pressure associated with the pulmonary hypertension may open an anatomically-patent foramen ovale, allowing entry of gas bubbles and fat emboli into the systemic arterial circulation.

Boothby and coworkers (Boothby and Lovelace, 1938; Boothby et al., 1940) demonstrated that partial denitrogenation of the body by preflight breathing of 100% oxygen gave significant protection against aeroembolism, and Evelyn (1941) presented evidence of the value of oxygen ventilation carried out for a sufficient length of time. Ferris et al. (1943) demonstrated that under the most stringent bends-producing conditions, preflight oxygen inhalation could prevent decompression sickness in highly susceptible individuals and that at the altitudes selected for the study (35000 ft or less), oxygen lack could be ruled out as a factor in producing the symptoms of decompression sickness. The value of oxygen inhalation in the prevention of bends after exposure to increased atmospheric pressure had already been stressed by von Schroetter (1906) many years before.

Frommer (1959) stated "Today we may say that the symptoms of decompression sickness result from the evolution of gaseous nitrogen, and possibly of other body gases, during environmental pressure changes. The symptoms are the effects of the influence of the gases in some incompletely understood manner, in adjacent or distant vascular and somatic tissue. It is speculative to say more than this."

That controversy exists in this area is shown by the fact that Mason (1962), in his study on aviation accident pathology, is of the opinion that it is unlikely that frank air embolism is an essential part of the decompression sickness syndrome. He believes that the main factor in the etiology of post-decompression shock is a generalized disruption of body cells which occurs in susceptible individuals due to expansion of gases within cells. Further, he states that disruption of fat cells is part of a generalized process and that the significance of fat emboli discovered at post mortem is merely that of being a convenient marker of such a process. It seems that this thesis is rather hypothetical. Good evidence that there is an essential difference between post-decompression shock resulting from exposure to reduced atmospheric pressure in aviators and to increased atmospheric pressure in divers is not available. Disruption of body cells can be caused by bubble formation; vasospasm, reflex action and sludge phenomena can all be secondary phenomena. Clinical and experimental evidence is much more in support of the thesis that the pathogenesis of decompression sickness is the same in both aviators and divers – that is, the consequences of bubble formation in the body.

3. Role of the Cardiovascular System in Decompression Sickness

The cardiovascular system is involved in many ways in decompression sickness. Since pathophysiological processes can start in many different organs of the body, several areas that are of importance in varying combinations in cases of decompression sickness will be identified and stressed here.

A. IMPAIRMENT OF TISSUE PERFUSION BY BUBBLES

There are several local effects of bubble formation. There is tissue damage by bubble expansion, capillary obstruction by intra- and extravascular bubbles, modification of local blood flow and increase of diffusion distances for tissue nutrients. These events lead to local effects characterized by hypoxia, acidosis, insufficient cellular nutrition and further limitation of inert gas removal by way of the circulating blood.

Lambertsen (1968) has emphasized that the pain of bends itself, associated with the processes mentioned above, may lead to the complex events of "reaction of pain", with the consequences of excessive sympathetic drive and if the bends are severe, to a generalized circulatory collapse from this reaction only; this additional sympathetic drive will aggravate the already limited inert gas exchange.

B. OBSTRUCTION OF THE PULMONARY CIRCULATION BY EMBOLI

One of the most serious manifestations of decompression sickness is termed 'the chokes'. It consists of substernal pain, a feeling of tightness in the chest and often rapid, shallow respiration. It is very likely that these symptoms are caused by intravascular gas bubbles mainly in the pulmonary arterioles and capillaries. Extensive gas embolization in the pulmonary circulation frequently progresses to neurocirculatory collapse.

It has been found experimentally that an important sign in decompression sickness is a rise in pulmonary artery pressure; this pressure may rise from normal to 55 mm Hg. In spite of a large increase in pulmonary artery pressure, the central venous pressure and left atrial pressure may remain unchanged for a long period of time. Soon after a significant rise in pulmonary artery pressure, the systemic arterial pressure will fail, presumably due to a low left cardiac output. Before the pulmonary artery pressure increases, bubbles may be seen in venous viewing cuvettes, migrating from the peripheral vascular bed.

Probably pulmonary hypertension and tachypnea are produced by mechanical blockage of the pulmonary vascular tree by gas bubbles. At the same time a large amount of pulmonary arteriolar spasm will be present. This adds significantly to the work load put on the heart. It has been shown that during recompression therapy the elevated pulmonary artery pressure drops rapidly.

Together with the pulmonary artery pressure rise and fall there is a rise and fall in the respiratory rate. Marked changes in the respiratory frequency can be utilized as a sign of decompression sickness. However, in experiments this sign wasnot as reliable as the presence of intravascular bubbles and pulmonary hypertension (Leverett *et al.*, 1963). Notably, pulmonary hypertension and tachypnea are signs of pulmonary emboli in general and are not specific for decompression sickness.

There is a marked difference in the severity of decompression sickness in man. The mere occurrence of bends pain indicates the presence of bubbles in the tissues and probably in the blood vessels. In most cases the intravascular bubbles are apparently eliminated by external respiration. When the bubble build-up is high in the pulmonary bed, pulmonary hypertension and tachypnea can result to a varying degree.

C. THE ROLE OF HYPOXIA

At high altitude, hypoxia will occur because of low oxygen tension; it may also be the result of pulmonary artery blockage. When hypoxia is severe, it results in lowering of cardiac output; when this occurs in cases of decompression sickness the symptoms will be more severe, compared to similar conditions with unaffected cardiac output. Many people with a poor myocardium will travel by air in the future. Even a slight reduction in oxygen supply in these individuals may lead to the onset of cardiac failure, which means a reduction in the potential for nitrogen transport and hence a greater risk of decompression sickness.

D. A DROP IN ARTERIAL PRESSURE MAY RESULT IN THE DEVELOPMENT OF BUBBLES ON THE ARTERIAL SIDE

In experiments on decompression sickness, arterial viewing cuvettes have been used in order to demonstrate bubbles in the arterial system. Usually bubbles in these cuvettes were seen in large quantities at the point that animals began showing evidence of circulatory failure with death intervening; this can be explained on the basis that the intra-arterial pressure is sufficiently high to keep bubbles invisible to some extent if they are present. So the arterial system, with its high pressure, acts as a protection against arterial bubble emboli.

E. ARTERIAL EMBOLI MAY OCCUR VIA ARTERIOVENOUS SHUNTS IN THE LUNGS AND VIA A PATENT FORAMEN OVALE

The existence of arteriovenous shunts in the normal lung has been the source of considerable confusion and controversy. Shunts have been looked for either by injecting particles of known size into the pulmonary arteries and by serial histologic studies (Strandness, 1969; Prinzmetal *et al.*, 1948) found that spherules up to $300\,\mu$ in diameter could be recovered from the pulmonary venous outflow. Niden and Aviado (1956) recovered glass beads varying in size from 60 to $420\,\mu$ in the dog; the number of beads recovered was increased by elevating the pulmonary artery pressure. Tobin and Zariquiey (1950) demostrated shunts up to $500\,\mu$ in diameter in the lungs of infants and adults.

Wagenvoort *et al.* (1964) disputed these reported findings because they were inconsistent with the findings of histologists. When the arteriovenous anastomoses have been found they were sparse and often of small caliber. Thus, such anastomoses may not be significant under normal conditions, yet quite a few will open up in case of embolization. Moreover, there is good reason to believe that small nitrogen emboli will pass through these arteriovenous shunts, especially when the pulmonary artery pressure rises. Furthermore, emboli may pass from the venous system to the arterial system via a patent foramen ovale.

4. At What Altitude Is Decompression Sickness Likely to Occur?

Before World War II, airplanes were not capable of attaining high altitudes, so aeroembolism in flight was not a problem. Physiologic studies therefore dealt mainly with the coincidental hypoxemia. The studies of Armstrong and Heim (1937), who systematically exposed humans to critical simulated altitudes brought general recognition of the fact that exposure to high altitudes caused symptoms of a nature similar to those of caisson disease. Armstrong (1939) pointed out that the basic physical mechanisms were the same, whether a subject ascended from 4 to 1 ata, or from 1 to 0.25 ata. However, these studies were fragmentary and incomplete and, at the time of the last world war, the true clinical nature and the significance as a problem in high altitude flying had not been evaluated. The maximum altitude below which aeroembolism will not occur in men is unknown. On the basis of equivalent gas volumes, Boycott et al. (1908) believed that a drop of approximately one-half of the original gas pressure would be safe whatever its value. Therefore, in aviation, a critical altitude of 18 000 ft above sea level (0.5 ata) would be set. Others have suggested that the critical altitude at which aeroembolism can occur in men will be 20 000 to 25 000 ft (0.45 to 0.37 ata). It will be impossible to give an exact level at which aeroembolism will occur, for many factors are involved in its development, such as rate of ascent, amount of nitrogen to be removed and condition of the cardiovascular system. Many reports are available in literature of cases of dysbarism occurring above 30 000 ft. Below 30 000 ft, the cases are fewer.

The lowest level at which a certain case of decompression sickness with post decompression shock occurred was at 18 500 ft, reported by Fryer (1963). In general, it can be expected that unless circulatory anomalies or serious overweight are present, Smedal's (1948) expectations will not be far from reality. He decided from the evidence of literature that very mild cases might occur in air crew exercising at 20 000 ft, that mild cases might occur at 23 000 ft under similar conditions and that no serious cases were to be expected below the latter altitude. However, one has to be aware of the exceptions that occur even in people expected to be healthy.

5. More Problems Can Be Expected in the Future

Probably more cases of decompression sickness will occur in the future because higher levels are necessary in air traffic for economical purposes. Dangers of decompression sickness and hypoxia are very closely correlated. The advent of jet aircraft has created a large population exposed to a significant decrease in atmospheric pressure in both training and operational situations. The number of persons exposed or potentially exposed to altitudes in excess of 30000 ft will be further increased with increase in air traffic and with the advent of supersonic aircraft. Inevitably this increased exposure will lead to more cases of dysbarism.

Flying has become so safe and convenient that many disabled people prefer to travel by this means. Of special importance is the fact that the number of patients with diseases of the cardiovascular system carried by air will be increasing. At the same time obesity is becoming a serious problem in our society; fatty tissue stores a large amount of nitrogen and fatty tissue is badly vascularized.

The degree of hypoxia at present day ordinary cruising altitudes, due to the reduction in cabin atmospheric pressure is mild. This degree of hypoxia is insufficient to affect healthy adults, but may be an embarrassment to passengers with impairment of the cardiovascular or respiratory systems. Beighton and Richards (1958) stated that as many as 5% of passengers on routine scheduled services are suffering from some form of disability, though less than 1% are self-declared invalids; 20% of the latter group are suffering from diseases of the cardiovascular and respiratory system.

During 1963, 1964, and 1965, 25 patients had been admitted to a hospital near London Airport; all had collapsed with conditions affecting their cardiovascular system, either during or immediately after a normal routine flight. The number of these cases will increase; we have to realize that a diseased cardiovascular system and some degree of hypoxia may mean that it is impossible for one to increase his cardiac output, so leading to cardiac failure. This also means that denitrogenation is diminished, with an increased risk of decompression sickness even at much lower levels than one would expect in otherwise healthy individuals.

6. Therapy

The aims of bends therapy include:
    diminution of bubble size
    acceleration of bubble resolution
    maintenance of tissue oxygenation.
The following therapeutic measures are of importance:
    compression to levels higher than 1 ata
    intravenous fluid therapy
    administration of a gas mixture containing 95% oxygen and 5% CO_2
    support of the circulatory system by cardiaca and isuprenaline
    sedatives and spasmolytics
    artificial ventilation.

Diffusion, the spontaneous movement of a gas from a region of high partial pressure to regions of lower partial pressure, is the fundamental process by which gas leaves the gas bubbles in decompression sickness and air embolism. Probably the most significant information about the decompression bubble is its diameter. The diameter will determine whether or not the bubble blocks a blood vessel, and it should determine the amount of tissue distortion or damage due to an extravascular bubble. In an experimental study of the factors in the resolution of tissue gas bubbles, Liew (1967) showed that bubbles became smaller and disappeared sooner at increased pressure; there was a great difference between bubble resolution during oxygen breathing at ambient pressure and at 3 ata. Electroencephalographical and electrocardiographical changes, produced by arterial air embolism in rabbits improved rapidly during compression therapy (Meijne *et al.*, 1963). So rapid recompression cannot be overemphasized, for regardless of the etiology of delayed decompression sickness, the sooner bubble formation and bubble size are reduced, the better should be the chance of complete recovery. The condition when cardiac failure and a concomitant drop in arterial pressure occurs is very serious.

The availability of recompression facilities for aviator's decompression sickness will be a major problem. It is remarkable that in diving it was known for many years that recompression to a higher level was necessary in the treatment of decompression sickness. In aviation medicine the first clinical case was not recompressed to higher atmospheric pressure levels until 1960, in spite of the fact that Behnke advised to do so in 1955. Donnell and Norton (1960) reported for the first time a case where recompression has been used as treatment for decompression sickness resulting from exposure to pressures less than 1 ata (43000 ft in altitude chamber). The patient was compressed to 165 ft; the serious condition with cardiovascular collapse and paralysis improved rapidly.

Bratt (1962) reported the treatment of a patient who had experienced neurocirculatory collapse during flight. Compression treatment to 6 ata resulted in dramatic improvement of the patient's condition. Cannon and Gould (1964) reported 4 cases with immediate relief of symptoms after compression to levels higher than 1 ata (3 ata maximum).

So compression therapy, eventually to 6 ata, is recommended as the treatment of choice for the neurocirculatory collapse of aviators decompression sickness. Six ata is in accordance with the United States Navy tables for the treatment of decompression sickness and air embolism; probably compression to 3 ata will be sufficient in most cases. Every attempt should be made to move the patient to a treatment chamber as quickly as possible. At present time 3 ata tables are used by United States Air Force in aviators.

Intravenous fluid administration may be necessary to compensate for fluid losses into tissues. Systemic hypoxia, within the range compatible with life of the organism, has no certain effect on capillary permeability. Severe and, so far as possible, total oxygen lack make the capillary wall permeable to protein and fluid as indicated by decreased effect of osmotic pressure of the plasma protein and by an increased filtration coefficient, respectively. Only in agonal or ante-mortem stages of asphyxia of anoxemia is there some slight evidence of increased capillary permeability. In shock, the possibility that generalized hypoxemia might increase capillary permeability has been considered on many occasions. So the effects on capillary permeability of arrested blood flow, and more specifically of hypoxia, are still uncertain and require more careful studies as to quantitative aspects and as to mechanism. When gas bubbles are reduced in size, however, perfusion may be restored in areas where it had been arrested before, and increased capillary permeability in several areas may be the result.

The administration of oxygen is necessary in order to provide as much oxygen to the tissues as possible and in order to make the nitrogen tension gradient between gas bubbles and surrounding tissues as great as possible. Administration of CO_2 is important in order to increase the blood flow to tissues.

When the blood pressure is low it is necessary to get information about the central venous pressure. When central venous pressure is low, fluid administration is of primary importance; when this pressure is high, cardiac failure will be the main disorder and support of the circulatory system by cardiaca and isuprenaline is indicated. Because of its dilatory effect on a large part of the circulatory system, the effect of isuprenaline (aleudrine) will be better than levophed or aramine; the last drugs have severe spastic effects on vessels and will be only second choice.

Sedatives may be necessary to control agitation; thereby oxygen consumption will be reduced as well as sympathetic drive caused by pain. Spasmolytics are indicated because in the presence of emboli, there always is a great degree of vascular spasm.

Artificial ventilation is indicated when respiration is insufficient.

7. Prevention

Generally, it can be stated that the risk of decompression sickness decreases when the amount of gases to be removed from the body is less and the condition of the cardiovascular system is optimum. Denitrogenation by oxygen inhalation decreases the risk of decompression sickness considerably. Overeating and lack of physical exercise have become an increasing problem in our society. Obesity, by increasing the weight of the body, increases the energy expenditure during physical activity which in most cases involves moving the body. The increased energy requirements increase the load on the circulatory system, and it is well known that obese individuals often show limited ability to perform physical work. Most patients with severe altitude sickness have been overweight. The significance of fat depots in the etiology of decompression sickness was suggested early in this century (Twort and Hill, 1910). All 4 cases reported by Cannon and Gould (1964) were overweight. Fryer's case (1963) was approximately 67 pounds overweight according to the Royal Air Force air crew standards. Philp and Gowdey (1964) found that in rats the incidence and severity of bends following prolonged exposures to compressed air was related to the amount of body fat regardless of the age of the animal. Very lean rats were more resistant to bends than normal rats. Repeated exposures to compressed air every 48 hr appeared to increase the risk of incurring and the severity of the bends. So weight reduction appears to be a most practical method of prevention.

It can be expected that a good cardio-pulmonary reserve will decrease the risk of decompression sickness. 'Physical fitness', defined as adequate cardiopulmonary reserve in flying personnel and much more in the average air traveller is frequently very poor. A training program in order to develop better physical conditioning (Cooper, 1968) can be advocated as a preventive measure. At this point it is of importance to stress the fact well known in working under increased pressure that young men from 18 to 26 years of age stand the work best. Furthermore, divers who have done deep dives when young, may become paralyzed at less depths in advanced years, probably because of an impairment of the circulation. There is good evidence that denitrogenation, weight reduction and physical fitness are the most important factors in the prevention of decompression sickness.

8. Summary

Several aspects of the problem of decompression sickness are discussed from the cardiovascular point of view. The cardiovascular system is of great importance in this disease because it is the system by which the nitrogen has to leave the body. The risk of decompression sickness will be higher when a large amount of nitrogen has to be removed (overweight!) and when the cardiovascular system is functioning at less than an optimum level. It can be expected that decompression sickness in aviation will occur more frequently in the future because of higher flying altitudes, more obesity, and cardiovascular systems functioning far from optimal.

References

Armstrong, H. G.: 1937, *J.A.M.A.* **109**, 417.
Armstrong, H. G.: 1939, *Principles and Practice of Aviation Medicine*, Williams and Wilkins, Baltimore, 1st ed. p. 496.
Behnke, A. R.: 1955, *Military Med.* **117**, 257.
Beighton, P. H. and Richards, P. R.: 1968, *Brit. Heart J.* **30**, 367.
Boothby, W. M. and Lovelace, W. R.: 1938, *J. Aviat. Med.* **9**, 172.
Boothby, W. M., Lovelace, W. R., and Benson, O. O.: 1940, *J. Aero. Soc. Amer.* **7**, 1.
Boycott, A. E., Damant, G. C. C., and Haldane, J. S.: 1908, *J. Hyg.* **8**, 342.
Bratt, H. R.: 1962, *Aerospace Med.* **33**, 358.
Cannon, P. and Gould, T. R.: 1964, *Brit. Med. J.* **1**, 282.
Cooper, K. H.: 1968, *J. Occupat. Med.* **10**, 636.
Donnell, A. M. and Norton, C. P.: 1960, *Aerospace Med.* **31**, 1004.
Evelyn, K.: 1941, Report Associate Committee Aviation Medical Research, National Research Council Canada, Ottawa, Canada.
Ferris, E. B., Webb, J. P., Ryder, H. W., *et al.*: 1943, Committee on Aviation Medicine, U.S. National Research Council, Washington, D.C.
Folkow, B., Heymans, C., and Neil, E.: 1965 in *Handbook of Physiology*, Vol. II: Respiration (ed. by W. F. Hamilton), American Physiological Society, Washington, D.C., p. 1787.
Frommer, J. R.: 1959, *U.S. Armed Forces Med. J.* **10**, 1292.
Fryer, D.I.: 1963, Memo 199, Flight Personnel Research Council, Royal Air Force, London, England.
Guyton, A. C.: 1963, in *Circulatory Physiology*, Saunders, Philadelphia, p. 301.
Hepburn, A. N.: 1968, *Aerospace Med.* **39**, 455.
Lambertsen, C. J.: 1968, *Aerospace Med.* **39**, 1086.

Leverett, S. D., Bitter, H. L., and McIver, R. G.: 1963, AF-SAM-TDR-63-1, U.S. Air Force Sch. Aerospace Med., Brooks AFB, Texas, U.S.A.

Liew, H. D. van: 1967, in *Proceedings Third Underwater Physiology Symposium* (ed. by C. J. Lambertsen), Williams and Wilkins, Baltimore, p. 191.

Mason, J. K.: 1962, in *Aviation Accident Pathology; A Study of Fatalities*, Butterworths, London, p. 168.

Meijne, N. G., Schoemaker, G., and Bulterijs, A. B.: 1963, *J. Cardiovasc. Surg.* **4**, 757.

Niden, A. H. and Aviado, D. M.: 1956, *Circ. Res.* **4**, 67.

Philp, R. B. and Gowdey, C. W.: 1964, *Aerospace Med.* **35**, 351.

Prinzmetal, M., Ormitz, E. M., Simkin, B., and Bergman, A. L.: 1948, *Amer. J. Physiol.* **152**, 48.

Schroetter, H. von: 1906, *Der Sauerstoff in der Phophylaxe und Therapie der Luftdruckerkrankungen*, Berlin.

Smedal, H. A.: 1948, reported by Fryer (1948).

Strandness, D. E., Jr.: 1969, in *Collateral Circulation in Clinical Surgery*, Saunders, London, p. 171.

Tobin, C. E. and Zariquiey, M. O.: 1950, *Proc. Soc. Exp. Biol. Med.* **75**, 827.

Twort, J. F. and Hill, L.: 1910, *J. Physiol.* **5**, 41.

Wagenvoort, C. A., Heath, D., and Edwards, J. E.: 1964, *The Pathology of the Pulmonary Vasculature*, C. C. Thomas, Springfield, p. 1.

FACTORS INFLUENCING THE TIME OF SAFE
UNCONSCIOUSNESS (TSU) FOR COMMERCIAL JET
PASSENGERS FOLLOWING CABIN DECOMPRESSION

J. G. GAUME

Douglas Aircraft Company, McDonnell Douglas Corporation, Long Beach, Calif., U.S.A.

1. Introduction

As a practical consideration, high altitude aircraft may not require passenger emergency oxygen. A decision in this matter cannot be based only on statistical analysis of the results of past aircraft sudden decompressions. To effect a valid decision, detailed physiological analyses, with emphasis on the passenger, are required. Many variables must be considered while performing the necessary analyses. Basically, the variables can be divided into two categories – physical, and physiological. In addition to facilitating a decision on the basic problem, these studies should point to a quick reference guide for passenger safety to be used by the flight crew in the event of sudden decompressions.

2. Discussion

A study to establish a 'time of safe unconsciousness' for passengers requires detailed consideration of physical and physiological variables. The physical variables, not necessarily in the order of importance are: rate of decompression, maximum cabin altitude, rate of aircraft descent, rate of cabin descent, elapsed times above certain altitudes (*i.e.*, 33 000 ft, 25 000 ft, 15 000 ft), final cruise altitude prior to landing, and elapsed time between critical altitudes and the return to a 'recovery' altitude. The last variable noted will vary as a function of the first six. The physiological variables are the changing partial pressure of oxygen in the atmosphere, alveoli, blood, and cells, the time spent in a critically hypoxic atmosphere, the partial pressure of oxygen at the final cruise altitude following descent, and the time to recovery of consciousness following unconsciousness due to hypoxia.

The criterion used in the past in trying to make the decision to delete passenger emergency oxygen has been the standard curves used to depict the 'time of useful consciousness (TUC)', as shown in Figure 1, for air crews who must perform a task in the aircraft, whether it is military or civilian. The passenger in a commercial jet is not performing an operational task. Therefore, the TUC curve need not and should not apply for passengers. Rather, 'the time to unconsciousness', although also inadequate, would be a more suitable guide for use by carriers and manufacturers in determining the seriousness of the hazard to the passenger (Figure 2, curve C). The standard TUC curve should apply only to the flight crew. It is well known that hypoxia due to decompression to high altitudes brings on unconsciousness more rapidly than merely

D. E. Busby (ed.), Recent Advances in Aerospace Medicine, 198–203. All Rights Reserved.
Copyright © 1970 by D. Reidel Publishing Company Dordrecht-Holland.

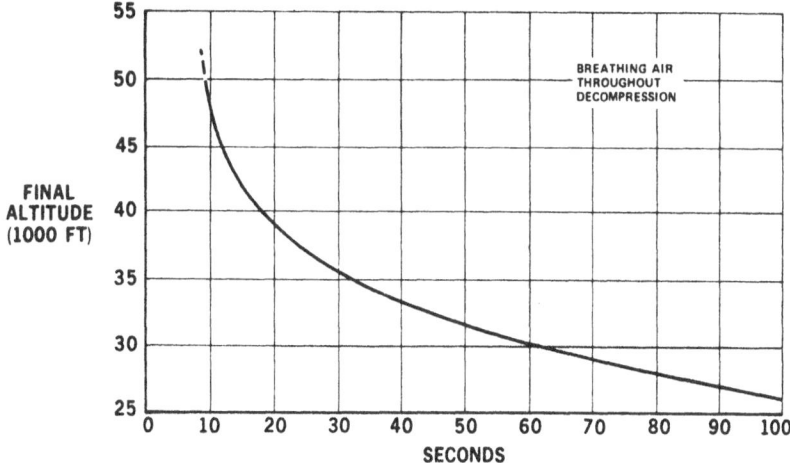

Fig. 1.   Time of useful consciousness (TUC) ([2]).

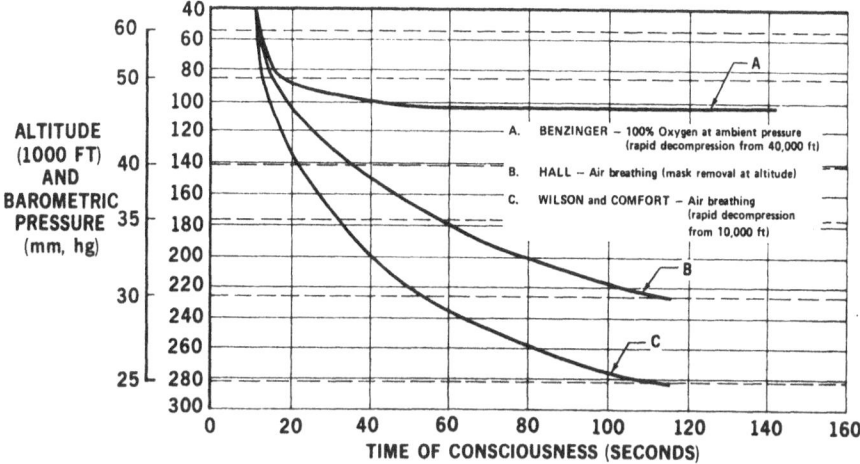

Fig. 2.   Time of consciousness with varying types of exposure at high altitude ([3]).

removing one's oxygen mask at the same equilibrium altitude. It is important, therefore, to consider not only how long it takes a passenger to become unconscious, but
also how long he is unconscious. For this reason, a new criterion is needed, and it is
suggested that this can be called the 'time of safe unconsciousness (TSU)' following
decompression.

It is also well known that short periods of unconsciousness due to hypoxia can be
well tolerated, but that longer periods are intolerable. Exact information as to how
long this type of unconsciousness can be safely tolerated is not available because of the
wide variability in individual tolerances and other factors, such as temperature.

A more accurate rule-of-thumb for safe exposure to decompression might be the
time the cabin altitude is above a given level. Most subjects who have been exposed
in altitude chambers can tolerate several minutes of hypoxia at altitudes up to 25 000

ft without becoming unconscious. Below 25000 ft is considered relatively safe without becoming unconscious. Also, below this altitude is considered relatively safe with regard to the syndromes of dysbarism, such as 'bends', 'chokes' and neurocirculatory collapse. Although these conditions have been known to occur below 25000 ft, they are not common below this level. Therefore, a better set of criteria for passenger safety would consider the following factors:

(1) Rate of decompression.
(2) Maximum cabin altitude, or equilibrium altitude.
(3) Time cabin is at maximum altitude.
(4) Time cabin altitude is above 25000 ft.
(5) Rate of descent.
(6) Final altitude.

These factors can be plotted on a graph indicating altitude and time. Simply stated, the degree of hazard is directly proportional to the time the passenger is unconscious, which is a function of the factors listed above. The safe altitude after a given decompression event is a function of the severity of the deprivation or loss of oxygen from the body, or the hypoxidosis. This is also determined by the six factors above. Whenever the partial pressure of oxygen in the atmosphere is reduced to a level below that in the lungs and blood, the oxygen flow in the lungs will be reversed; that is, oxygen will diffuse from the pulmonary capillaries to the alveoli and will be lost to the atmosphere during expiration. When the atmospheric partial pressure of oxygen is lower than that in the blood, oxygen will not be absorbed on inspiration. This reverse diffusion will continue until equilibrium is established between the atmosphere and the blood. The rate of reverse diffusion is dependent on the atmospheric partial pressure of oxygen, which in turn, is dependent on the maximum altitude change above 33000 ft. Time to unconsciousness and time of unconsciousness will depend on the magnitude of the oxygen loss from the blood. The rapidity and degree of recovery of adequate blood oxygenation will depend on the partial pressure of oxygen in the atmosphere of the aircraft as it descends and after it levels off following descent.

If the maximum cabin altitude during decompression is 35000 ft or more, it is questionable whether passengers would survive the hypoxia without brain damage if the aircraft levels off at 15000 feet after descent. At 15000 ft the ambient partial pressure of oxygen is less than 90 mm Hg. After the severe loss of oxygen from the blood that would occur in the first 2 min after the cabin altitude exceeded 35000 ft, it is questionable if this partial pressure of oxygen would suffice for complete and unharmed recovery. For these reasons, in a decompression occurring from an 8000 ft cabin altitude, it is desirable and mandatory that the cabin altitude be maintained below 25000 ft, or permitted to exceed that level for only a minute or two before descending below this altitude.

The higher the maximum altitude above 25000 ft, the more critical is the need to descend more rapidly. If above 25000 ft too long it will be necessary to descend below 15000 ft, perhaps as low as 5000 ft, and to land as quickly as possible. The interactions of the variables involved make it quite difficult to determine exact criteria. However, if cabin altitude does not exceed 25000 ft at any time, and a normal descent is made to 12000 ft, this profile may be adequately safe. Twenty-five thousand feet may be considered as a critical altitude when a subject ascends to and remains at that altitude. If decompressed to higher altitudes, this 'safe' level may no longer be considered as such because the recovery time after receiving 'adequate' oxygen found at 15000 ft may be too long to be safe. There can always be exceptions in the case of cardiopulmonary disease and other pathophysiological factors which enter into the determination of individual safety among passengers. The analysis of passenger health performed

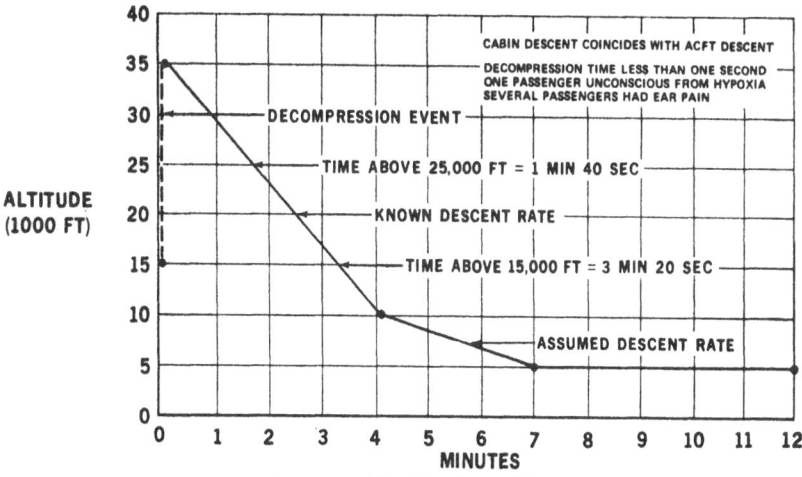

Fig. 3. Cabin altitude profile.

by Emery *et al.* (1965) [1] for the supersonic transport revealed that approximately 10% of the passenger list would be affected by potentially significant cardiorespiratory disease.

Figure 3 shows an example of the method of estimating the times that a decompressed cabin is above certain critical altitudes. In this actual case, all passengers survived with only relatively minor effects. The time-history explains why. It should be noted that the rate of descent was more rapid than 'normal', and that the final altitude of 5000 ft provided adequate oxygenation for rapid recovery of the one unconscious passenger. By plotting other known decompression events in a similar manner, a data bank can be accumulated which eventually would make it possible to judge the average TSU for any given decompression event. Such events can then be related to pressure system failures of different origins and time histories, and if that decompression event and recovery will be within the tolerable limits of the TSU.

Figure 4 shows two theoretical examples of an aircraft cruising at 42000 ft, with a 25000 ft^3 cabin decompressed from 8000 ft altitude as a result of hole sizes of approximately 9.0 ft^2 and 0.90 ft^2, respectively. The more rapid decompression (to 42000 ft) could be quite serious for any passenger without oxygen, whereas the slower decompression is most likely survivable without physiological damage even though the aircraft should level off at 15000 ft. Following the rapid decompression to 42000 ft,

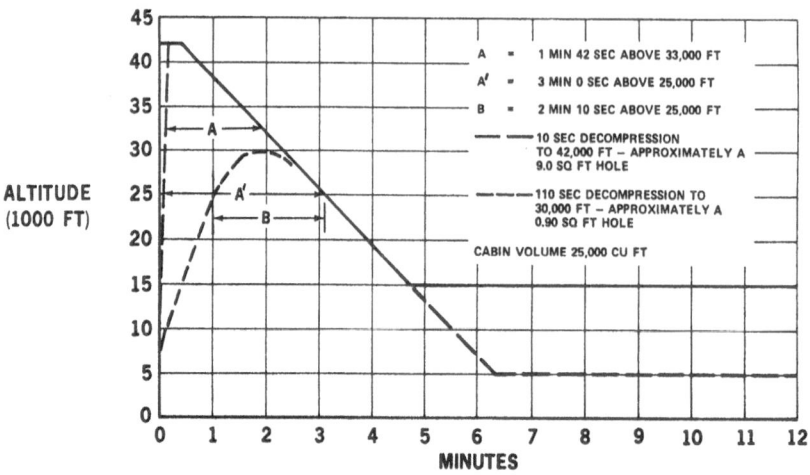

Fig. 4.   Critical altitudes vs. time.

aircraft should descend to 5000 ft for final cruise altitude for adequate recovery of unconscious passengers, terrain permitting.

In all examples, a constant or average rate of descent has been assumed. In Figure 4, a 10-sec decompression plus a 17-sec pilot reaction time has also been assumed.

The cabin stay time above certain altitudes (e.g., 25000 ft) can be obtained mathematically for a very rapid decompression, if one assumes a constant rate of descent, by using the formula:

$$T_{25} = (H_0 - H_{25})/\bar{R}$$

where $\bar{R}$ is the constant rate of descent, H_0 is the cruising altitude of the aircraft, and H_{25} is 25000 ft.

Where the decompression is slow (Figure 4, B) the time above 25000 ft may be solved for by using the equation:

$$T_{25} = T_2 - T_1$$

where T_{25}=time cabin is above 25000 ft, T_1=time required for the cabin to reach 25000 ft from the start of the decompression, and T_2=time the aircraft is above 25000 ft. If sufficient data are available for a given decompression event, the cabin altitude profile can be plotted, and the T-factors can be read directly from the graph.

The rate of descent for an aircraft is a function of time. Therefore, by using realistic values for descent rate, initial altitude prior to descent, hole size, etc., the time above other critical altitudes (e.g., 15000 ft) can be determined. Also, if these values are known or assumed, the descent time to an adequate recovery altitude can be solved for and specified. If the specified time cannot be met by a particular aircraft because of structural damage or other reason, the passengers must rely on an emergency oxygen system for survival without physiological damage.

3. Conclusions

In the event of an aircraft cabin decompression, it is suggested that a quick-reference guide for pilots to determine the safety of passengers be established as the time the cabin is above 25000 ft altitude. A relatively safe time may be considered as 1 min 40 sec to 2 min. The passengers may become unconscious due to other influential factors, such as decompression rate, maximum cabin altitude, rate of descent, and final cruise altitude. To be more accurate in determining the TSU, these factors must all be considered, assuming healthy passengers. Finally, a plea must be made for the collection of better data on decompression events which will occur in the future, so that the TSU can be determined more accurately.

References

[1] Emery J. A., Burrows, A. A., and Collier, D. R., Jr.: 1965, Advanced Biotechnology Rept. 61 Douglas Aircraft Company, Long Beach, Calif., U.S.A.
[2] 1964, *Bioastronautics Data Book* (ed. by P. Webb), NASA-SP-3006, National Aeronautics and Space Administration, Washington, D.C.
[3] 1968, *Flight Surgeon's Guide*, AFP-161-18, U.S. Air Force, Washington, D.C.

GAS EXCHANGE AT LOW AMBIENT PRESSURE

M. E. SLUIJTER

Wilhelmina Hospital, University of Amsterdam, Amsterdam, The Netherlands

Consider man's gas exchange when air is breathed. Inspired air contains about 21% oxygen ($F_{I_{O_2}}$) which, at the sea-level pressure of 160 mm Hg (P_B), exerts a partial pressure of 159 mm Hg ($P_{I_{O_2}}$). At the alveolar level, the O_2 concentration is less, due to the presence of water vapor (partial pressure 47 mm Hg) and of carbon dioxide (CO_2) in the alveoli, and to the fact that O_2 is being continually removed from the alveoli. Therefore, the difference between the inspired ($P_{I_{O_2}}$) and alveolar ($P_{A_{O_2}}$) partial pressures of oxygen will depend upon ventilation on one hand and the uptake of O_2 by the body on the other. The $P_{A_{O_2}}$ can be calculated with the alveolar gas equation:

$$P_{A_{O_2}} = F_{I_{O_2}}(P_B - 47) - P_{A_{CO_2}}\left[F_{I_{O_2}} + \frac{1 - F_{I_{O_2}}}{R^*}\right]$$

Using this equation, the $P_{A_{O_2}}$ can be calculated for different ambient pressures, yielding data such as shown in Figure 1. The three lower lines represent the values for $P_{A_{CO_2}}$-values of 30, 40 and 50 mm Hg respectively.

From the alveoli, O_2 is transmitted to the arterial blood. Here the partial pressure is slightly lower than in the alveoli since not all the venous blood passes through the alveoli. Part of the blood shunts from the right to the left side of the heart without being oxygenated. Normally this quantity amounts to 1 to 2% of the total circulatory flow. It is usually responsible for an alveolo-arterial oxygen gradient of not more than a few mm Hg.

Therefore, it can be said that the pressure limit of airline pressure cabins, which is 575 mm Hg, is quite safe for normal people. Due to the flat shape of the upper part of the oxyhemoglobin dissociation curve, an arterial oxygen partial pressure ($P_{a_{O_2}}$) of better than 60 mm Hg can be considered as satisfactory. Under this condition, around 90% of the hemoglobin is saturated with oxygen.

However, there are a few 'buts' which should be mentioned. First, not all passengers have normal lungs. Some elderly people can be expected to suffer from obstructive respiratory disease. At low ambient pressure this will affect the $P_{A_{O_2}}$ in two ways. These people may have an elevated $P_{A_{CO_2}}$ and, as shown above, this has a direct effect upon the concentration of oxygen in the alveoli. Also these people are known to shunt a higher proportion of venous blood from the right to the left side of their circulation, thus increasing the alveolo-arterial oxygen tension gradient.

If one considers, for example, a person with mild respiratory obstructive disease having a $P_{a_{CO_2}}$ of 50 mm Hg and a 10% shunt, then it is easy to calculate the effect of

---

* Respiratory exchange ratio.

D. E. Busby (ed.), Recent Advances in Aerospace Medicine, 204–207. All Rights Reserved.
Copyright © 1970 by D. Reidel Publishing Company, Dordrecht-Holland.

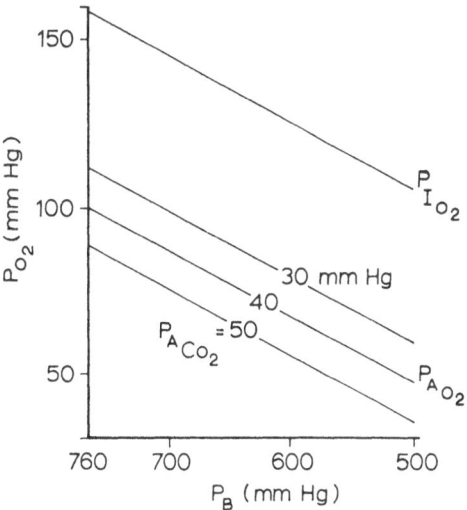

Fig. 1. P_{AO_2} calculated for different ambient pressures and P_{ACO_2} levels. Upper line: P_{IO_2} at different levels of ambient pressure. Three lower lines: P_{AO_2} at different levels of ambient pressure, for P_{ACO_2} of 30, 40 and 50 mm Hg.

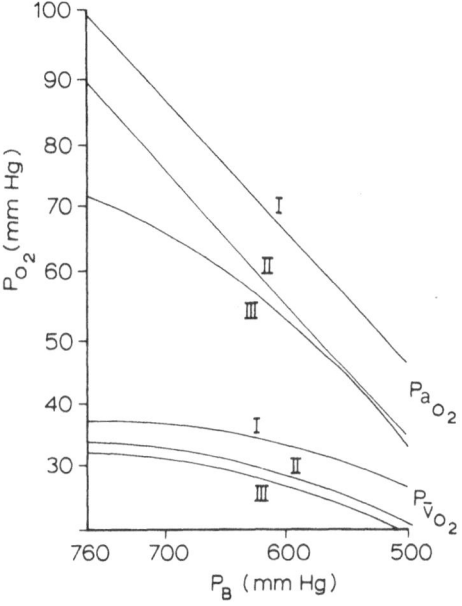

Fig. 2. P_{aO_2} and $P_{\bar{v}O_2}$ as related to ambient pressure, P_{aCO_2} and degree of venous-arterial (right-to left) shunting – (I) $P_{aCO_2} = 40$ mm Hg $R-L$ shunt $= 0\%$; (II) $P_{aCO_2} = 50$ mm Hg, $R-L$ shunt $= 0\%$; (III) $P_{aCO_2} = 50$ mm Hg, $R-L$ shunt $= 10\%$.

these deviations on the P_{aO_2}. Such a person is likely to have few subjective symptoms and lead a normal life. It can be seen in Figure 2 that ambient pressures, which are considered to be normal for pressure cabins, now result in P_{aO_2}-levels which are in the steep part of the oxyhemoglobin dissociation curve. Of more interest than the P_{aO_2}

is the mixed venous oxygen partial pressure ($P_{\bar{v}_{O_2}}$), which is indicative of the lowest tension at which oxygen is offered to the cell. If a normal arteriovenous oxygen difference of 6 vol % is assumed, the result can be calculated. The values are given in the three lower curves of Figure 2. Here also it can be seen that people with mild respiratory disease have a very narrow safety margin of oxygenation when travelling in an airplane. Indeed, it can be expected that a number of passengers have to compensate slightly for a level of oxygenation which is not quite sufficient. This compensation takes place in the form of an increase in cardiac output, resulting in a decrease of the arteriovenous O_2 difference.

A second factor which should be taken into account, is smoking. Smoking produces carbon monoxide (CO), and carbon monoxide is known to be a highly potent toxic agent when the $P_{I_{O_2}}$ is below normal. In heavy smokers, it can be found that up to 15% of the total amount of hemoglobin is bound to CO. This value corresponds with a P_{aco} in the blood of 0.08 mm Hg. If we now take this heavy smoker to an ambient pressure of 600 mm Hg, his $P_{A_{O_2}}$ will decrease to about 65 mm Hg. If he continues smoking, and so maintains a high level of $P_{I_{co}}$, the P_{aco} will now be sufficient to bind 20% of the available hemoglobin instead of 15%. In itself this would be of little consequence, but apart from combining with hemoglobin CO shifts the oxyhemoglobin dissociation curve to the left. Oxygen is therefore delivered to the cell at a tension which is 6 to 9 mm Hg lower than without the presence of CO in the example just given. To compensate for this low $P_{\bar{v}_{O_2}}$, the cardiac output would have to increase with a factor of the order of magnitude of 1.5 to 2. It is unlikely that this will take place, so that the tissues will remain slightly but definitely lacking O_2. This is because cardiac compensation is known to be poor during CO-poisoning, due to the fact that the $P_{a_{O_2}}$ is not affected.

From what has been said above, it becomes clear that when air is breathed the lower limit of safety has been reached at 575 mm Hg ambient pressure. Below this limit we enter into a level in which compensated hypoxia exists, which may be symptomless and hard to define with objective signs, but which is nevertheless a reality.

At lower ambient pressures, O_2-breathing is generally resorted to. This first involves the process of denitrogenation. The nitrogen (N_2), which is in solution in the tissues, is transported to the lungs and excreted. Theoretically, this might give rise to diffusion hypoxia, the N_2 displacing the O_2 molecules from the alveoli. This process is well known to anesthesiologists, since it is an important cause of hypoxia during the first 5 to 10 min following nitrous oxide anaesthesia. Since the solubility coefficient of N_2 is low, this will hardly play a role during increasing altitude, provided that O_2-breathing is commenced in good time and the decrease in the ambient pressure is not too fast.

Once denitrogenation has taken place, very low ambient pressures can be tolerated without the danger of hypoxia. Safety will now largely depend upon the fit of the face mask. A conventional mask may easily leak as much as 40%. This would still be quite satisfactory to use as an emergency mask in airplanes which fly at an altitude of about 8000 m. Even with a maximal leak it would then still provide for a $P_{A_{O_2}}$ of about

120 mm Hg. At higher altitudes, however, the more elaborate and more expensive type of mask can provide safety. These masks are not so easy to apply and to use properly without some practice and instruction.

A general remark should be added to what has been presented above. Given certain circumstances one may predict a P_{aO_2} and a $P_{\bar{v}O_2}$, and one may predict the oxygen tensions which prevail in Krogh's tissue cylinder. One may not predict the behaviour of tissue circulation itself, however, and therefore the radius of the tissue cylinder. This will largely depend on the quantity of circulating nor-adrenaline and on the tone of the sympathetic nervous system. If there is a lot of circulating nor-adrenaline, the path of a fraction of the blood may be changed from capillaries to arteriovenous shunts, in which the blood does not exchange gas with the cells. Thus the radius of the tissue cylinder may increase considerably, and parts of a tissue may become hypoxic in the absence of deviations of the arterial or even of the mixed venous O_2 content. This is not only true for the exchange of O_2, but also for the exchange of N_2. Nitrogen is an inert gas, and the behaviour of an inert gas in the body can now be predicted accurately with the aid of electrical analogue computers. This has also been done successfully for most volatile anesthetics. Each tissue group is represented by an electrical resistance connected to a condenser, blood flow being analogue to conductivity, and the product of tissue mass and solubility being analogous to capacity. If tissue circulation were uniform, such an analogue computer could provide us in a simple way with valuable data on the conditions which lead to nitrogen bubble formation. However, if the level of circulating noradrenaline is high, a tissue cannot be represented by a simple resistance coupled to a condenser, but only by a whole group of those units in parallel.

These theoretical considerations may explain why similar decompression circumstances may lead to problems from bubble formation in tissues at altitude on one day, and yet give no trouble on the next. It is interesting to note that the use of α-adrenergic blocking substances is very successful in the treatment of fat embolism. One cannot consider such a treatment for decompression sickness at this time, since recompression therapy is in fact quite simple and satisfactory. However, when it comes to explaining the symptomatology of decompression sickness, the importance of tissue circulation must always be kept in mind.

OXYGEN TOLERANCES AND ADVERSE REACTIONS

A. R. BEHNKE

2865 Jackson St., San Francisco, Calif., U.S.A.

1. Introduction

Clinical applications of oxygen (O_2) at pressure higher than 1 ata cannot be separated from long-standing inhalation of O_2 to expedite decompression of divers and to treat decompression sickness. Were it not for the apparent freedom of thousands of young men from residual injury following exposures to O_2 at elevated pressures, one would not be justified, in view of the toxic effects on nervous and pulmonary tissue (time-pressure dependent), in prosecuting clinical application without first conducting long-term tolerance tests and observations on life-span of exposed animals. However, this statement is tempered by lack of knowledge of long-term daily exposures at therapeutic levels (3 ata or less). A serious consideration is that such chronic exposures may be conducive, as observed in animals at pressures of 4 ata and higher, to both focal and large areas of neuronal necrosis involving mid-brain and spinal cord. Such neuronal deficit may be covert over long periods of time and escape routine examination. Another deterrent to hyperbaric therapy, apart from lack of knowledge as to the specific etiology underlying convulsive seizures and pulmonary damage, is variability of time in onset of adverse reactions to O_2. This paper will serve to recapitulate some experience derived from exposure of man and animals to inhalation of O_2 at higher pressures.

2. Earlier Test Data (1932–1935)

In 1932 Naval Medical Officers were afforded the opportunity to conduct hyperbaric investigations on animals and man in the newly-installed pressure chamber at the Harvard School of Public Health. At the time the perspicacious investigations of Bert (1878), and the observations of Smith (1899) had established in animals the toxicity of O_2 for the nervous system and the lungs. Their findings did not encourage Naval application. However, in view of the theoretical value of O_2 in promoting nitrogen (N_2) elimination from the tissues of divers and in the treatment of decompression sickness, it appeared worthwhile to determine the duration of the apparent latent period of well-being prior to onset of adverse effects.

A. ANIMAL EXPERIMENTS

In tests of several hours in duration at pressures of 4 to 6 ata, it appeared that pulmonary injury might well nullify the value of hyperbaric O_2 in diving. The liver-like consistency of entire lobes of the lungs presented an alarming appearance. However, following the gentle inflation suggested by Drinker, the lungs assumed a normal appearance, devoid of 'hemorrhagic' areas; grossly, there was no edema. Pulmonary injury, when it did occur at the higher pressures (3 to 6 ata), was secondary in onset

D. E. Busby (ed.), Recent Advances in Aerospace Medicine, 208–225. All Rights Reserved.
Copyright © 1970 by D. Reidel Publishing Company, Dordrecht-Holland.

to nervous manifestations. In any case, the pulmonary injury did not appear to be proportional to, nor was it compounded by the elevated pressure.

Tests on small animals confirmed the regular occurrence of epileptiform seizures at pressures of 4 ata and higher, and served to focus on a unique derangement of respiration in later stages, characterized by primitive gasping – an irregular type of breathing prior to respiratory failure due to spasmodic contractions of the diaphragm. Subsequently the experiments of Jamieson (1966) showed that cortical damage, as revealed by the electroencephalogram, appeared early. Biochemically, enzymes in brain tissues concerned in carbohydrate metabolism, such as succinic oxidase, are poisoned by O_2 and, in the case of the succinic dehydrogenase component, the poisoning is irreversible.

Hyperbaric O_2 (6 ata) administered daily to the dog until the onset of the seizure, when the dog was switched to air, was tolerated for at least a month without gross injury (Table I). In contrast to wide variability of initial symptoms in man (however, in man, O_2 inhalation would be terminated usually prior to convulsion), it is apparent that the latent period preceding the onset of convulsion increased about three-fold

TABLE I

Latent period preceding onset of O_2-induced convulsions at 6 ata during the course of repeated exposures of a dog[a]

Time (min)										
July, 1935	8	11	10	12.5	13	14.5	12.5	10	11	10
August, 1935	14	13	15.5	13.5	14.5	22	23.5	26.5	21.5	22.5
	22.5	24.5	27.5	23	24					

[a] Dog remained in good condition throughout the test period as observed in running ability and gain of 1.1 kg (Weight 6.3 kg).

during the course of the tests. The dog remained in good condition during the course of, and following 34 seizures as observed in running ability and gain of 1.1 kg (weight 6.3 kg) in weight. At autopsy, the brain and the lungs were grossly normal.

The grand mal type of seizure need not be described in detail. It is sufficient to invite attention to violent contractions of the diaphragm and labored breathing prior to seizure. At this time the dog may be rigid and in a dazed condition (subsequently designated as 'dazzle' in Donald's (1947) description of his divers). The pupils are widely dilated and do not react to light. Recovery is rapid following onset of air-breathing. Initially during recovery, the dog walks tremulously with a broad base. Vision appears to be completely lost at this time (pupils remain dilated and do not react to light) but is restored in about 10 to 20 min. There is no pharmacologic or other agent which can so drastically disrupt body economy, and yet be followed by apparently complete recovery. Repeated seizures in close succession give rise to chronic paralysis in survivors.

Although diurnal seizures separated by several hours may not be attended by gross injury, there is greatly heightened excitability of the entire nervous system. The reflex excitability of the spinal cord mimics the response to strychnine. Visual, auditory, and tactile stimuli provoke tetanic contractions of major muscle groups. Inhibition of antagonist muscles, as in strychnine poisoning, is abolished. The body becomes rigid, eyes turn outward, extremities are spread apart, and opisthotonus is marked. Spastic contraction of the diaphragm stops respiration. Even with a shift to air, tetanic contractions may recur 4 to 12 times/min in response to auditory and tactile stimuli. Apparently the second seizure serves to abolish cortical dominance, which is not wholly restored during the interval following the initial seizure. These striking manifestations relate to tonic, clonic, and tetanic seizures, to spasmodic contractions of the diaphragm, paralysis of respiration, and to persistent bradycardia.

In contrast to the susceptibility of the nervous system, the heart is remarkably resistant to injury. Bradycardia (pulse rate 80/min compared with a pre-test rate of 120/min in the unanesthetized dog) is a striking feature of hyperbaric oxygen exposure. Cardiac function in the anesthetized dog may be maintained for periods as long as 90 min following respiratory paralysis. Under these circumstances pulmonary blood is adequately oxygenated despite the absence of lung movement. Accumulation of carbon dioxide (CO_2) however, in a closed breathing system to levels above 250 mm Hg brings about asphyxial death. Noteworthy is the ability of the heart to sustain widely fluctuating levels of blood pressure during the period of cumulative hypercarbia.

The inseparability of CO_2 from O_2 reactions has given rise to controversial interpretation. One 'school' placed emphasis on the CO_2-mediated increase in cerebral blood flow as the factor chiefly responsible for augmented toxicity. The classical experiments of Shaw et al. (1934) and subsequently of Lambertsen (1953) will be cited later in this paper. It suffices to state here that the O_2-potentiating effect of CO_2 is specific and not related to a lowering of pH per se. Thus, in an experiment at 4 ata (O_2), the pH of venous blood of the dog was lowered to 6.9 by intravenous infusion of 1000 ml of 1 N (10%) lactic acid. This procedure was not followed by convulsions, which routinely occurred when the dog inhaled a CO_2-enriched atmosphere.

B. TESTS ON MAN

Although some aspects of the animal derangements were of concern, there was no serious deterrent to the initial objective of definition of the relatively safe latent period prior to functional disruption. Favorable features were the latent period of well-being and unmistakable signs of impending incapacitation, and the rapidly reversible nature of adverse manifestations. Earlier tests on man were, however, terminated by syncope (an unusual reaction) or by seizure at the relatively high pressure of 4 ata.

At 3 ata, in a well-lighted chamber, tests were usually terminated during the fourth hour of O_2 inhalation. Onset of end-point symptoms may be abrupt (Table II). There is a sharp rise on both systolic and diastolic pressure, a reversal of bradycardia, tubular vision followed by amblyopia (Figure 1E) and, at times, a subjective feeling of impending collapse.

Subsequently, hyperbaric O_2 was inhaled routinely (as high as 3 ata) by U.S. Navy

TABLE II

Circulatory and visual effects of O_2 at 3 ata during the course of one test
(Behnke *et al.*, 1936)

Gas	Time (min)	Blood pressure mm Hg	Pulse rate beats/min	Visual acuity % Decrease	Time of negative after-image (sec)	Remarks
Air	O⁻	132/86	96	0	–	
O_2	55	115/90	75	3	8	
	117	114/88	63	20	18	Facial pallor
	145	124/84	57	28	18	
	177	138/102	57	26	18	
	190	120/94	63	–	–	
	205	Period of well-being terminated				Numbness of fingers and toes
		Decreased field of vision				
	209	150/104	75	60	20	
	212	–	81	Amblyopia		
	213	Off oxygen				
Air	12	140/92	81	40	7	

divers during decompression (U.S.S. Squalus salvage operations), and for the treatment of decompression sickness. In diving operations which involve work, and so are conducive to CO_2 retention, the inhalation of O_2 has been rigidly curtailed, chiefly as a result of tests by Yarbrough *et al.* (1947) and the extensive and convincing experiments in the Royal Navy conducted by Donald (1947) and Haldane (1941) during World War II.

TABLE III

O_2 tolerance in 272 exposures of men at rest in the
dry chamber, and underwater at 60, 80, and 100 ft
(Yarbrough *et al.*, 1947)

Dry chamber Depth (Equiv. ft)	Pressure (ata)	Number of tests	Test duration (min) 120	60	< 60
60	2.82	20	20	–	–
80	3.42	46	10	10	26
100	4.03	26	–	3	23
Underwater					
60	2.82	107	11	64	32
80	3.42	53	–	5	48
100	4.03	20	–	1	19

% Reactions terminating tests: nausea (40), twitching (21), vertigo (17), visual (6), restlessness (6), numbness (6), convulsions (4)

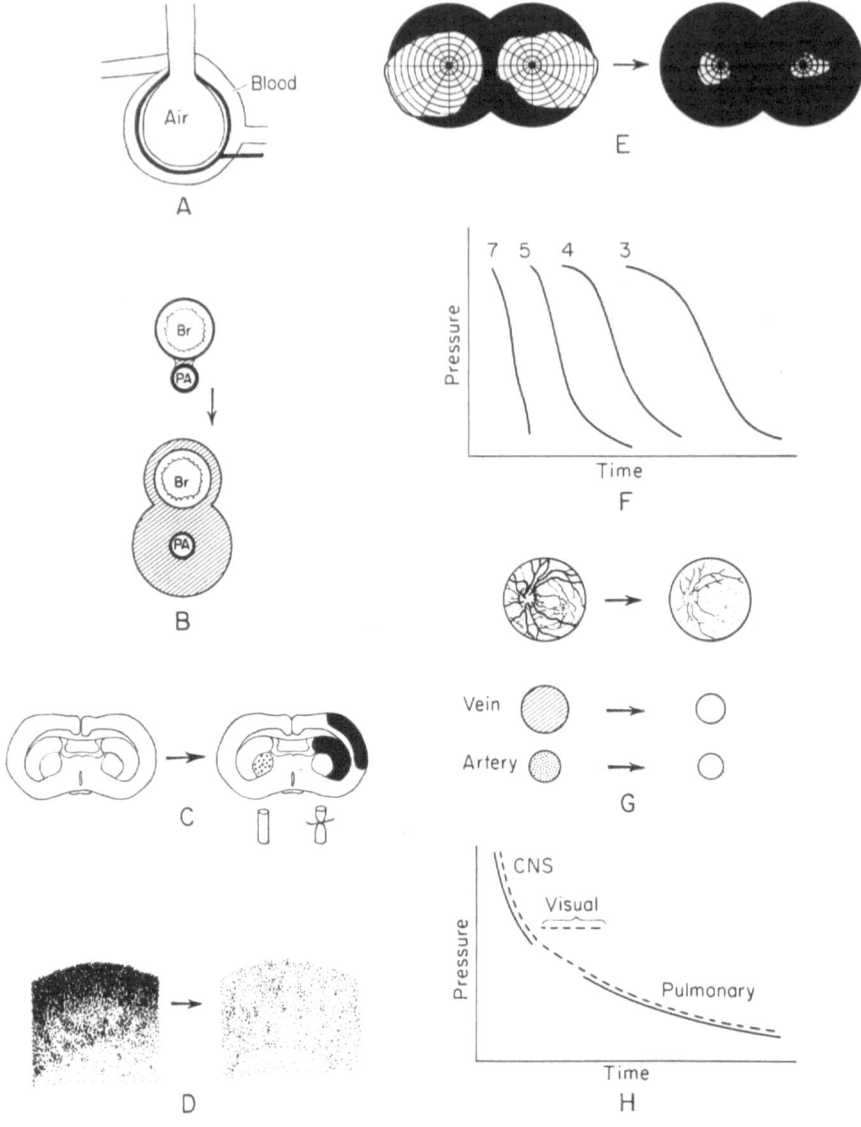

Fig. 1. Panel of sketches depicting adverse effects of hyperbaric O_2 with references to specific investigations.

A. A progressive thickening of the air-blood barrier in the O_2-exposed rat lung, from normal of 1.5 μ, to 3 μ, after 3 days (98.5% O_2, 1 ata) was due primarily to enlargement of the interstitial space by accumulation of edema (Kistler *et al.*, 1967).

B. Development of interstitial edema. Fluid appears first in the interstitial connective tissue compartment around vessels and airways (Staub *et al.*, 1967).

C. The different location in coronal sections of the rat brain produced by hypoxia (shaded area), and hyperbaria (dotted area), following ligation of one carotid artery. Exposure of the rat to hypoxia produces extensive damage to layers of the cortex on the ligated side; following exposure to hyperbaria, necrosis is observed in the globus pallidus on the side contralateral to ligations. Damage to myelin in the cerebral peduncles by hyperbaria is offered as a reasonable explanation for the severe spastic paralysis observed in rats (from Balentine *et al.*, 1966).

3. Later Tests and Investigations

More than 1000 hyperbaric O_2 tests during and following World War II have confirmed earlier findings in regard to man at rest. Attention has been focused on limitations and adverse effects. Wide individual variability, chiefly underwater and during exercise, has severely restricted the inhalation of O_2 under these conditions. Essential data are presented in Tables III, IV and V. It should be pointed out that following

TABLE IV

Variability in O_2 tolerance of 36 physically-fit men breathing through a mouthpiece in the dry chamber at 3.13 ata (Equiv. 90 ft) (Donald, 1947)

Number of exposures	Tolerance time (min)	Signs and symptoms at end-point (number of men affected)
12	6 to 17	Lip twitching (23), vertigo (5),
11	17 to 27	nausea (4), convulsions (3), drow-
5	30 to 35	siness, numbness, confusion, visual,
8	50 to 96	auditory, hallucinations, stupefaction, and epigastric aura (4)

TABLE V

Variation in O_2 tolerance time of a diver[a] in the wet tank exposed to end-point (2 to 3 times weekly) over a period of 90 days at 70 ft (3.12 ata) (Donald, 1947)

Duration of each exposure (min)[b]								End-point: Signs-symptoms
7	41	96	12	48	125	21	61	Lip twitching, nausea, au-
23	62	27	67	28	148	78	28	ditory, visual hallucinations,
82	31	37	86					stupefaction ('dazzle')

[a] Diver won a middleweight boxing championship during the period of exposure
[b] Not arranged in consecutive order

D. On the left, section of the normal adrenal gland of the rat. The zona fasciculata of the cortex contains large amounts of lipid (black); On the right, section of the gland of a rat exposed to hyperbaric oxygen. The zona fasciculata and the zona reticularis are enlarged. Strikingly, lipid is depleted from these portions of the cortex. Recovery from a hyperbaric oxygen exposure when the animal is replaced in air, is accompanied by restoration of lipid (Bean, 1955).

E. Perimetric measurements before and after 3.5 hr of oxygen inhalation by a healthy, young man at 3 ata (Behnke et al., 1936).

F. Effect on beta-wave response on the electroretinogram of continuous exposure to O_2 pressures of 7 to 3 ata. At 3 ata the latent period before the onset of beta-wave decline is about 100 min, and at 7 ata, decline begins after only 20 min exposure, see Table IX (Noel, 1962).

G. Upper graphs show diagrammatically normal caliber retinal vessels (left), and the severe vasoconstriction (right) of the vessels in the retina of a premature infant exposed to 70% O_2 (1 ata) for 4 days (Patz, 1968).

Lower graphs depict the mean decrease in size of arteries (19%) and veins (28%) of the retina in young adults who inhaled O_2 at a pressure of 3 ata (Saltzman et al., 1965).

H. The time-pressure hyperbaric O_2 tolerance curve indicates the dichotomy between pulmonary response observed after longer exposures to relatively low pressures of O_2, and central nervous system reactions observed at higher pressures. The effects of hyperbaric O_2 on the visual system (cells, blood vessels) can be represented as a time-pressure continuum which bridges the dichotomy between central nervous system and pulmonary functions (Behnke, based on data in Table IX).

extensive employment of oxygen rebreathing apparatus (e.g., Lambertsen's equipment) during World War II, there has been no gross cumulative or residual impairment.

A. EXPERIMENTAL DATA ON MAN (U.S. NAVY, 1938–1945)

Tests at the Experimental Diving Unit showed that in 20 exposures to O_2 in the dry chamber at rest (2.82 ata, 60 ft equiv.), symptoms did not terminate tests within a period of 2 hr. However, at the same depth underwater, 32 of the 107 exposures were terminated prior to 60 min (Table III). The average duration of exposure was 32 min (range 8 to 58 min). Two seizures occurred, one at 13 min, the other at 24 min.

At a pressure of 3.42 ata (80 ft), 74 of the 99 exposures to O_2 were terminated prior to 60 min; at a pressure of 4.03 ata (100 ft), 43 of the 46 exposures were less than 60 min.

Moderate work could be undertaken safely at depths of 30 ft or less. At this depth, in 35 tests adverse symptoms supervened in two divers at 87 and 111 min, respectively. At greater depths, it was not feasible to breathe O_2 during exercise underwater.

B. RESULTS OF ROUTINE 'O_2 TOLERANCE TEST'

(Data compiled by Dr. M. W. Goodman, U.S. Navy Deep Sea Diving School, 1951 to 1961)

Of the 1388 exposures of 30 min in duration to O_2 at a pressure of 2.82 ata (27.8 psi, 60 ft equiv.), reactions were observed in 14 examinees, 5 of whom had seizures. Subsequently, in accord with the 'low pressure' O_2 treatment tables, 20-min periods of O_2 inhalation interspersed with 5-min intervals on air, have been well tolerated during the course of hundreds of treatments. In our own series of 135 cases of decompression sickness treated with hyperbaric O_2 and air-spaced intervals, there have been no adverse reactions.

C. O_2-INDUCED CONVULSIONS IN MAN

Donald (1947) has summarized his extensive experience with convulsive phenomena in man. "The most important aspect of oxygen poisoning is the intoxication of the central nervous system. It seems that the whole cerebrospinal axis is involved. The twitching of muscles is definitely subcortical in origin, and the sensitivity of the facial nerve to tapping would indicate that even the most peripheral components are affected. Meanwhile the cortex is also being poisoned, and in a number of cases phenomena exactly similar to epileptic auras occur which are presumably due to cortical dysfunction. In some cases, severe muscle twitching, and even convulsions, may be precipitated without any such aura being reported. The more peripheral motor discharges may predominate throughout and even cause generalized jactitations without electrical or clinical evidence of cortical disturbance. In other cases, non-convulsant cortical disturbances may cause symptoms of such severity that the exposure is discontinued. The remarkable individual variation in reaction to unphysiological tensions of oxygen is again emphasized", (Tables IV and V). It is reiterated that up to the time of seizure or other adverse effects, there may exist not only apparent normality but also feelings of stimulation and alertness (an adrenergic response?).

In a follow-up of Donald's (1947) subjects continued over a period of three years, there was no overt effect on neurological integrity, intellectual ability, or personality. Furthermore, the marked bradycardia recorded (pulse rate 35 to 50 beats/min), particularly after exposures to 60 ft (2.82 ata), has not been accompanied by any irregularity in cardiac rhythm, nor has there been any evidence of chronic injury to the cardiovascular system.

D. O_2-INDUCED PARALYSIS AND CENTRAL NERVOUS SYSTEM HISTOPATHOLOGY IN RATS

It would be a serious omission not to point out that extensive lesions causing paralysis or death can be produced in the thalamus, mid-brain, spinal cord and other areas of the central nervous system by as few as 4 to 9 successive daily exposures of 1-hr duration at 4.88 ata (Balentine and Gutsche, 1966). The neurologic injury comprises both focal necrosis and complete or partial necrosis of nuclear groups, with damage to myelin, axons, and glia within the area of grey matter involved. The lesions are not those characterized by hypoxia produced in rats by exposure to low oxygen tension (Figure 1c). In hypoxia, motor nuclei of cranial nerves were frequently found to be involved; in hyperbaric exposure sensory nuclei were predominantly injured.

Important is the finding that the rats which showed lesions had convulsions; un-anesthetized rats which did not develop seizures within the 1-hr period of exposure did not develop paralysis. In contrast, anesthetized rats following a single 0.5 hr exposure in an atmosphere (4.88 ata) containing 95% O_2 and 2% CO_2 developed severe paralysis. It should be noted that 2% CO_2 at the high pressure is equivalent to 9.8% at 1 ata. These experiments are cited to show that severe functional and morphologic injury is possible at high pressures. Furthermore, irrespective of the nature of the derangements in electron transfer pathways and oxidative phosphorylation, the O_2 effect is time-pressure dependent for nervous tissue above an ill-defined minimal pressure level.

E. RESPIRATORY EFFECTS OF O_2 AT 4 ATA AND HIGHER

In man, dysrythmic breathing, choking sensations, and even temporary inspiratory arrest (5 ata) have been reported. Reference has been made to the jerky, inspiratory gasps observed in the unanesthetized dog. In the barbiturate-anesthetized dog it is possible to suppress peripheral motor activity and to observe what best may be described as 'convulsive respiration'. The O_2-induced seizure is restricted to violent contractions of the muscles of the neck and thorax. The seizures are synchronous with inspiratory gasps, which progressively become weaker to terminate in apnea.

Mention has been made of the experiments of Jamieson (1966) in which bioelectric signals (electromyogram) from the diaphragm of urethan-anesthetized rats, and cortical (electroencephalogram) activity were recorded. Cortical damage induced by hyperbaric O_2 appeared much earlier than derangement of the respiratory pathway as seen on the electromyogram. As in the dog, respiration increased in depth (the characteristic labored breathing). This response developed into a gasping pattern synchronous with vigorous bursts of bioelectrical activity. Such activity continued despite failure of ventilation in damaged lungs. Respiratory depression and failure were also observed in the absence of appreciable lung damage. As in the dog, the heart beats, characterized by bradycardia, persisted for as long as 1 hr after respiratory failure ensued.

F. RESPIRATORY EFFECTS IN MAN AT PRESSURES LESS THAN 3 ATA

Despite edema and hemorrhagic consolidation observed chiefly in the lungs of small animals exposed to hyperbaric O_2, there has been in healthy man a virtual absence of pulmonary complications from hyperbaria. No exacerbation of subclinical respiratory infection has been reported in divers who inhaled O_2 for periods of several hours or longer (up to 3 ata) in the treatment of decompression sickness. In over 1000 experiments (1.9 to 4.68 ata) reported by Donald (1947), the end-point was anchored to signs and symptoms referrable to the nervous system. Chest examinations revealed only negative findings. However, there may be some respiratory distress at relatively low pressures if inhalation of O_2 is continuous and prolonged.

In earlier tests at 1 ata, subjects lying prone, which was conducive to shallow breathing, complained of pulmonary irritation within a period of 4 hr (Behnke et al., 1935). At higher pressures (to 3 ata), with subjects in a sitting position, there were never irritative symptoms during the same time period. In carefully monitored tests (Clark and Lambertsen, 1967; Fisher et al., 1968), it was observed that healthy men could breathe O_2 (2 ata) for about 8 hr before their vital capacity decreased significantly. Between 8 to 12 hr, burning sensation on deep inhalation, cough, and dyspnea were progressive. Complete recovery supervened after about 24 hr.

At 1 ata the most frequent complaint associated with continuous O_2 inhalation is substernal distress of variable intensity, which may supervene during exposures as short as 4 and as long as 74 hr. Typical findings are those of Comroe et al., (1945) who reported that 28 of 34 healthy men developed substernal distress intensified by inspiration during an average period of 14 hr (range, 4 to 24 hr). The symptoms were never alarming and disappeared within 12 hr after change to air-breathing. However, there was accentuation of the pulmonary irritation during the recovery period by deep inspiration, breathing of cold air, and inhalation of tobacco smoke. One of the 4 subjects developed unusual degrees of fatigue; joint pains and crackling sensations were also reported after 24 hr.

The tests of Caldwell et al., (1966) are noteworthy for the extended period of time that 4 volunteers were able to breathe 98% O_2 (1 ata), in a chamber, 30, 48, 60, and 74 hr, respectively. The fall in vital capacity was rapidly progressive after 60 hr; this was associated with a decrease in pulmonary diffusing capacity. The adverse effects were not readily reversible following the prolonged exposures. Frank illness was reported during the course of inhalation of 90% O_2 (1 ata) between 48 to 65 hr attended by nausea and vomiting (Becker-Freyseng and Clamann, 1950). Dyspnea, pains in the knee joints, and paresthesia in fingers and toes supervened. The term, 'poisoning', appears to be applicable to the more severe pulmonary symptoms which may arise following prolonged exposure to high concentrations of O_2 at relatively low pressures.

G. INTERSTITIAL EDEMA – THE INITIAL PATHOLOGIC DERANGEMENT

The prime target of the 'direct' effect of O_2 on the lungs appears now to be not alveolar epithelium but pulmonary capillary endothelium. The injury initially produced by O_2 is the same as that following capillary damage induced by injection of alloxan as described by Staub *et al.* (1967). These authors pointed out that fluid first appears in interstitial connective tissue around vessels and airways (Figure 1B). Alveolar wall thickening begins after the interstitial compartment has been filled. A similar description pertains to the effect of O_2 on the rat lung exposed for 48 to 72 hr at 1 ata (98.5% O_2). From definitive electron microscopic observations (Kistler *et al.*, 1967), there was progressive thickening of the air-blood barrier due primarily to enlargement of the interstitial space by accumulation of edema, which was replaced secondarily by cells and fibrin (Figure 1A). "The primary cellular damage was located in endothelial cells which underwent cytoplasmic changes and, finally, fragmentation. In contrast, the damage to the epithelial lining of alveoli was relatively scarce compared to the extensive endothelial changes" (Kistler *et al.*, 1967). This investigator has observed fluid distention of perivascular space and, notably, engorged lymphatics, in the lungs of dogs exposed to O_2 inhalation at 4 ata for periods up to 4 hr. The bronchi were 'dry' and there was no obstruction of airways.

In man, the substernal distress which accompanies deep inspiration, associated with an unproductive cough, may well be an expression of an incipient 'wet' perivascular space. The decreased vital capacity and pulmonary compliance observed in man are not associated with atelectasis or fluid in alveoli.

Mention should be made of chronic pulmonary lesions in rats living in compressed air (4 ata; O_2, 635 mm Hg) for periods up to 3 months. In the classical experiments of Bennett and Smith (1934), perivascular edema appeared after 3 days of exposure. Subsequently, there was hyalinization of the large pulmonary arteries and pulmonary hypertension.

In decompression sickness, intravascular bubbles in the pulmonary vessels are associated with pulmonary arterial hypertension. Diagnostic of bubbles is substernal distress and 'dry' paroxysmal coughing, which may also have a common etiology in interstitial edema.

H. PARADOXICAL REACTIONS TO O_2 AT 1 ATA OR LESS

Some remarkable and unanticipated neuropsychic responses have attended inhalation of O_2 under certain conditions at relatively low pressures. An abrupt switch to O_2 following a period of hypoxia may result in mental confusion, cardiovascular collapse, and seizures of short duration. These responses have been observed not only in emphysematous patients but in aviators and divers. Essentially, when a person is hypoxic and is then abruptly supplied with an abundance of O_2, his condition may rapidly worsen; in severe cases there may be clonic muscular spasms or unconsciousness for as long as 30 sec. On the other hand, the condition may be transient or pass unnoticed unless brought to light by special tests. At a simulated altitude of 20000 ft

(0.46 ata), 52 subjects rendered hypoxic by breathing air for periods of 4 to 5 min were given pure O_2 to breathe (Latham, 1951). A paradoxical reaction was demonstrated in 13 of the 52 subjects. Chronic hypoxemic patients during the initial stage of O_2 therapy may become drowsy and even stuporous under conditions of CO_2 retention. Presumably, the abrupt relief of hypoxemia provided by O_2 inhalation inhibits powerful chemoreflexes from the aortic arch and carotid bodies. Administration of O_2 in graded amounts serves to prevent the untoward reactions.

I. EFFECTS ON MAN AND ANIMALS OF CHRONIC HYPERBARIC O_2 EXPOSURE

What should have been the most important section of this paper will be disposed of, because of lack of knowledge, by a few sentences and a meager table. There are virtually no repetitive daily exposures of individuals at hyperbaric O_2 levels employed in diving or in therapy (*e.g.*, at 2.5 ata). Such measure would serve to eliminate the hazard of decompression sickness and chronic avascular bone necrosis, and to ensure economic stability of a now excessively costly industrial operation. However, the possibility of low grade, but cumulative brain damage is a deterrent to daily O_2 inhalation by tunnel workers at pressures of 2 to 2.8 ata for periods of not more than 2 hr.

Some information on chronic tolerance to oxygen comes as a collateral benefit from recent work by Jacobs (1969), Winter (1967), and their co-workers. These investigators found a paradoxical improvement in cerebral function and in well being of patients

TABLE VI

Trend of chronic O_2 tolerance of man and several species following daily exposures to O_2 at therapeutic levels

	Pressure (ata)	Schedule (daily)	Air interval (hr)	Exposures (number or duration)
Elderly men	2.5	1.5 hr × 2	10.5	150–450
Rat	3.0	1.0 hr × 6	2	28 days
Dog	3.0	1.0 hr × 4	1	30 days
Rabbit	2.0[a]	1.0 hr × 6	3	20 days
Pig	2.0[b]	2.0 hr × 4	4	24 hr

[a] Exposure at 3.0 ata for 2 hr were attended by hyperpnea, gasping respiration, and death.
[b] Some animals showed respiratory distress after 20 hr and it was necessary to lower the pressure to 1.5 ata.

who manifested senile deterioration. Oxygen was inhaled twice daily for 90-min periods at 2.5 ata; total number of treatments ranged from 150 to 435 (Table VI).

In chronic animal exposures to pressures of 3 ata and less, there is a wide difference in tolerance between several species. The rat tolerates 6 one-hr daily exposures at 3 ata for 28 days; for the rabbit, such an exposure induces pulmonary injury, and surprisingly, the pig is even more sensitive (Table VI). It is apparent that there is a pressing requirement to investigate long term hyperbaric O_2 exposures at therapeutic O_2 levels. In small animals, detection of subtle derangements in central nervous system morphology by sophisticated techniques would be a prime objective.

4. Factors Influencing Variability of Response to Hyperbaric O_2

A. ROLE OF CO_2

The level of CO_2 in the lungs, blood, and fixed tissues, may be the chief determinant underlying the wide variability in individual response to a stable alveolar O_2 pressure. One mechanism to explain the CO_2 synergism is vascular dilatation and increased blood flow, notably through such organs as the brain. In 1933, Hill showed that convulsions were induced in various species more rapidly and at lower O_2 pressures when CO_2 was added to the inhalation mixture. In the experiments of Shaw et al. (1934), it was possible to quantify the CO_2 action. In anesthetized dogs two criteria, fall in blood pressure and onset of seizures, signalized the adverse effect of O_2 at 4 ata. If alveolar CO_2 was lowered to a level of 22-27 mm Hg by hyperventilation in a Drinker respirator, adverse responses did not supervene during the 2.5 to 3-hr test period. On the other hand, elevation of alveolar pCO_2 to 60–68 mm Hg by administration of CO_2-enriched oxygen, was attended by a fall in blood pressure in 7 to 20 min and by seizures in 57 to 78 min (Table VII). The unequivocal data of Lambertsen et al. (1953) showed that in male subjects the O_2 pressure in venous blood returning

TABLE VII

Alveolar CO_2 level and O_2 toxicity (dogs) (Shaw et al., 1934)

Inhaled oxygen tension mm Hg	Alveolar CO_2 tension mm Hg	Duration of exposure (min)	Time (min) of onset of	
			Fall in blood pressure	Seizures
2986	22[a]	164	–	–
3000	22[a]	180	–	–
3018	27[a]	159	152	–
2935	60[b]	124	20	57
2935	68[b]	133	10	64
190	85[b]	150	–	–

[a] Hyperventilation of anesthetized dog in Drinker respirator
[b] CO_2 added to inhaled O_2.

from the brain relative to a fixed pressure of inhaled oxygen (3.5 ata), could be increased ten-fold by addition of CO_2 to the inhaled O_2 (Table VIII). Since CO_2 tensions in lungs and tissues may fluctuate over a wide range, it is difficult to regulate the partial pressure of O_2 in the capillaries and tissues. Response to a given ambient O_2 tension is variable because the effective tissue O_2 tension is variable.

In view of the striking potentiation of the adverse effects of oxygen by CO_2, we have substantial reason to explain the greater toxicity of O_2 in the wet chamber com-

TABLE VIII

Variation of O_2 pressure in venous blood in relation to constant levels of inhaled O_2, and the effect of added CO_2 in elevating venous O_2 tensions

A. Man[a]

Inhaled oxygen pressure (ata)	Venous oxygen tension (mm Hg)
3.5	75
3.5 (+2% (O_2))	1000

B. Man[b]

Estimated tissue oxygenation at 3.5 ata (Air) (O_2),

Tissue	Venous oxygen tension (mm Hg)	
	Breathing air	Breathing oxygen
Heart	21	40
Brain	35	50
Muscle	36	300
Kidney	63	1543

C. Dog[c]

Inhaled oxygen pressure (ata)	Mixed venous O_2 tension (mm Hg)
3.89	533 (90–1200)

[a] Lambertsen et al., 1953.
[b] Lambertsen, 1965.
[c] Behnke et al., 1935.

pared with the dry environment, and especially the greatly reduced O_2 tolerance associated with exercise. Indeed Lanphier (1963) was impressed by the high incidence of O_2 poisoning during work underwater when divers breathed O_2-N_2 mixtures through a SCUBA mouthpiece. Pulmonary ventilation in response to exercise underwater was inadequate for the elimination of CO_2. In one group of 17 divers the mean (end-tidal volume) partial pressure of CO_2 during exercise was 55 mm Hg; the highest value (70 mm Hg) pertained to a diver especially sensitive to the neurologic disturbances induced by O_2. The divers were unaware of CO_2 retention and seemingly acquired some degree of tolerance for higher CO_2 tensions which rendered them susceptible to O_2.

Since the blood flow to various organs and their O_2 requirements differ greatly, there is no way to control the O_2 supply at the cellular level. The high extraction rate of heart muscle for O_2 carried in blood would greatly lower the tissue O_2 tension compared with the low extraction rate in skeletal muscle (Table VIIIB). These highly fluctuating metabolic, circulatory, and pH factors serve to explain in part at least, variation in individual susceptibility.

B. INFLUENCE OF HORMONES

It is certain that adrenal, thyroid, and pituitary hormones augment the neurotoxic action of O_2 (Bean, 1955), and serve to shorten the latent period of comparative well-being. Subjectively, the inhalation of O_2 gives rise to an adrenergic response. Furthermore, the apprehensive individual, in contrast to the phlegmatic person, empirically appears to be much more susceptible to the untoward reactions associated with inhalation of hyperbaric O_2. Experimentally, it has been demonstrated that hyperbaric O_2 exerts a stimulating effect on the sympathetic nervous system (Edström and Röchert, 1961). Ganglionic blocking agents, for example, have been found to reduce both pulmonary damage as well as convulsions (Johnson and Bean, 1957). It has been confirmed that inhalation of hyperbaric O_2 is associated with adrenal hypertrophy in the rat and depletion of steroids (Figure 1D). Recovery following hyperbaric O_2 exposure is attended by a return to normal appearance of histologic morphology of the gland. Adrenalectomy serves to offer appreciable protection against O_2 toxicity; under these conditions, the injection of epinephrine aggravates the symptoms of O_2 poisoning.

Individual variation in response to O_2 inhalation, notably in the pressure range of 2.5 to 3.5 ata, can be attributed in large measure to the factors enumerated, namely, variable levels of CO_2 in the lungs, blood, and fixed tissue, exercise, metabolic state of the individual, and endocrine factors involving the adrenal and other glands, and sympathetic pathways.

C. MODIFICATION OF O_2 TOXICITY BY SURGICAL INTERVENTION

Clinically, there is a durable impression that hypoxemic patients tolerate unusually high pulmonary O_2 tensions. Experimentally, a right-to-left surgical shunt which largely prevents elevation of arterial O_2 tension when dogs are exposed to hyperbaric O_2 (2.5 ata), serves not only to prevent convulsions but also reduce the extent of pulmonary damage and delay onset of death (Winter et al., 1967). The question arises as to whether or not the protective effect of venous admixture is mediated centrally for example, by neuro-humoral factors, or locally by reason of reduced O_2 pressure which spares vascular endothelium. Thomas et al. (1969) have done much to clarify this problem. Their ingenious surgical techniques made possible two types of lung perfusion relative to a constant alveolar O_2 tension (3 ata) firstly, with arterialized blood, and secondly, with predominantly mixed venous blood. Further O_2 inhalation consisted of repeated exposures (60 to 120) of dogs (4 times daily, 1-hr O_2 and 1-hr air). This procedure practically eliminated convulsive seizures as well as respiratory distress and insufficiency.

It was found that perfusion of the lungs with 'low O_2' blood (pulmonary venous oxygen tension from 90 to 640 mm Hg) protected the lungs; perfusion with 'high O_2' blood (pulmonary venous oxygen tension from 1650 to 1970 mm Hg) damaged the lungs. Essentially, the histologic pulmonary changes in the face of constant pressure of inhaled O_2 (3 ata) were proportional to the level of pulmonary venous O_2. It would appear that the lungs, by surgical procedure, were protected in the same manner as the heart with its high extraction rate, namely, by the creation of a low O_2 tension in the milieu of tissue.

5. Time-Pressure Relationship of OHP and Visual Cells

Noel (1962) and Bridges (1967) demonstrated progressive functional and pathologic derangements in a homogeneous cell population closely identified over a wide range with time of exposure and level of O_2 pressure. Heretofore, it has not been possible to show a continuum on a time-pressure plot of injury either to the lungs or to the nervous system. Both morphologic and functional dichotomy tend to separate the responses of the two systems relative to high and lower pressure. The visual cells of the rabbit provide the homogeneous cellular matrix which reacts to O_2 in a striking parallelism to the adverse reactions (time and pressure-dependent) in man.

The visual system (including its vascular elements) is especially sensitive to O_2 (Figure 1E). In the premature infant, vasoconstriction and 'reactive' proliferation of blood vessels characterize retro-lental fibroplasia (Figure 1G). A second lesion of the eye has been identified in the nerve fiber layer of the retina of dogs, characterized by cytoid bodies, which reflect segmental degeneration of axons. The third impairment is functional disruption and death of visual cells.

The electroretinogram (ERG) is the electrical response to a flash of light recorded by an electrode in contact with the cornea or inserted into the anterior chamber of the eye. Continued exposure of the rabbit to an O_2 pressure of 1 ata or higher results in severe attenuation or disappearance of the ERG whether or not systemic effects are evident. At pressures of several atmospheres the onset of O_2 poisoning is reflected by the depression and subsequent extinction of the beta-wave component of the ERG (Figure 1F). The tolerance time for O_2 inhalation in man (3 ata) coincides with the onset of ERG (beta-wave decline) in the rabbit. The data in Table IX show the

TABLE IX

Response of a visual cell population (rabbit) to increased oxygen pressure
(Noel, 1958)

Oxygen pressure (ata)	Visual cell death	
	Duration of exposure (min)	Cell death
0.50	12 days	none
0.55 to 0.60	7 days	in 50% of animals
1.0	40 hr	in 100% of animals
	Duration of latent period prior to beta wave decline in the electroretinogram (min)	
3	100	
4	80	
5	60	
7	20	

continuity of untoward responses of the visual system during the course of long exposures at relatively low pressures and short exposures at pressures as high as 7 atmospheres (Figure 1H).

Recovery of beta-wave sensitivity starts in a few minutes after onset of air-breathing. "It proceeded at almost constant rate until 75% of the control amplitude had been regained. This required from 30 to 90 min. Recovery of the remaining deficit occurred slowly, and 3 to 6 hr were generally needed until the ERG was the same as prior to exposure." Recovery was delayed when the exposure was prolonged beyond the time of occurrence of a marked decrease in the beta-wave. It then often required more than 24 hr and it was occasionally incomplete. Of 6 animals exposed to approximately 3 ata for 5 to $6\frac{1}{2}$ hr (beta-wave decline starting at about 2 hr); 4 showed death of a small fraction of the visual cell population indicating the irreversibility of the changes incurred during exposure".

6. Etiology of O_2 Poisoning – A Biochemical Wilderness

Incapacitating procedures which suppress metabolism or restrict normal function (adrenalectomy, thyroidectomy, hypothermia) and various substances have been demonstrated to improve tolerance of small animals to hyperbaric O_2. Thus, certain monoamine oxidase inhibitors (pargyline, iproniazid) provide significant protection in the rat from neurologic manifestations of O_2 toxicity (Blenkarn et al., 1969). Likewise, succinate with its high adenosine triphosphate (ATP) capacity is protective, again for the rat. The dosage of succinate required, however, is large (1400 mg/kg), and requires infusion of large volumes of hypertonic fluid in fasted animals. Regulation of acid-base balance by such substances as tris-buffer (THAM) and sodium lactate for more complicated reasons (Felig, 1965) appear to be more applicable to man.

Heretofore, it has not been possible to discover any effect on any isolated enzyme system which occurs with sufficient rapidity to explain the time of onset of convulsive seizures. Furthermore, in vitro tissue slices of brain are exposed to far greater tensions of O_2 than those which in vivo are restricted by blood flow and diffusion. Chance et al. (1966) have recognized the temporal discrepancy between immediate adverse reactions and the more extended time required to inactivate sulfhydryl groups of dehydrogenases. They point to their observations that O_2-induced oxidation of pyridine nucleotide in mitochondria may account for early symptomatology, specifically convulsions. However, this finding pertains to the effect of O_2 pressures well above any therapeutic level. Straub (1967), for example, was able to show that there was no difference between the O_2 effect at 3 ata compared with that at normal pressure, in reduction of nucleotide (NAD) in mitochondria of rat liver. Further, in view of relatively high concentrations of substrate, one would tend to focus on enzymes with their lower concentrations (by a factor of one thousand or more), which are known to be highly sensitive to hyperbaric O_2. The chapter by Wood (1969) and the review by Haugaard (1968) summarize current knowledge. A biochemical statement of 'recovery' time for enzymes sensitive to hyperbaric O_2 would be welcome.

In any case, the biochemical wilderness can be left to the prescient investigators trained and equipped to unravel devious metabolic pathways. Until 'normalase' is isolated and crystallized, we must depend upon the rapid regeneration of this elusive substance when O_2 is replaced by air. In the meantime, by properly spacing the intervals of O_2 and air inhalation, we may extend O_2 tolerance manyfold.

References

Balentine, J. D. and Gutsche, B. B.: 1966, *Amer. J. Path.* **48**, 107.

Bean, J. W.: 1955, in *Proceedings First Underwater Physiology Symposium*, NAS/NRC Publ. 377, National Academy of Sciences – National Research Council, Washington, D.C., p. 13.

Becker-Freyseng, H. and Clamann, H. G.: 1950, in *German Aviation Medicine in World War II*. U.S. Government Printing Office, Washington, D.C., Vol. I, p. 493.

Behnke, A. R., Shaw, L. A., Shilling, C. W., *et al.*: 1934, *Amer. J. Physiol.* **107**, 13.

Behnke, A. R., Johnson, F. S., Poppen, J. R., and Motley, E. P.: 1935, *Amer. J. Physiol.* **110**, 565.

Behnke, A. R., Forbes, H. S., and Motley, E. P.: 1936, *Amer. J. Physiol.* **114**, 436.

Bennett, G. A. and Smith, F. J. C.: 1934, *J. Exp. Med.* **59**, 181.

Bert, P.: 1878, *La Pression Barométrique*, Masson, Paris.

Blenkarn, G. D., Schanberg, S. M., and Saltzman, H. A.: 1969, *J. Pharmacol. Exp. Therap.* **166**, 346.

Bridges, W. Z.: 1966, *Arch. Ophthalmol.* **75**, 812.

Caldwell, P. R. B., Lee, W. L., Jr., Schildkraut, H. S., and Archibald, E. R.: 1966, *J. Appl. Physiol.* **21**, 1477.

Chance, B., Jamieson, D., and Williamson, J. R.: 1966, in *Proceedings Third International Conference on Hyperbaric Medicine*, NAS/NRC Publ. 1404, National Academy of Sciences – National Research Council, Washington, D.C., p. 15.

Clark, J. M. and Lambertsen, C. J.: 1967, in *Proceedings Third Underwater Physiology Symposium*, Williams & Wilkins, Baltimore, p. 439.

Comroe, J. H., Jr., Dripps, R. D., Dumke, P. R. and Deming, M.: 1945, *J.A.M.A.* **128**, 710.

Criswick, V. G. and Harris, G. S.: 1967, *Arch. Ophthalmol.* **78**, 788.

Donald, K. W.: 1947, *Brit. J. Med.* **1**, 722.

Edström, J. E. and Röchert, H.: 1961, *Acta Physiol. Scand.* **55**, 255.

Felig, P.: 1965, *Aerospace Med.* **36**, 658.

Fisher, A. B., Hyde, R. W., Puy, R. J. M., *et al.*: 1968, *J. Appl. Physiol.* **24**, 529.

Haldane, J. B. S.: 1941, *Nature* **148**, 458.

Haugaard, N.: 1968, *Physiol. Rev.* **48**, 311.

Hill, L.: 1933, *Quart. J. Exp. Physiol.* **23**, 49.

Jacobs, E. A., Winter, P. M., Alvis, H. J., and Small, S. M.: 1969, in *Proceedings Fourth International Congress on Hyperbaric Medicine*, Sapporo, Japan, p. 67.

Jamieson, D.: 1966, in *Proceedings Third International Conference on Hyperbaric Medicine*, NAS/NRC Publ. 1404, National Academy of Sciences – National Research Council, Washington, D.C., p. 89.

Kistler, G. S., Caldwell, P. R. B., and Weibel, E. R.: 1967, *J. Cell Biol.* **33**, 605.

Lambertsen, C. J.: 1953, *J. Appl. Physiol.* **5**, 471.

Lambertsen, C. J.: 1965, in *Handbook of Physiology*, Section 3: *Respiration*, Vol. II., American Physiological Society, Washington, D.C., p. 1027.

Lanphier, E. H.: 1963, in *Proceedings Second Underwater Physiology Symposium* NAS/NRC Publ. 1181, National Academy of Sciences – National Research Council, Washington, D.C., p. 124.

Latham, F.: 1951, *Lancet* **1**, 77.

Noel, W. K.: 1962, in *Environmental Effects on Consciousness* (ed. by K. E. Schaefer), Macmillan, New York, p. 3.

Patz, A.: 1968, *Trans. Amer. Ophthal. Soc.* **66**, 941.

Saltzman, H. A.: 1965, in *Monographs of the Surgical Sciences*, Williams & Wilkins, Baltimore.

Shaw, L. A., Behnke, A. R., and Messer, A. C.: 1934, *Amer. J. Physiol.* **108**, 652.

Smith, J. L.: 1899, *J. Physiol.* **24**, 19.

Staub, N. C., Nagano, H., and Pearce, M. L.: 1967, *J. Appl. Physiol.* **22**, 227.

Straub, J. P.: 1967, *Nature* **215**, 1196.

Thomas, A. N., Ketchum, S. A. III, Hall, A. D., and Zubrin, J. R.: 1969, *Proceedings Fourth International Congress on Hyperbaric Medicine*, Sapporo, Japan, p. 9.

Winter, P. M., Gupta, R. K., Michalaski, A. H., and Lanphier, E. H.: 1967, *J. Appl. Physiol.* **23**, 954.

Wood, J. D.: 1969, in *Physiology and Medicine of Diving and Compressed Air Work* (ed. by P. B. Bennett and D. H. Elliott), Williams & Wilkins, Baltimore, p. 113.

Yarbrough, O. D., Welham, W., Brinton, E. S., and Behnke, A. R.: 1947, Experimental Diving Unit, Rept. No. 1, Project X-337, Washington Navy Yard, Washington, D.C.

OSCILLATIONS IN EXPIRATORY GAS FLOW
DURING PERFORMANCE OF FORCED VITAL CAPACITY

D. H. GLAISTER

R.A.F. Institute of Aviation Medicine, Farnborough, Hants., U.K.

1. Introduction

When water was made to flow through a thin-walled latex rubber tube immersed in a tank of water, oscillations in flow occurred when the pressure at the downstream end of the tube was less than the surrounding hydrostatic pressure. High-speed cine-photography showed that the central portion of the tube first started to narrow. The narrowing then became more pronounced and moved downstream until complete closure occurred when the constriction reached the downstream end (Figure 1). At this point, flow ceased. The tube then reopened and the sequence was repeated, the frequency of repetition being of the order of 2 to 10 cps.

During a forceful expiration, similar pressure relationships develop within the thorax. This is explained on the basis that, while the same pressure is applied externally to the alveoli as to the airways, the internal pressure drops with distance due to flow resistance, so generating a transmural pressure difference which tends to collapse the larger airways. Any reduction in calibre which results increases the resistance to flow, and so increases the closing pressure. Additionally, if air-flow is laminar, the Bernoulli effect leads to the development of a low pressure zone within the constriction which will also further its development. If complete closure does occur, then cessation of flow will lead to equalization of pressures and the elastic airways will reopen. The cycle could then be repeated.

McWilliam *et al.* (1966) predicted the development of a constriction at the junction of the intrathoracic and extrathoracic portions of the trachea during forced expiration, and commented that "a stable throat is unlikely to be formed... collapse cannot be maintained continuously and flow oscillates". These investigators observed oscillation in rubber tube models, but were unable to obtain evidence of similar oscillation in man. Earlier, Fry and Hyatt (1960) had likened the intrathoracic airways to Starling resistors (collapsible tubes in pressure chambers) and stated that "under certain conditions this type of system will become unstable so that the flow will oscillate".

The presence of cartilage does not prevent narrowing of the larger airways, for such narrowing has been seen in man during coughing (Holden and Ardran, 1957; Marshall and Holden, 1963), and complete closure of the trachea has been demonstrated in isolated specimens (Dekker and Groen, 1957). In this case the pressure required to close the trachea was only one-seventh of that recorded within the esophagus in the present investigation (70 mm Hg).

The factors which govern the maximum attainable expiratory flow become of importance under conditions where resistance to flow is increased by some additional

D. E. Busby (ed.), Recent Advances in Aerospace Medicine, 226–232. All Rights Reserved.
Copyright © 1970 by D. Reidel Publishing Company, Dordrecht - Holland.

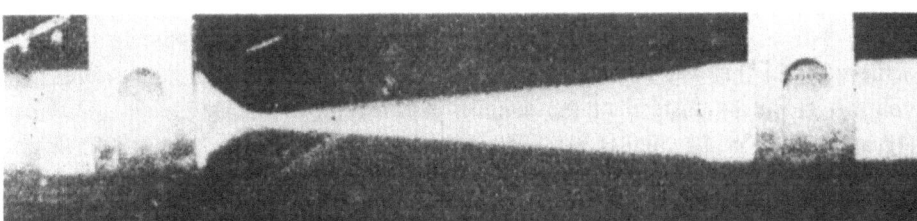

Fig. 1. Frames from high-speed cine film illustrating oscillatory behaviour of a thin-walled latex tube 1 cm in diameter when water flows through it and the outlet pressure is less than the 5 cm water hydrostatic pressure which surrounds it. (A) tube fully open. (B) constriction forms. (C) constriction develops and moves downstream. (D) tube closed at downstream end. Sequence repeats at 3 cps.

mechanism. While the commonest circumstance is obstructive disease of the airways, of particular relevance to environmental medicine is the breathing of dense gas mixtures, such as sulfur hexafluoride or air under increased pressure, and ultimately the breathing of a liquid which would be needed to increase man's tolerance to acceleration by eliminating all gas from the thoracic cavity.

2. Method

Flow-volume curves were recorded during forced vital capacity manoeuvres using an Electro/Med Model 780 waterless spirometer. This instrument gives electrical volume and, by differentiation, flow outputs. Its frequency response is stated to be flat to 50 cps and its resonant frequency was 42.5 cps. Preliminary studies showed that flow rates of 15 1/sec. could be achieved within 60 msec of the start of a forced expiratory effort. Thus, if an X-Y plotter were to be used for recording flow-volume curves, a writing speed in excess of that of any available instrument would be required. This problem was overcome by recording the flow and volume signals on magnetic tape at 30 in/sec, and then replaying on to a Bryans Autoplotter Model 22020 at $3\frac{3}{4}$ in/sec. This gave the plotter an effective writing speed of 30 ft/sec on either axis, and the ability faithfully to reproduce oscillations of up to 40 cps with an amplitude of up to 6 cm.

For each recording of forced vital capacity, the subject inspired maximally and then expired maximally and as forcibly as possible into the spirometer. It was found that vibration of the flexible low-resistance tubing supplied with the instrument could induce artefactual oscillations in the flow record, so the subject was either connected directly to the spirometer or through a length of 2 in internal diameter rigid brass tube. The natural resonant frequency of this pipe was calculated to be 70 cps. At maximal flow rates the back pressure induced by the recording system was less than one centimeter of water.

3. Results and Discussion

Figure 2 shows three flow-volume curves obtained from a subject breathing air at normal atmospheric pressure. The X-axis was displaced between recordings to aid clarity. After one litre of gas had been expired, a peak flow of some 15 1/sec was achieved, and this was followed by a flow which decayed to zero at residual lung volume. However, instead of the smooth exponential decline classically described (Hyatt et al, 1958; Fry and Hyatt, 1960; Schilder et al, 1963), oscillations in flow rate were apparent. When this subject repeated the manoeuvre in a compression chamber at a total pressure of 4 ata, peak flows were decreased and the curves became more irregular, but oscillations at the original frequency of 9 cps were still seen (Figure 3).

Figure 4 shows similar recordings from another subject at normal atmospheric pressure, and here oscillations are seen to persist throughout most of the vital capacity (most obvious in the second of the three records). The frequency of oscillation was constant, hence independent of lung volume, averaging 11.4 cps. The apparent closing up of the flow peaks with diminishing lung volume is due to the decreasing flow rate

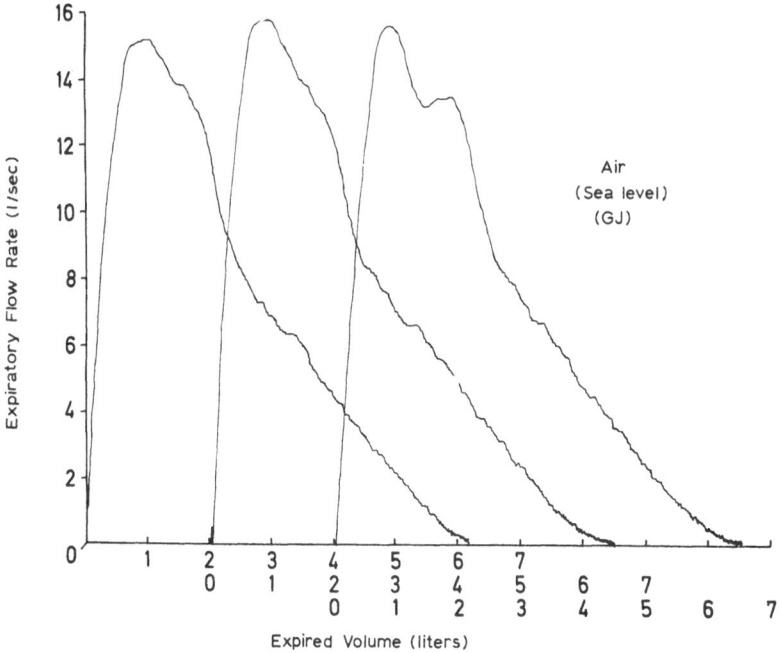

Fig. 2.   Expiratory flow-volume curves obtained during three forced vital capacities with subject breathing air. The X-axis has been shifted between each recording.

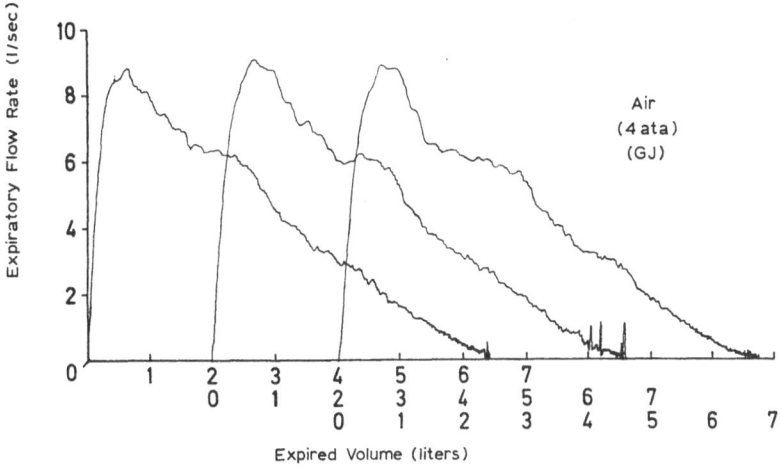

Fig. 3.   As Figure 2 but with the subject breathing air at a pressure of 4 ata. Up to 3 low frequency oscillations are visible in each recording and on these are superimposed higher frequency components.

with subsequent compression of the X-axis. Figure 5 shows recordings from this subject performing at a pressure of 4 ata, and Figure 6 his performance following a vital capacity breath of sulfur hexafluoride. This procedure gave the expired gas a density about 4.5 times that when breathing air and, as expected, the result was very similar to that obtained with air at a pressure of 4 ata.

Recordings of forced vital capacities from 2 subjects breathing air at 1 and 4 ata and from 3 subjects breathing air and sulfur hexafluoride were transferred to punched tape and submitted to Fourier analysis on an I.C.L. 1907 computer. The relative amplitudes of frequency components from 5 to 35 cps, obtained from one subject

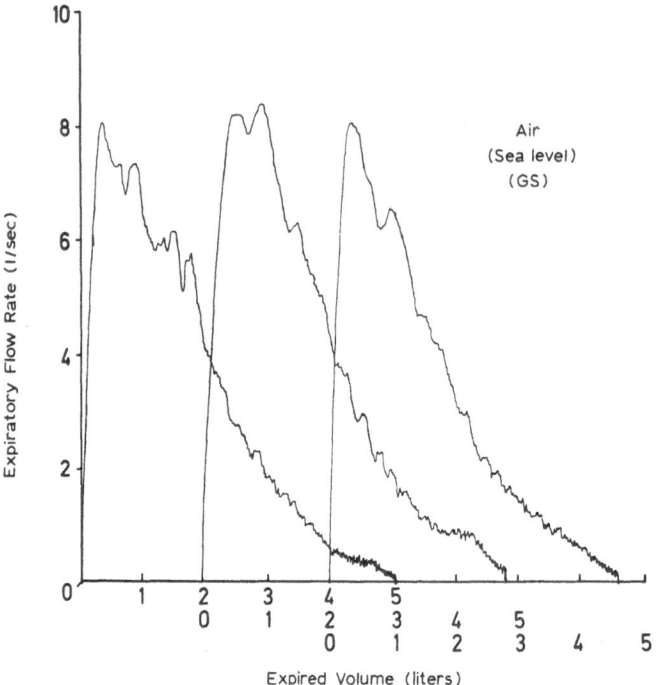

Fig. 4.   Expiratory flow-volume curves from a second subject breathing air at atmospheric pressure. Obvious oscillations are present, and in the second recording these persist throughout most of the vital capacity.

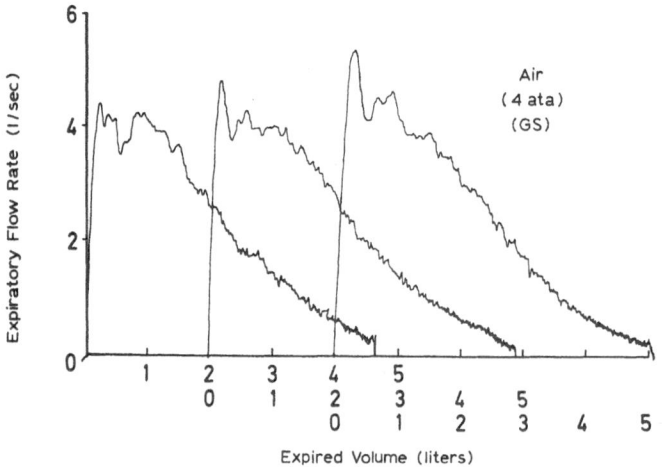

Fig. 5.   As Figure 4, but with subject breathing air at a pressure of 4 ata.

breathing air at the differing pressures, are shown in Figure 7. Each histogram is based on the average of three manoeuvres. A base line analysis showed that the noise contribution fell from a relative amplitude of 0.3 at 5 to 10 cps, to an average amplitude of 0.1 from 11 to 35 cps. At one atmosphere (left hand panel, Figure 7), the relative amplitude fell with increasing frequency to approach the noise level at 35 cps. At a pressure of 4 ata, there was an increase in the higher frequency components and their

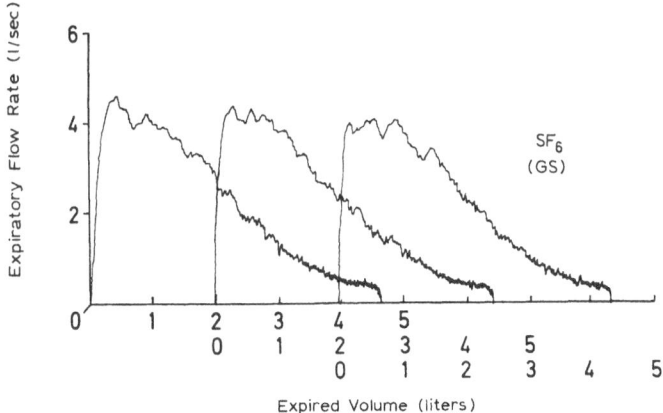

Fig. 6.   As Figure 4, but following a maximal inspiration of sulphur hexafluoride.

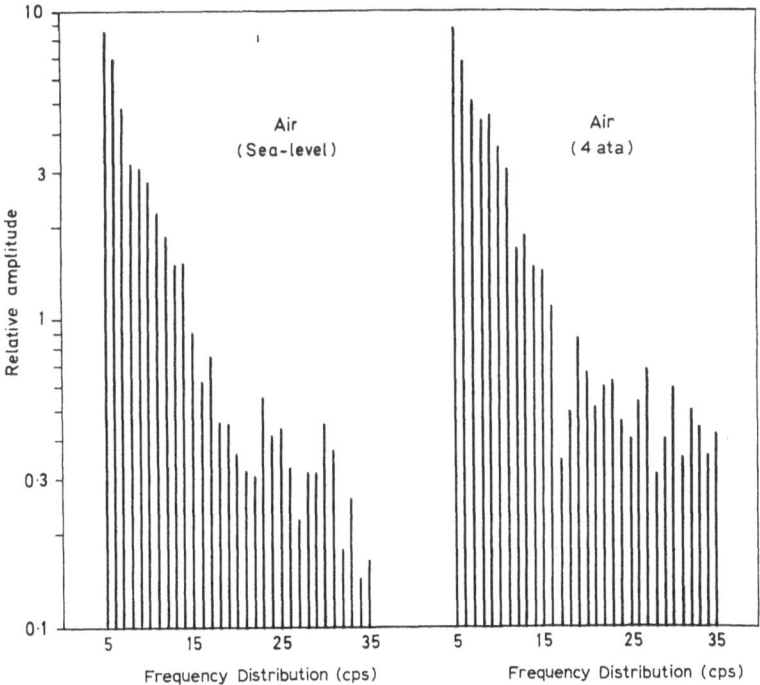

Fig. 7.   Frequency distributions obtained by Fourier analysis of curves illustrated in Figures 4 and 5. The relative amplitude of components above 15 cps is increased by breathing the denser atmosphere.

amplitude tended to flatten out at a value of about 0.4. While these differences were quite small, they were seen consistently, and a similar increase in the high frequency components was seen when sulfur hexafluoride was breathed.

Towards the end of the second forced vital capacity manoeuvre illustrated in Figure 3, the subject coughed three times. Coughs were preceded by a brief cessation of expiratory flow, and resulted in a flow rate several times the maximum which could be attained by voluntary effort at that lung volume. Thus, the low flows seen towards the end of the manoeuvre were not simply the outcome of inefficient muscle action. It appears that initial closure of the glottis causes airways to open as airway pressures equalize. Subsequent opening of the glottis permits a greatly increased gas flow, though this must be transient as airways soon close again. In the present experiments coughing was often seen when subjects breathed air at increased pressure, or sulfur hexafluoride, but was rarely seen when air was breathed at atmospheric pressure.

4. Conclusions

The observation of oscillation in air flow supports the concept that airways may behave like Starling resistors and become unstable during expiration. If oscillations result from cyclic alterations in airway calibre, then the oscillation which is seen to occur at 8 to 11 cps must occur is a common airway, or in a number of airways oscillating in phase. The simplest explanation is that these oscillations are taking place in the intrathoracic portion of the trachea. In this respect the studies of Hamosh and Luchsinger (1968), on isolated, liquid-filled lungs are of interest. They noted intermittent flow as saline drained from the lung, and motion pictures showed that all the extra-pulmonary airways were oscillating. Further studies are required to determine if the same phenomena can be seen with air.

When a dense gas is breathed, the pressure drop along the airways increases and the point at which collapse will tend to occur will move upstream. In this way a greater number of smaller airways will become involved and the frequency of oscillation would be expected to rise. However, individual airways need not oscillate in phase. Inspection of the recordings suggests that the larger airways are still oscillating, and at a frequency apparently unaffected by gas density. It seems that the properties of the airway wall may be more important than those of the flowing gas in determining their dynamic behaviour, and that each portion of the airway has its characteristic frequency of oscillation.

References

Dekker, E. and Groen, J.: 1957, *Lancet* **1**, 1064.
Fry, D. L. and Hyatt, R. E.: 1960, *Amer. J. Physiol.* **29**, 672.
Hamosh, P. and Luchsinger, P. C.: 1968, *J. Appl. Physiol.* **25**, 485.
Holden, W. S. and Ardran, G. M.: 1957, *J. Fac. Radiol. (Lond.)* **8**, 267.
Hyatt, R. E., Schilder, D. P., and Fry, D. L.: 1958, *J. Appl. Physiol.* **13**, 331.
McWilliam, R., Nightingale, J. M., and Kinnier-Wilson, A. B.: 1966, *Med. Biol. Eng.* **4**, 555.
Marshall, R. and Holden, W. S.: 1963, *Thorax* **18**, 54.
Schilder, D. P., Roberts, A., and Fry, D. L.: 1963, *J. Clin. Invest.* **42**, 1705.

SECTION IV

MAN IN HIS KINETIC ENVIRONMENT

DYNAMIC CROSS-COUPLING IN THE SEMICIRCULAR CANALS

G. MELVILL JONES

Defence Research Board, Aviation Medical Research Unit,
Dept. of Physiology, McGill University, Montréal, Québec, Canada

1. Introduction

The physical response of a semicircular canal to rotational movement in its own plane is the outcome of continuous interplay between forces due to inertia and viscosity of the contained fluid and elasticity of the cupula. When the head rotates relative to an already rotating platform, the interactions of these three variables in a set of three orthogonal canals is rather complex. Various authors have examined these interactions using a variety of analytical methods. Groen (1961) has examined the matter in terms of the physical properties of a spinning top. On the other hand, several authors have examined the cross-coupling effects in terms of the Coriolis forces which are applied to the mass of fluid contained in the canals when one canal is brought into and out of the plane of rotation. Peters' (1969) analyses are particularly valuable since he compared the analysis of Coriolis forces with component vector analysis and showed that the two methods of analysis yield identical conclusions about patterns of mechanical end-organ response.

The present article does not repeat these detailed analytical treatments, but rather aims to examine the functional nature of cross-coupled responses in terms which it is hoped may be understandable by those who are unfamiliar with the relevent methods of analysis. For this, it is helpful to examine first the response of a simplified model comprising only one circular canal and without introduction of forces due to cupular elasticity; that is, considering the fluid displacement in a circular tube which has no transducing cupular system interfering with the flow pattern of response.

Before proceeding, however, it should be forcefully pointed out that adverse dynamic cross-coupling in the canal system which forms the basis of this article, arises only when time has permitted the elastic restoring force due to cupular deflection to have played a material part in the overall response of the end-organ. In natural life it seems that the everyday patterns of head movement fall within the frequency band which does not permit the intrusion either of elastic cupular restoration or delayed fluid displacement due to the inertial-viscous time constant (Melvill Jones and Milsum, 1965). Thus it seems likely that significant adverse effects due to dynamic cross-coupling in the canals does not normally occur in natural life. The effects are specific to particular, unnatural, man-made, movement environments such as those of flight and space, and hence the detection and amelioration of these powerful adverse effects becomes a matter which holds especial significance in the science of aviation medicine.

D. E. Busby (ed.), Recent Advances in Aerospace Medicine, 235–248. All Rights Reserved.
Copyright © 1970 by D. Reidel Publishing Company, Dordrecht-Holland.

2. Mechanical End-Organ Response

A. SINGLE CIRCULAR CANAL WITH NO CUPULA

In this simple model, an angular acceleration in the plane of the canal, from rest to say 60 deg/sec, would result in a volume displacement of fluid round the canal circuit which would at all times be proportional to the instantaneous angular velocity of the platform, always assuming the inertia/viscosity time constant to be insignificantly small (van Egmond *et al.*, 1949; Mayne, 1950; Melvill Jones and Milsum, 1965).

In the present context, it is important to appreciate that in the absence of a cupular restoring force, the physical response of this system, namely volume displacement of fluid round the circuit, would continue to register 60 deg/sec angular velocity as long as this steady rotation continued in the plane of the circular tube. This feature can easily be demonstrated by filling a plastic transparent tube of about ½ in diameter with silicone fluid of about 50 centipois viscosity containing a few flecks of visible indicator having approximately the same density as the contained fluid and then joining the two ends after exclusion of any bubbles of air. If such a mechanical ana-logue of a canal is rotated in its own plane, one can see how the fluid displaces by an amount always proportional to the angular velocity achieved, returning to its original position when the rotation is stopped.

Figure 1 illustrates this phenomenon using the notation of a vector of angular velocity, having direction oriented along the axis of rotation and magnitude propor-tional to the length of the arrowed line. The usual convention is adopted here, in which an arrow denotes clockwise rotation as viewed when looking along the arrow in its direction of 'flight'. Thus the arrow in the left hand diagram of Figure 1 denotes angular velocity vector of response about a vertical axis (clockwise when looking along the arrow) having a speed proportional to arrow length. On arresting rotation, the contained fluid would return to its original position in the canal and hence the vector representing response would also return to zero.

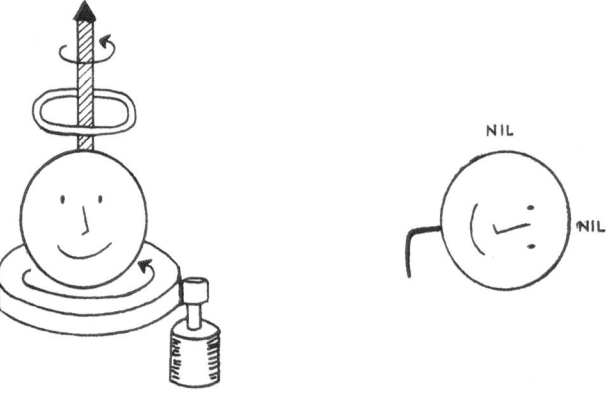

Fig. 1.   Response of a single circular canal containing fluid, but no cupula. The large vertical arrow denotes the angular velocity vector of response; direction along the axis of rotation (clockwise looking along the arrow) and magnitude proportional to length.

If during maintained rotation of the platform which carries this canal, the canal is itself turned through a right angle about an axis perpendicular to that of the rotating platform, then the canal's actual rotation in its own plane must be decelerated to zero angular velocity (see right hand diagram in Figure 1). As before, the angular deceleration must drive the fluid back to its starting point, and again this phenomenon can easily be seen with the simple mechanical analogue canal described above. Note particularly that in Figure 1 a circular tube containing fluid without the presence of an elastic cupula is still being considered.

If the above conclusion is true for one unobstructed circular canal, then it is equally true for each of three similar orthogonal (right angular) canals. Hence, with proper trigonometric resolution of rotational velocity vectors associated with the separate canal responses, such a three-canal system should yield the correct vector (direction and magnitude) of head angular velocity relative to space, provided there were no forces due to cupular elasticity. Such a system would act as a good 'DC' 3-D angular speedometer which would function equally well on Earth and in space.

B. SINGLE CANAL WITH CUPULAR ELASTICITY

Now consider a similar maneuver, again applied to a single canal, but this time with

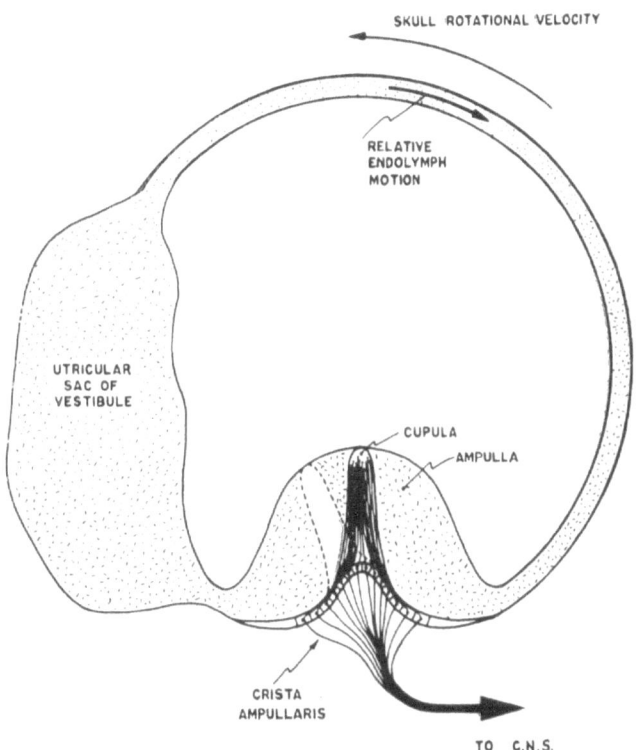

Fig. 2.   Displacement of the elastic cupula due to circulation of fluid in the canal.
(Mevill Jones and Milsum, 1965.)

introduction of forces due to cupular elasticity. Figure 2 is a diagrammatic representation of a semicircular canal, and illustrates how relative circulation of contained
fluid deflects the water-tight, swing-door cupula, so that cupular elasticity tends to
return the fluid with a force proportional to the angle of cupular deflection and
hence also to the angle of fluid displacement around the canal. The new situation is
represented diagrammatically in Figure 3, which uses similar notation to that in
Figure 1. At rest the response is zero. Then with sudden acceleration to 60 deg/sec
angular velocity in the plane of the canal, there is volume displacement of fluid round
the canal circuit, and hence cupular deviation proportional to the instantaneous
angular velocity of the canal. A vector develops as indicated in the top left diagram of
the figure. However, on assuming a constant angular velocity of 60 deg/sec, cupular
elasticity this time forces the fluid exponentially back whence it came, with a time
constant in man of about 15 to 20 sec. After, say, 10 sec the vector of response
becomes reduced somewhat as in the second diagram of Figure 3. After 1 to 2 min
(about four-time constants) the system then incorrectly registers essentially zero
angular velocity of response.

Now consider the situation on turning this model, with cupular elasticity built in,
through a right angle. As before, the canal's actual rotation in its own plane then
becomes decelerated to zero angular velocity. Consequently, inertial forces must
drive the fluid in the canal, this time away from, rather than towards the zero position.
Hence a response is generated, registering angular velocity in the new plane adopted
by the canal. Since the cupula is now deflected in a direction opposite to that in the

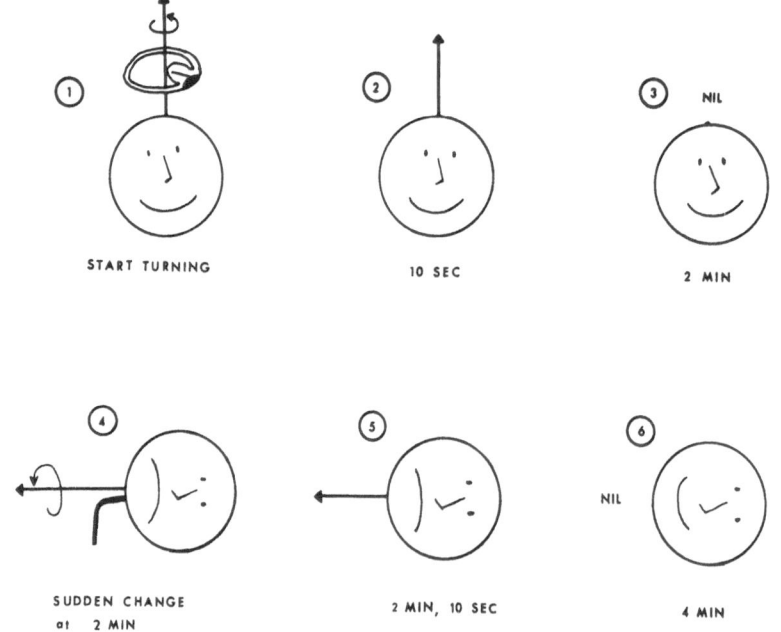

Fig. 3.   Response of a *single* canal *with* its elastic watertight cupula. Rotation of the platform is
initiated at (1) and maintained throughout.

first diagram of Figure 1 (relative to the head) we have to draw the vector of response as indicated in the fourth diagram of Figure 3. This vector thus represents what is familiarly known as 'post-rotational sensation'. However, owing to having turned the head through one right angle, the direction of post-rotational sensation must be carried through one right angle also. Note incidently that in these specific circumstances, this single canal system generates 'sensation' of rotational velocity in a plane which is at right angles to both those of the platform rotation and the transient head rotation (rotation of head from erect to shoulder positions). With cupular elasticity, this post-rotational vector of angular velocity response will decay exponentially, until after about four time constants, there will be zero response about all axes (sixth diagram in Figure 3).

C. COMPLETE CANAL SYSTEM

Thus far, only the case of a single lateral canal has been considered; first, without cupular elasticity, and second, with the introduction of cupular elastic restoring forces. Now consider the response pattern after introduction of the vertical canals. It can be shown that for the purpose of analysis, the two vertical canals can be replaced by a single hypothetical canal in the sagittal plane. This feature is indicated diagrammatically in Figure 4 in which two orthogonal canals, one horizontal and one

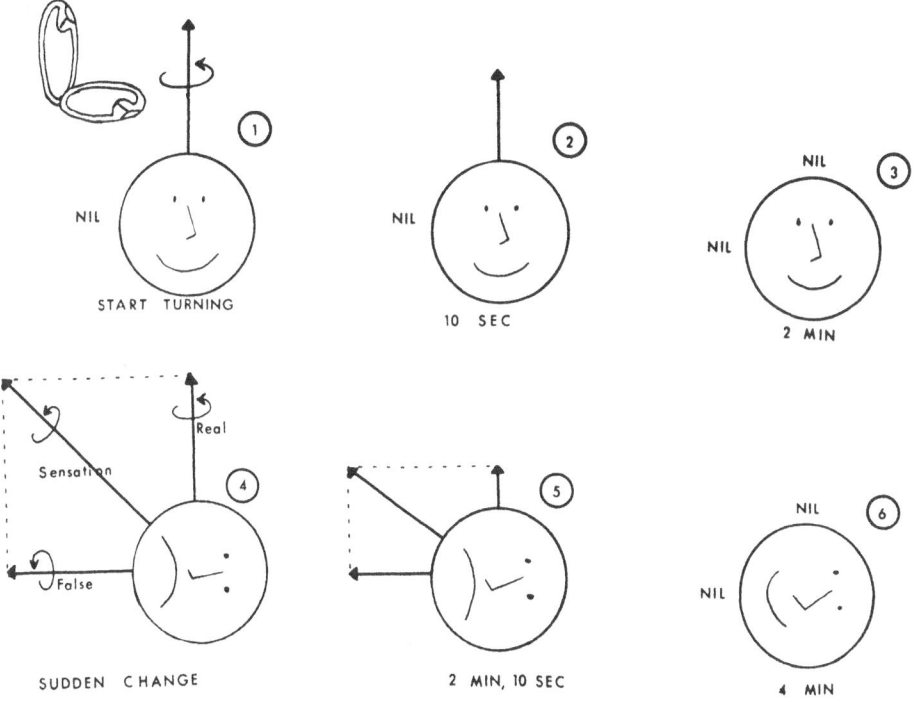

Fig. 4. Combined response of horizontal and vertical canals when the head is suddenly moved from erect to shoulder positions during a prolonged turn started at (1) and maintained constant throughout the rest of the maneuver. Note particularly that in this sequence the head is maintained erect until the initial canal response has died away completely and then turned sharply over on to the left shoulder.

vertical in the sagittal plane, are considered with cupular elasticity introduced in both canals, and symbolized in the figure by diagrammatic illustration of ampullae in the canals. As before, with head erect the whole system is suddenly accelerated in a horizontal plane from rest to say 60 deg/sec. A single vector of angular velocity response emerges at right angles to the horizontal canal since the vertical canal illustrated in the figure is not yet rotated in its own plane. Again with time, due to cupular restoration, the vector of response decays exponentially through the second and third diagrams to register nil response after about four time constants of rotation, suggested in this case as 1 to 2 min.

Now the subject quickly turns his head about a fore-aft axis and through a right angle, until it rests on his left shoulder. Immediately, as in Figure 3, a vector of post-rotational response develops. But in Figure 4, which includes the vertical canal system, an additional vector of response arises due to bringing the vertical canals into the plane of rotation as a result of turning the head through a right angle. The new response in the vertical canals is correctly related to the real rotation. But a response which corresponds to that illustrated in Figure 3 represents the simultaneous false post-rotational response introduced in the lateral canals for the reasons described above.

If these two responses, the real one introduced in the vertical canals, and the false one in the lateral canals, are relayed to the brain stem as equally valid indications of head angular velocity, and assuming trigonometric resolution in the brain stem, the message received by the brain will be represented by the vectorial sum of these two response components. The outcome is illustrated in the third diagram of Figure 4 as the diagonal vector labelled as sensation. The meaningful characteristic of this vectorially combined response would then be of an angular velocity of rotation in a plane at right angles to the indicated vector, having magnitude equal to $\sqrt{2} \times 60 = 85$ deg/sec. This value is arrived at since the length of the resultant vector is that of a hypotenuse of an isosceles, right-angled triangle of sides representing the original 60 deg/sec angular velocity of turn. Again, as before, cupular elasticity will reduce the relevent vectors to zero over an exponential time course.

A complicating factor is encountered in the different rates of cupular restoration attributed to vertical and horizontal canals; response to vertical canal excitation decays considerably faster than that of the lateral canals (Melvill Jones *et al.*, 1964). Thus, the vectors of response about the two orthogonal axes will decay at different rates as indicated in the fifth diagram of Figure 4. Note that in this case the summed response vector not only changes in magnitude, but also in direction relative to the head, moving progressively towards the vector of response having the longest time constant of decay, namely, that pertaining to the lateral canals.

It should be noted that Figures 1, 3 and 4 consider only the case of sudden movement of the head from an erect to a shoulder position. Of course, during rotational movement of the head from erect to shoulder positions, the head is moving with angular velocity in the frontal plane, for which there would be a third vector of response directed into the picture at right angles to both the primary and secondary responses indicated in the fourth diagram of Figure 4. During such head movement, therefore, the total response must be represented by the vectorial sum of all three orthogonal vectors. Accordingly, the more complicated case of slow head movement from erect to shoulder position would invoke a resultant vector which was substantially changing in both direction and magnitude. The real case is then somewhat further complicated by time permitting cupular restoration in all three axes and the solutions for particular cases of real movement must thus be individually calculated. Probably the best approach to useful solution of the general case is analogue simulation, as has been adopted by Young *et al.* (1966).

3. Response of the Whole Organism

For the engineer, analogue simulation of the mechanical end-organ response is a relatively simple matter. But simulation of the whole biological system is much more difficult. First one may inquire, with what fidelity is the physical end-organ response relayed in the neural afferent system to the brain stem.

A. FIDELITY OF NEURAL RESPONSE

Figure 5 illustrates the unit response of a single nerve cell in the medial vestibular nucleus of a cat shown experimentally to be specifically lateral-canal dependent. The

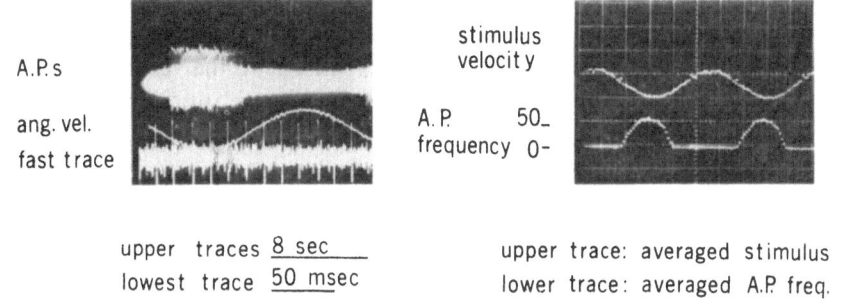

upper traces <u>8 sec</u>   upper trace: averaged stimulus
lowest trace <u>50 msec</u>   lower trace: averaged A.P. freq.

Fig. 5.   Unit neural response obtained from the medial vestibular nucleus of a cat during sinusoidal rotational stimulation of 65 deg/sec angular velocity amplitude and 16 sec period. Original records on left and computer-averaged records (16 cycles) on right. The lowest record on left shows the single unit action potentials displayed during a single fast sweep of the oscilloscope. The averaged record on right has been written out twice to aid visual interpretation of the record.

record was obtained during sinusoidal rotational oscillation of the cat in the plane of the lateral canals. The record indicates that, at least for this cell, the frequency of firing was closely related to the mechanical response of the end-organ, since it was more or less sinusoidally modulated in phase with stimulus angular velocity. Furthermore, Figure 6 illustrates the response of a similar unit to post-rotational stimulation. Just as would be expected from the mechanical response characteristics of the canal endolymph-cupular system, at the moment of stopping rotation the cell burst into high frequency firing, which then decayed exponentially to the steady state condition.

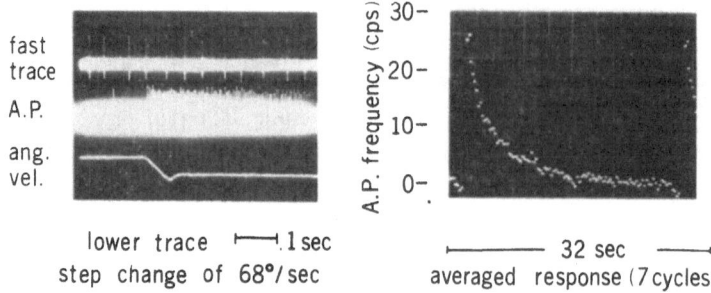

lower trace ⊢——⊣ 1 sec   ⊢——————— 32 sec ——⊣
step change of 68°/sec   averaged response (7 cycles)

Fig. 6.   Post-rotational response of a similar neural unit to that in Figure 5. At the moment of arresting a prolonged steady turn the cell burst into vigorous activity and thereafter the firing frequency decayed exponentially to its original resting level.

From experiments such as these (Melvill Jones, 1967), it seems reasonable to assume that at least thus far in the chain of events (receiving station in the brain stem), the neural signal probably does approximate mechanical response of the end-organ.

Moreover, it is well established that in many circumstances angular velocity stimulation of the semicircular canals will induce compensatory ocular nystagmus as a reflex response operating in the sense which will lead to auto-stabilization of the image of the outside world on the retina of the eye (Hallpike and Hood, 1952). Thus, referring to Figure 3, sudden rotation of the head in the plane of the lateral semicircular canals tends to induce compensatory horizontal nystagmus, the slow phase (compensatory) angular velocity of which closely relates to the vector of response as indicated in diagrams 1, 2 and 3 of this figure. On initiating a steady rotation, horizontal nystagmus develops with a slow phase angular velocity which decays exponentially with time over a time course defined by the time constant of relevant cupular restoration.

Turning now to the lower diagrams in Figure 4, we might anticipate that the pattern of compensatory nystagmus should parallel the pattern of response vector development and decay indicated in the figure. Initially, on suddenly turning the head on to the left shoulder whilst maintaining a continued turn about the vertical axis, we have already seen that the vector of end-organ response should be diagonal, at 45 deg to both the real and false responses from the vertical and horizontal canals respectively. This conclusion would suggest that compensatory nystagmus would operate in a plane at right angles to the resultant vector; that is, diagonally at 45 deg to the sagittal plane. In order to examine the validity of this suggestion, it would be possible, as has been done by Guedry and Montague (1961), to make objective measurements of nystagmus in both vertical and horizontal planes and subsequently to vectorially summate the angular velocity components of slow phase nystagmus in these two planes. However, an alternative method yielding more direct results occurred to the author, using the simple radial-line disc illustrated in Figure 7. When the image of such a disc is made to slip on the retina, then lines parallel to the direction of image slip stand out strongly against all other lines and provide a clear indication of the plane in which such slip is occurring (Melvill Jones and Drazin, 1962). This plane may be indicated by the observer, using markers illustrated in the figure located on a transparent disc, free to move concentrically with the radial line disc and attached to a suitable sensing poten-tiometer. Figure 8 illustrates the results obtained from one subject seated in a small

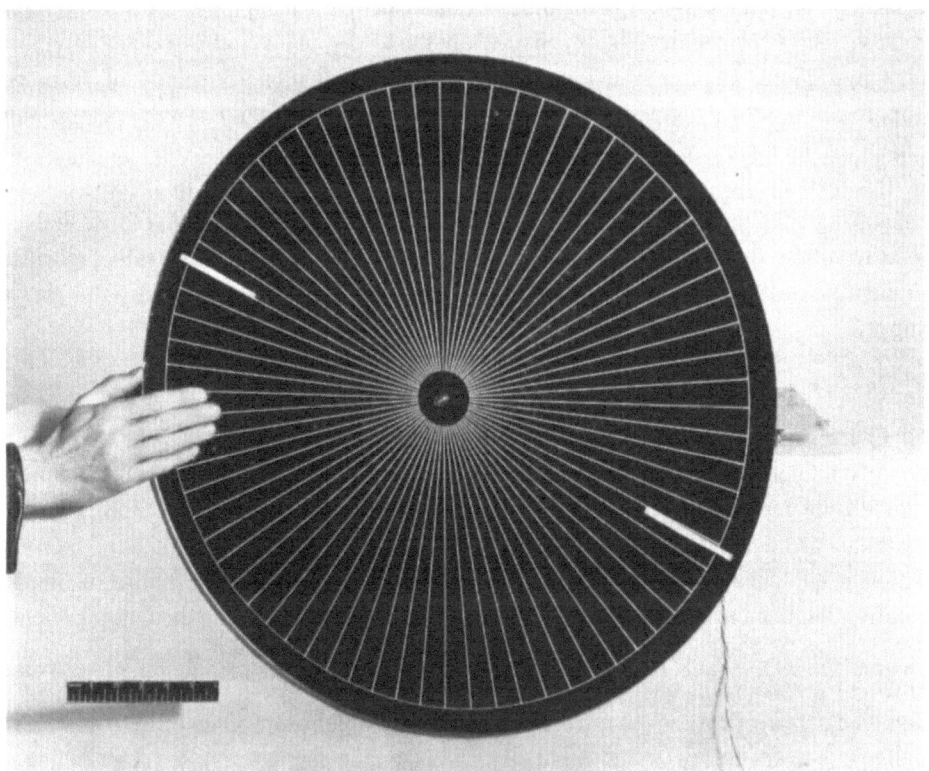

Fig. 7.   The radial-line disc apparatus.

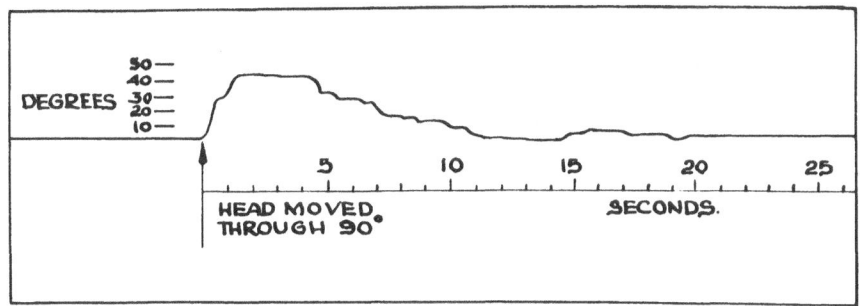

Fig. 8.   Plane of ocular nystagmus after suddenly moving the head from erect to shoulder positions during maintained body rotation (as in Figure 4). Ordinate gives angle between the plane of nystagmus and the yaw ('horizontal') plane of the head.

rotating room in front of the large radial-line disc in which the white lines were illumined from behind in the absence of any other illumination in the room. The subject, seated in front of this disc, was rotated with head erect about a vertical axis for a duration sufficient for all sensation of rotation to die away. He then suddenly rotated his head on to the left shoulder whilst looking at the disc, being required to indicate the lines which appeared to stand out as the result of the induced nystagmus. As can be seen in the figure, at the moment of rotating the head on to the left shoulder, relative image slip occurred in approximately the 45 deg plane, indicating that involuntary nystagmus was generated in this plane. Subsequently, the plane of response apparently moved progressively towards the plane of the lateral canals, presumably reflecting the increased rate of cupular restoration in the vertical canals as suggested in the fifth diagram of Figure 4. Similar results were observed in three subjects, suggesting that in these circumstances the basic oculomotor response does indeed tend to follow the vectorial sum of the separate signals, one real, one false, received in neurological components of the brain stem from the afferent vestibular nerve supply.

B. INFLUENCE OF OPTOKINETIC FIXATION

Of course, in an experiment such as this, the oculomotor response must be significantly influenced by optokinetic fixation reflexes. It has been shown, for example, that during recovery from an aerodynamic spin, the final outcome is the result of dynamic canal cross-coupling together with the influence of optokinetic fixation which itself turns out to have differential effects according to the plane of image rotation relative to the eye (Melvill Jones, 1965). Figure 9 shows the three components of nystagmoid response in the eye of a pilot recovering from an eight-turn spin. During the spin, rotational movement occurred about all three axes, whilst recovery involved arrest of rotational movement together with change of attitude from essentially nose-down to horizontal flight. It can be seen in the figure that at the moment of recovery, post-rotational effects in the yaw and pitch planes were largely eliminated in the oculomotor system by powerful visual fixation. But post-rotational effects in the roll or frontal plane continued almost unimpeded by visual fixation, which appears to

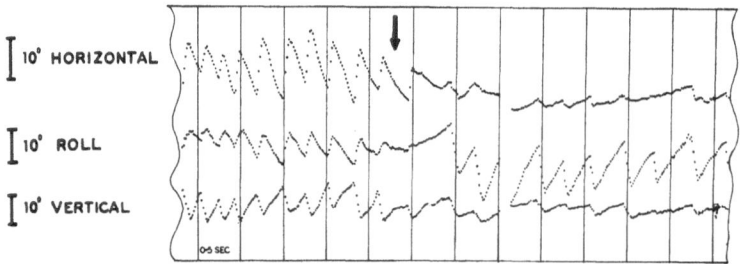

Fig. 9.   Three-dimensional record of oculomotor response in a subject recovering from an eight turn aerodynamic spin. The arrow indicates the moment of spin recovery. (Reproduced from Figure 8 in Melvill Jones, 1964.)

be particularly weak in this plane (Melvill Jones, 1966). The result in this case must be substantial blurring of the image of the horizon due to image slip at an angular velocity quantitatively indicated by the slopes of slow phase components of rotational (torsional) nystagmus shown in the middle trace of the record.

C. ADDITIONAL COMPLICATING FACTORS

Guedry and Montague (1961) have shown that the sensation of response to dynamic cross-coupling stimuli does not necessarily conform with the mechanical response of the end-organ. For example, one might expect that quick rotation of the head onto the left shoulder as in Figure 4 would induce a sensation similar to, but reversed relative to that associated with returning the head to the erect position after complete equilibration to the head-on-shoulder position. In practice, this was not the case. Possibly, some of the anomalies might be attributable to differential effects of the direction of the prevailing gravitational vector upon the time course of sensation decay during continued rotation. For example, Benson and Bodin (1966) state that the "rate of decay of inappropriate post-rotational responses is greater when the linear acceleration is co-planar with the stimulated canals and least when normal to the plane of the canals".

Further features which must play a significant part in the overall biological response are the adaptive and habituation characteristics of the overall system. Malcolm and Melvill Jones (1970), for example, made extensive quantitative determinations of adaptive characteristics in the vestibular system which indicate that there is a tendency for any signal other than that of zero angular velocity to return towards the zero condition at a rate directly dependent on the magnitude of the signal. This term apparently operates independently of, and simultaneously to any signal decay due to end-organ mechanics. On a longer time scale, habituation effects can occur such that with repeated excitation of similar kind, the response of the whole biological, system will become progressively modified from one response to the next. Thus, experiments in the Pensacola slow rotating room (Guedry and Graybiel, 1962) have shown that repeated influence of dynamic cross-coupling effects upon the canals leads to radical modification of vestibulo-ocular responses, probably in such a way as to re-establish automatic stabilization of the eye in the special rotating room environment. Indeed the vestibulo-ocular response modification induced in this way is long-lasting, and apparently rehabituation to the natural environment is necessary after release from the rotating room.

Thus, one can see that it is by no means sufficient to calculate the mechanical response of the canal system due to dynamic cross-coupling effects, and assume that this will predict in a simple way the response of the whole biological system. In reality, it seems that the actual response associated with a complicated real-life situation in flight or space is unlikely to be accurately predictable in terms of current knowledge; experimental investigation of the whole system in the real environment remains the only safe method for determining the real response to a discrete environmental situation.

4. Amelioration of Cross-Coupling Effects

The effects of dynamic cross-coupling of the canals tend to be so troublesome and complex that it would be a great advantage to evolve methods by which they might be ameliorated. In this connection, we might possibly obtain assistance from the experience of the inertial guidance engineer who is confronted with the problem of guiding his rocket system from inertial-sensing elements which in essence have many characteristics similar to those of the biological vestibular system. An important step in simplification of the inertial guidance system is stabilization of the platform on which the system lies. Essentially this involves some form of inertia-sensed feed-back which, whenever an error signal arises, generates platform movements such as to null out that signal. With the platform inertially stabilized, cross-coupling effects such as those discussed above could be greatly ameliorated.

In this context, it is intriguing to find that the overall biological system is provided with strong vestibulo-collic (neck-muscle) reflexes tending, sometimes with remarkable precision, to generate automatic stabilization of the head during body movement. It is well known, for example, that the pigeon when rotated establishes good ocular stabilization by vestibulo-collic reflexes which in many situations virtually completely counteract imposed body rotational movement. The familar head nystagmus of the pigeon comprises a slow phase head movement during which the head is held stationary relative to space whilst the body rotates underneath it, the quick phase movement (saccade) repositioning the head relative to space so that intermittent head stabilization is achieved. It should be noted particularly that, as pointed out by Melvill Jones and Milsum (1965), and subsequently quantatized by Outerbridge (1969), such a mechanism is fundamentally different from vestibulo-ocular reflex stabilization of the eye in that the sensing system of canals is located in the skull but not in the eye. Thus, whereas canal stimulation will generate an appropriate angular velocity of compensatory slow phase eye movement, in the case of head stabilization, a canal signal will generate head movement which nulls out the canal signal which produced it. The vestibulo-collic system therefore functions as an 'error control system', basing its response upon geometrically determined feed-back from the canals. Complete head stabilization must be associated with zero output from the canal. In practice, of course, good head stabilization must be achieved as a result of small error signals in the canals in order to establish activation of the feed-back loop.

Such head stabilization occurs about all three axes and there is little doubt that this form of inertial stabilization of the sensing platform, namely the skull, must substantially reduce the incidence of misleading dynamic canal cross-coupling. The question arises: does inertial head stabilization occur in man? It is, of course, well-known clinically that pathological conditions in the neck can generate substantial interference with the whole of the vestibulo-postural system in man. Thus, dizziness and even head nystagmus will result from interference from dorsal root inflow at the level of the first cervical segments (Philipszoon, 1962). It seems highly probable that the neck-on-body system plays a potentially important part in man's orientation. Figure 10 is a record which illustrates that automatic vestibular head stabilization does indeed play an active functional role in man. The records are obtained from experiments of Outerbridge and Melvill Jones (1967) in which human subjects were rotated on a turntable with head free. On suddenly stopping prolonged, steady rotation, post-rotational nystagmus of the eyes is observed together with substantial decaying post-rotational head nystagmus. The subject was quite unaware of the presence of such head nystagmus. Yet it can be seen that the response was sufficient to materially

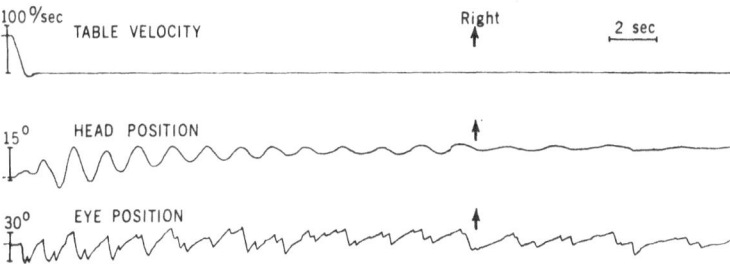

Fig. 10. Involuntary post-rotational head nystagmus generated in man by suddenly stopping a prolonged, steady body rotation. The vestibulo-collic response intermittently reduced the canal signal which is reflected in the slope of concurrent slow phase ocular nystagmus. (Outerbridge, 1969).

assist the oculomotor component of compensatory rotation. The implications of these effects in the context of the overall system are examined in theoretical and experimental detail by Outerbridge (1969), but for the present purpose it will suffice to draw the conclusion that substantial amelioration of dynamic cross-coupling effects in the canals will result if such automatic stabilization of the head occurs.

A. THE AEROSPACE ENVIRONMENT

To what extent can we take advantage of such effects in the aerospace environment? Returning to the experimental investigation of human factors in the aerodynamic spin (Melvill Jones, 1965), it seemed possible that by limiting degrees of freedom in which canal stimulation could occur during the active part of the spin, this measure of inertial stabilization of the head would stand to reduce very considerably the deleterious effects of cross-coupling in canals. To this end, spinning trials were conducted in which the pilot attempted to maintain his head erect relative to the outside visible horizon, despite oscillatory motion of the aircraft in all three planes throughout the spin. In these circumstances, the problem of recovery after a prolonged spinning maneuver was greatly facilitated, presumably due to amelioration of the cross-coupling effects along the lines discussed above. Possibly this approach might be extended to other situations, for example, instrument flying in difficult weather conditions. Perhaps a conscious effort to maintain the head attitude constant relative to the artificial horizon might stand to outweigh the disadvantages of attempting to do so, by amelioration of much more serious effects of dynamic cross-coupling in the canals.

References

Benson, A. J. and Bodin, M. A.: 1966, *Aerospace Med.* **37**, 889.

van Egmond, A. A. J., Groen, J. J., and Jongkees, L. B. W.: 1949, *J. Physiol.* **110**, 1.

Groen, J. J.: 1961, *Confin. Neurol.* **21**, 454.

Guedry, F. E. and Montague, E. K.: 1961, *Aerospace Med.* **32**, 487.

Guedry, F. E. and Graybiel, A.: 1962, *J. Appl. Physiol.* **17**, 398.

Hallpike, C. S. and Hood, J. D.: 1952, *Proc. Roy. Soc. London, Ser. B* **141**, 216.

Malcolm, R. and Melvill Jones, G.: 1970, *Acta Otolaryng.* (in press).

Mayne, R.: 1950, *J. Comp. Physiol. Psychol.* **43**, 309.

Melvill Jones, G.: 1964, *Acta Otolaryng.* **56**, 619.

Melvill Jones, G.: 1965, *Aerospace Med.* **38**, 976.

Melvill Jones, G.: 1966, *Aerospace Med.* **39**, 172.

Melvill Jones, G.: 1967, in *Proceedings Third Symposium on the Role of the Vestibular Organs in Space Exploration*, NASA-SP-152, National Aeronautics and Space Administration, Washington, D.C., pp. 169–180.

Melvill Jones, G., Barry, W., and Kowalsky, N.: 1964, *Aerospace Med.* **35**, 984.

Melvill Jones, G. and Drazin, D. H.: 1962, in *Human Problems of Supersonic and Hypersonic Flight* (ed. by Barbour and Whittingham), Pergamon Press, London, pp. 134–151.

Melvill Jones, G. and Milsum, J. H.: 1965, *IEEE Trans. Biomed. Eng.* **12**, 54.

Outerbridge, J.: 1969, *Experimental and Theoretical Study of Reflex Vestibular Control of Eye and Head Movement*, Doctoral Thesis, McGill University, Montreal, Canada.

Outerbridge, J. and Melvill Jones, G.: 1967, in *Proceedings Annual Meeting Aerospace Medical Association*, Washington, D.C., pp. 312–313.

Peters, R. A.: 1969, NASA-CR-1309, National Aeronautics and Space Administration, Washington, D.C.

Philipszoon, A. J.: 1962, *Pract. Otorhinelaryng.* **24**, 193.

Weaver, R. S.: 1965, *Acta Otolaryng. Suppl.* **205**.

Young, L. R., Meiry, J. L., and Li, Y. T.: 1966, in *Proceedings Second Symposium on The Role of the Vestibular Organs in Space Exploration*. NASA-SP-115, National Aeronautics and Space Administration, Washington, D.C., pp. 217–227.

INTERACTIONS BETWEEN SEMICIRCULAR
CANALS AND GRAVIRECEPTORS

A. J. BENSON

R.A.F. Institute of Aviation Medicine, Farnborough, Hants., U.K.

1. Introduction

Early in the history of powered flight, the importance to the pilot of the sense of equilibrium was recognized. As this sensory modality is subserved principally by the receptors of the vestibular apparatus, it became the fashion to perform rotatory tests on potential aviators, and if the duration of their nystagmic response fell within certain limits they were accepted for flying training. However, towards the end of World War I, it became apparent that when pilots were deprived of visual orientational cues for more than about half a minute, they were unable to maintain their equilibrium in the air. As Head (1920) and others were quick to recognize, in the flight environment false or inadequate signals from the vestibular end-organs were more likely to give rise to illusory than veridical perceptions of aircraft attitude and motion – they were an important cause of spatial disorientation and the loss of control which this might engender.

With the perspective of half a century we can now see truth in both these points of view. When motion occurs with a time course which is within the physiological range of the vestibular receptors, signals from these specialized sense organs stimulated by linear and angular accelerations, aid aircraft control. This has been demonstrated in a number of studies where the quality of operator control has been compared in fixed and moving base simulators (Perry and Naish, 1964; Fraser, 1966). In contrast, when the temporal pattern of the motion is outside the physiological range of vestibular receptors or is of unfamiliar duration and magnitude, control may be degraded by spatial disorientation, by involuntary motor responses, or by impaired visibility of aircraft instruments within the aircraft cockpit. Other papers presented in this symposium elaborate on these points.

Following the functional and anatomical differentiation of the vestibular apparatus, so clearly laid down by Magnus and his colleagues in the 1920s (Magnus, 1926), it had become customary to consider separately the contributions of semicircular canals and the otolith organs, which in turn transduce angular and linear accelerations. But in flight, as on the ground, angular motion is frequently co-existent with a change in linear acceleration. Experiments conducted in a number of centers have shown that it is not possible to predict with accuracy the response of an individual to a complex motion stimulus by consideration of the separate contributions of the angular and linear components of the stimulus. Nearly all the studies of the interactions between angular and linear accelerations – of interactions between semicircular canal and gravireceptor signals – have been carried out using simple stimuli, for such interactions must be understood before the responses engendered by motion with six degrees of freedom can be adequately synthesized.

In this discussion of the interaction of canals and otoliths, or rather canals and gravireceptors, for linear accelerations frequently stimulate mechanoreceptors other than those of the otolithic maculae, examples are drawn from two types of experiments: those in which canal and gravireceptor signals are antagonistic, and those in which the information from these receptors is synergistic.

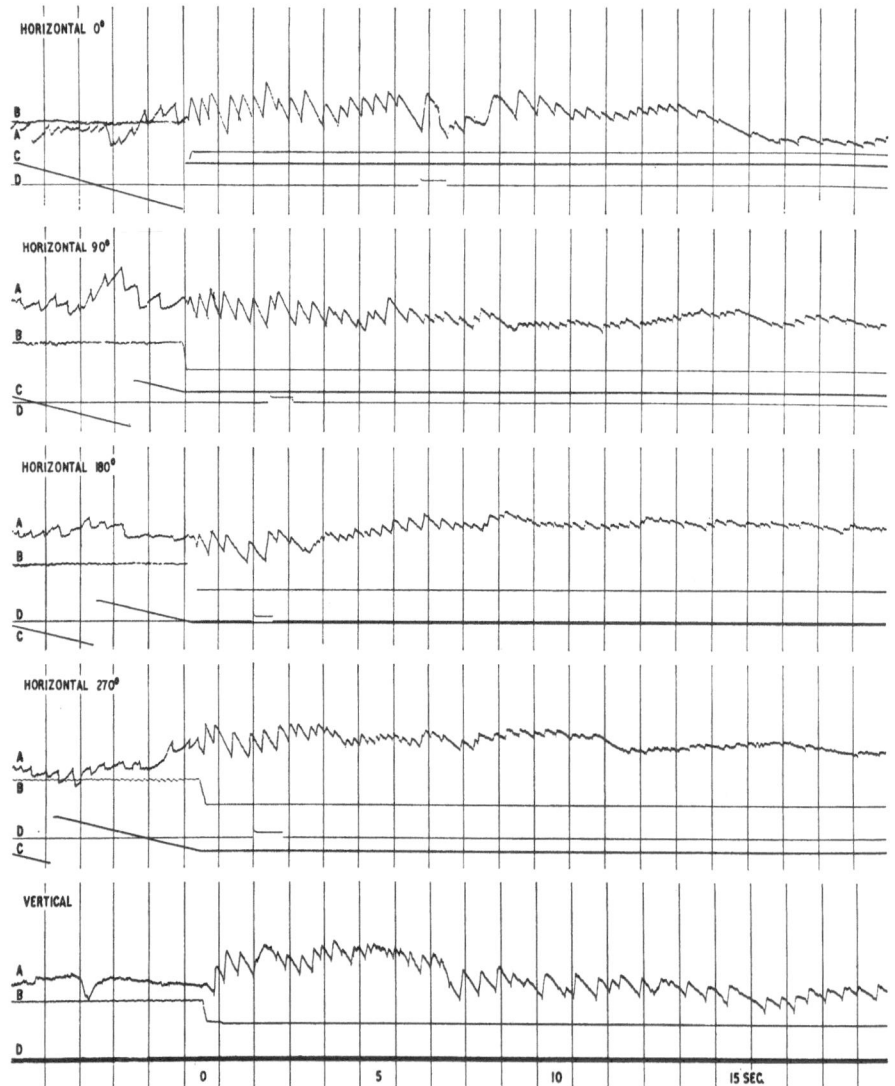

Fig. 1.   Records from one subject showing the more rapid decay of nystagmus, following a 60 deg/sec stopping stimulus, when the axis of rotation was horizontal than when it was vertical. The four stopping positions were supine (0 deg), right side down (90 deg), prone (180 deg) and left side down (270 deg). The traces are: *A*, lateral eye position; *B*, angular velocity of rotation; *C*, stretcher position; *D*, subject's marker to indicate disappearance of after-sensation (after Benson and Bodin, 1965).

2. Antagonistic Information from Canals and Gravireceptors

Clear indication of the suppression of the inappropriate nystagmus and sensations of turning by veridical gravireceptor signals was provided by Guedry (1966), Correia and Guedry (1964), Benson and Bodin (1965, 1966b). Both these groups of workers compared the responses following rotation about a subject's longitudinal (z) axis when the axis of rotation was vertical and when it was horizontal.

Figure 1 shows a typical record of the lateral nystagmus produced by a stopping stimulus of 60 deg/sec. Irrespective of the position in which the rotating stretcher was stopped, when the axis of rotation was horizontal the nystagmus died away more rapidly than when the axis of rotation was vertical. Measurement of the velocity of the slow phase component of the nystagmus revealed that the mean time constant of decay (Π/Δ) was 17.8 sec when the axis of rotation was vertical, and 8.5 sec when it was horizontal (Figure 2). The subjects' orientation to gravity (*e.g.*, prone, supine, left or right side down) following rotation about the horizontal axis has no consistent influence on the rate of nystagmus decay. The suppression of after-sensations was even

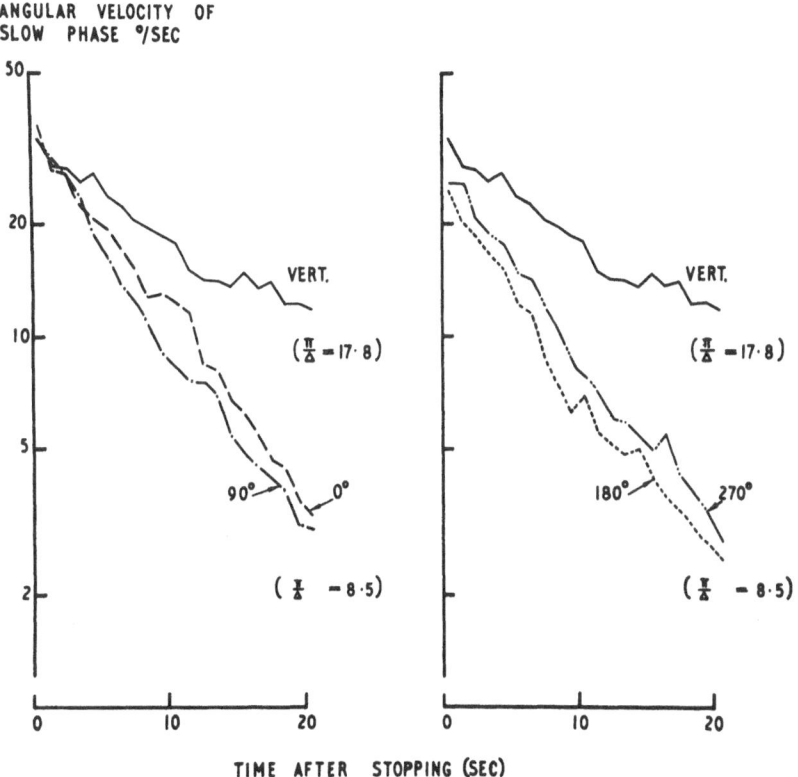

Fig. 2.   Pattern of decay of post-rotational nystagmus in the four horizontal positions, and when the axis of rotation was vertical (as Figure 1). Angular velocity of slow phase of nystagmus is plotted on a logarithmic ordinate scale. Π/Δ values indicate the time constant of decay in seconds. Mean values from 11 subjects (after Benson and Bodin, 1965).

more impressive when the rotation axis was vertical; the mean duration of the illusory sensations of turning was 20.2 sec but only 4.9 sec when the rotational axis was horizontal.

During rotation about a horizontal axis, a sustained per-rotational nystagmus is observed (Guedry, 1966; Benson and Bodin, 1966a; Janeke, 1968; Saito *et al.*, 1968) and is due to the stimulation of vestibular receptors by the rotation, with respect to the subject, of the linear acceleration vector (Guedry, 1966; Benson *et al.*, 1967; Correia and Money, 1968). Thus the stopping of rotation about a horizontal axis involves an angular acceleration and the contemporaneous cessation of rotation of the linear acceleration vector.

A simpler experimental situation is provided by a device (Figure 3) which allows the subject to be given a stopping stimulus and then, when all angular motion in the

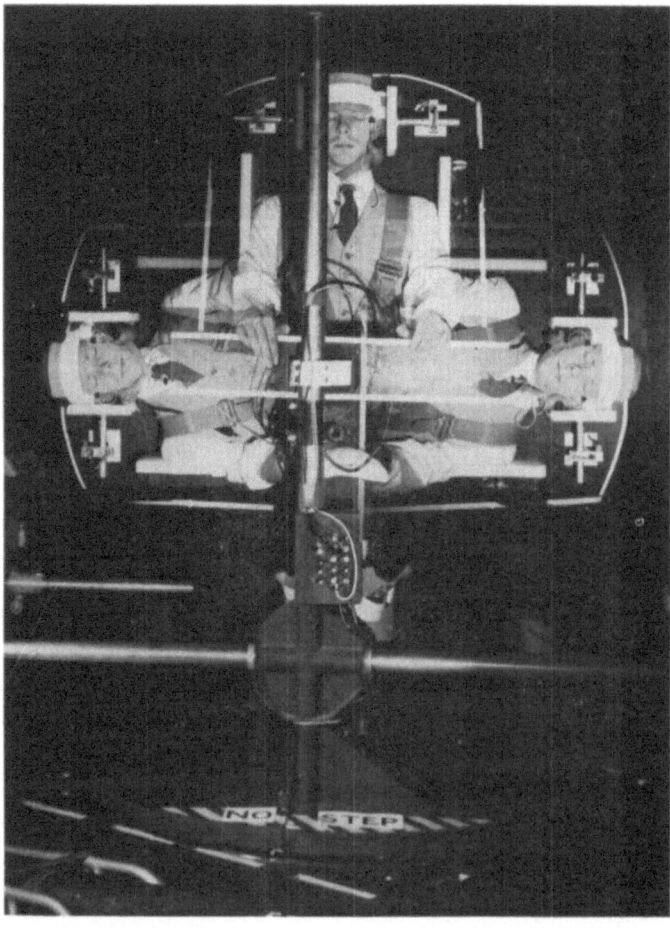

Fig. 3.   Multiple exposure photograph to show the vertical position in which the subject was rotated, and the right and left side down positions to which he was moved shortly after the turntable was stopped (after Benson and Bodin, 1966b.)

longitudinal (z) body axis has ceased, reorientated to gravity. Figure 4 shows that when the subject was moved to a left or right side down position within 2 to 3 sec of the stopping stimulus, the rate of decay of the post-rotational nystagmus was almost twice as great as that which was observed when he remained in the initial, head vertical position. As with horizontal axis rotation, the after-sensations showed proportionately greater suppression than the nystagmus when cupular restoration was allowed to occur in the presence of gravireceptor information, which contradicted the erroneous

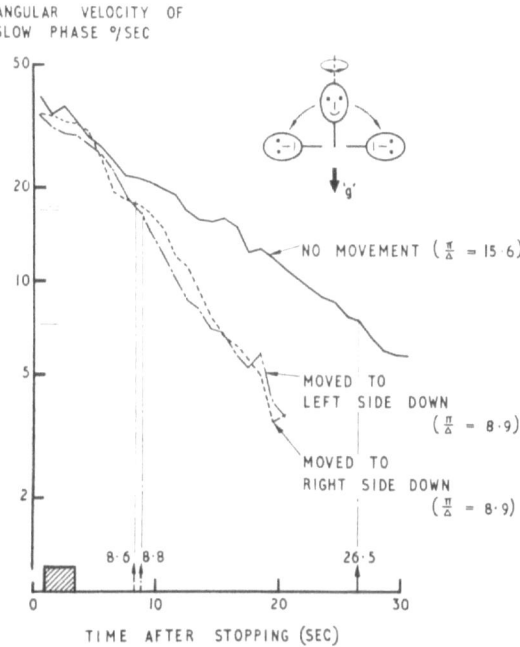

Fig. 4.   Comparison of the decay of post-rotational nystagmus when the subject was moved to the right or left side down position shortly after stopping, and when he remained in the vertical position. The shaded block on the abscissa indicates the time at which the subject's orientation to the vertical was changed. Figures on the abscissa show the duration of the after-sensations in the different experimental conditions. Mean values from 8 subjects (after Benson and Bodin, 1966b).

signal of rotation engendered by the ampullary receptors of the lateral canals. It is worthy of note that the nystagmus slow phase velocity at the time at which the after-sensations disappeared was significantly ($P=0.01$) higher when the head was horizontal than when it was vertical.

The dissociation of sensation and nystagmus, which has been observed in other experimental situations (Benson, 1967), implies that the inhibition brought about by gravireceptors does not act at a common center in the afferent projection from the canals, but rather at separate neural centers which are involved specifically in the relay of ampullary signals to oculomotor nuclei and the sensory cortex. The inhibition of post-rotational nystagmus by gravireceptor signals cannot be described by a simple subtractive or proportional function, for there was no sudden reduction of slow phase eye velocity coincident with the appearance of the antagonistic otolithic signals on moving the subject from the vertical to the horizontal position. Furthermore, when the subject was returned to the vertical position nystagmus velocity did not increase in intensity; there was only a restoration of its rate of decay to a value comparable to that which was observed when there was no reorientation to gravity in the post-rotational period (Figure 5).

It would thus appear that gravireceptor inhibition increases in intensity as an

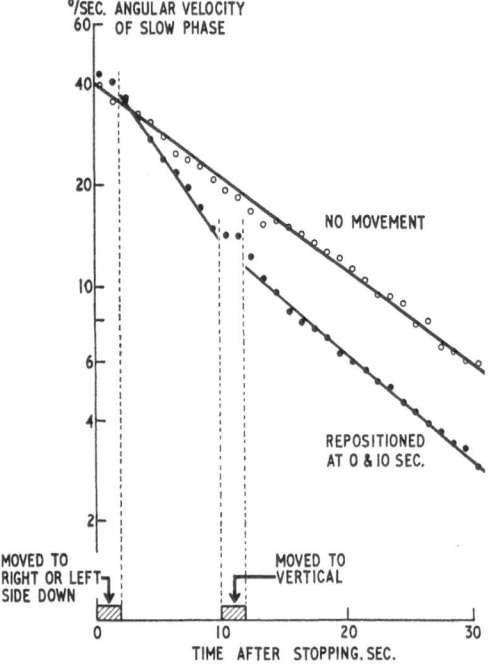

Fig. 5. Effect on post-rotational nystagmus of returning the subject to the vertical position 10 sec after having been placed in the right and left lateral position following a stopping stimulus. Mean values from 6 subjects.

exponential function of time. The time constant of this function is dependent upon the intensity of signals from otoliths and other gravireceptors, and upon their significance in relationship to concurrent signals from ampullary receptors. As gravireceptor inhibition is associated with a reduction in the magnitude of a secondary postrotatory nystagmus (Figure 6), it is considered that the attenuation of the canal response is more likely to be brought about by recurrent inhibitory connections (Benson, 1966), than by an augmentation of the 'adaptive' mechanism which is considered to be responsible for the secondary response (Collins, 1968; Young, 1968; Malcolm and Melvill Jones, 1969).

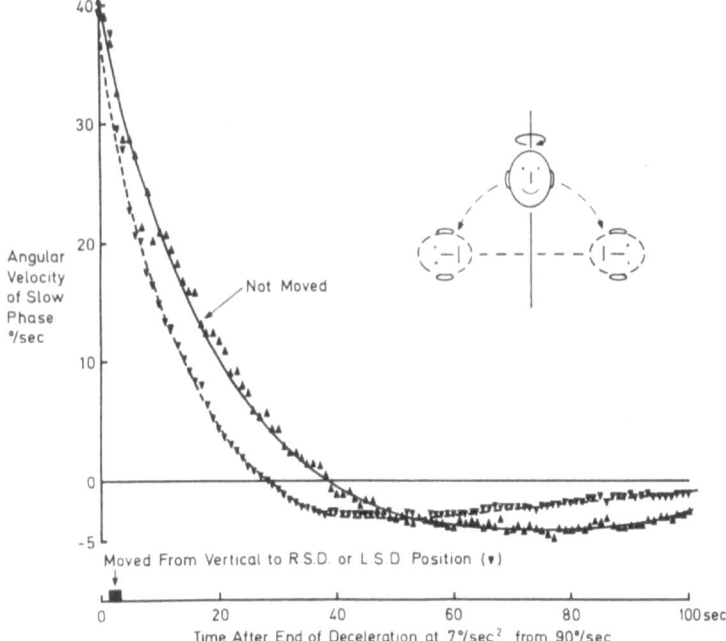

Fig. 6. The pattern of primary and secondary nystagmus, following deceleration at 7 deg/sec² from 90 deg/sec to 0 deg/sec, when the subject was moved to the right or left lateral position shortly after rotation stopped and when he remained in the vertical position. Note linear ordinate and extended time scale. Mean values from 6 subjects.

3. Synergistic Information from Canals and Gravireceptors

In everyday life, angular movements of the head are normally of short duration and are correctly transduced by the semicircular canal receptors. In addition, for head movements other than in the horizontal plane, there is adequate stimulation of receptors of the otolithic maculae consequent to the changed orientation of the head to gravity. Information on the ways in which veridical canal and otolith signals interact has been obtained with the aid of a new, high torque turntable (Figure 7). The dynamic response of the vestibular system to sinusoidal angular oscillations having a peak angular velocity of ± 30 deg/sec was determined over a frequency range of 0.01 Hz to 2.0 Hz. Lateral eye movements were recorded by conventional DC electro-oculography with the eyes closed. From the eye movement records, it was possible to measure the peak slow phase eye velocity during each half cycle. The gain or amplitude ratio of the vestibulo-ocular reflex was determined by dividing the mean modulus peak eye velocity by the peak turntable velocity. Phase shift was obtained by comparison of the time during each half cycle at which eye velocity was zero with zero stimulus velocity. The techniques employed were similar to those of Hixon and Niven (1961) and Meiry (1966).

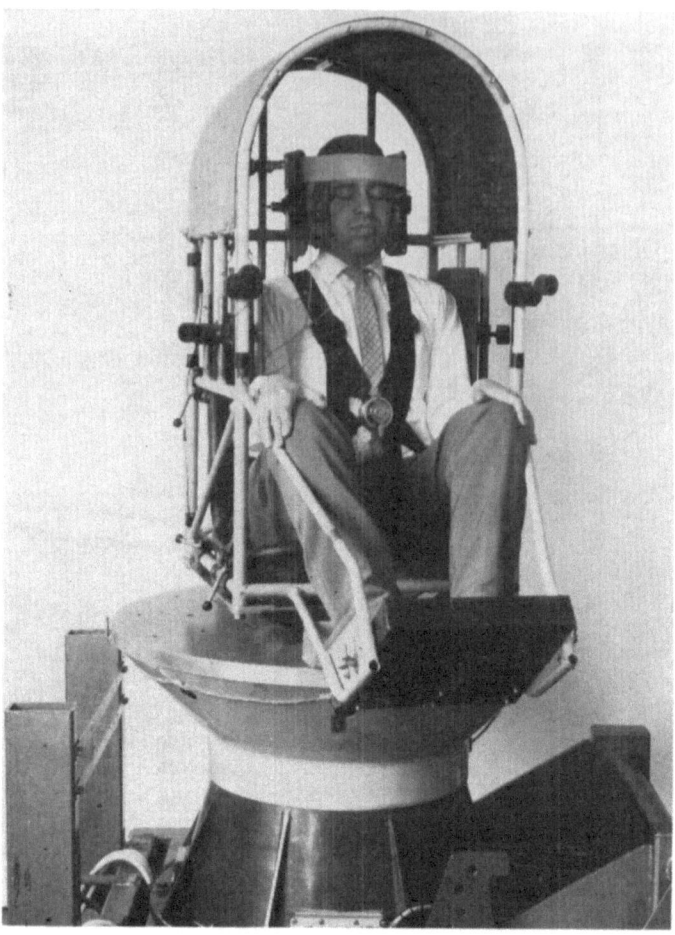

Fig. 7a.   Photograph of high torque (200 Lb.ft) turntable, with axis of rotation vertical. The subject was restrained by a four strap harness, feet and brow straps, and adjustable head and shoulder plates. Not shown are knee straps and a dental bite carried on an adjustable cross member.

Figure 8 shows the mean gain and phase shift data obtained from nine subjects. When the axis of rotation was vertical, the characteristic reduction in phase advance of the compensatory eye movements and increase in gain were observed as the frequency of the stimulus was increased from 0.01 Hz to 0.5 Hz. The effect of concomitant gravireceptor stimulation was studied by turning the turntable and the subject through 90 deg so that the axis of rotation was horizontal. In this mode, it was found that the phase error was significantly ($P < 0.05$) altered. At low frequencies (0.01 Hz to 0.05 Hz) the phase advance was less than when the axis of rotation was vertical, while at 0.2 Hz and 0.5 Hz there was a small, but significant, increase in phase error. On average, the peak eye velocity was slightly higher when the axis of rotation was horizontal than vertical, but this effect was not sufficiently consistent to

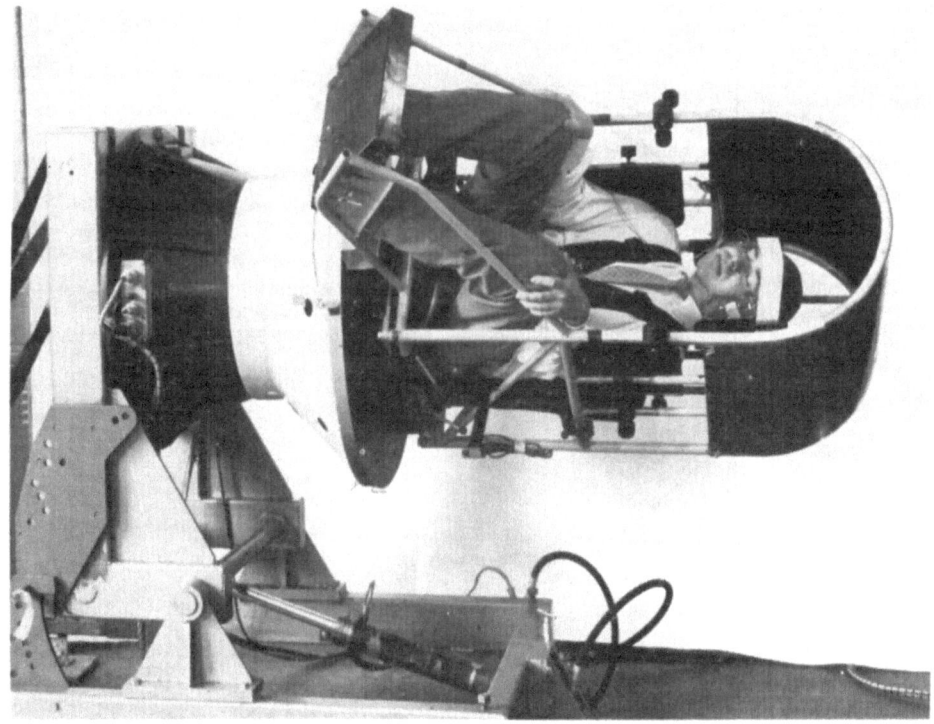

Fig. 7b. As Fig. 7a, but with the table jacked through 90° so that the axis of rotation was horizontal.

be statistically significant. At the low frequencies, rotation of the linear acceleration vector not only reduced the phase error of the compensatory eye movement, but also introduced a modulation of eye velocity which was related to the orientation of the head to gravity (Figure 9). Maxima and minima of the modulating wave form occurred when the subject was close to the left or right side down position (*i.e.*, when the transverse (y) axis of the skull lay in the gravitational vertical). This finding is in accord with other experimental studies (Guedry, 1966; Niven *et al.*, 1965; Benson, 1966; Steer, 1967; Benson, 1968) of the nystagmus evoked by a rotating linear acceleration vector in the absence of angular accelerations.

It is of particular significance that the response obtained during horizontal axis oscillation showed an alteration in phase of the fundamental wave form, which of itself was modulated by higher frequency components attributable to rotation of the gravity vector. Thus the overall response, observed during horizontal axis oscillation, cannot be accounted for by the algebraic summation of the basic canal response (as recorded during vertical axis oscillation) and the nystagmus generated by the rotating linear acceleration vector. Therefore, it is necessary to postulate that the reduced phase error in the presence of gravireceptor stimulation is caused by the central integration of canal and gravireceptor signals.

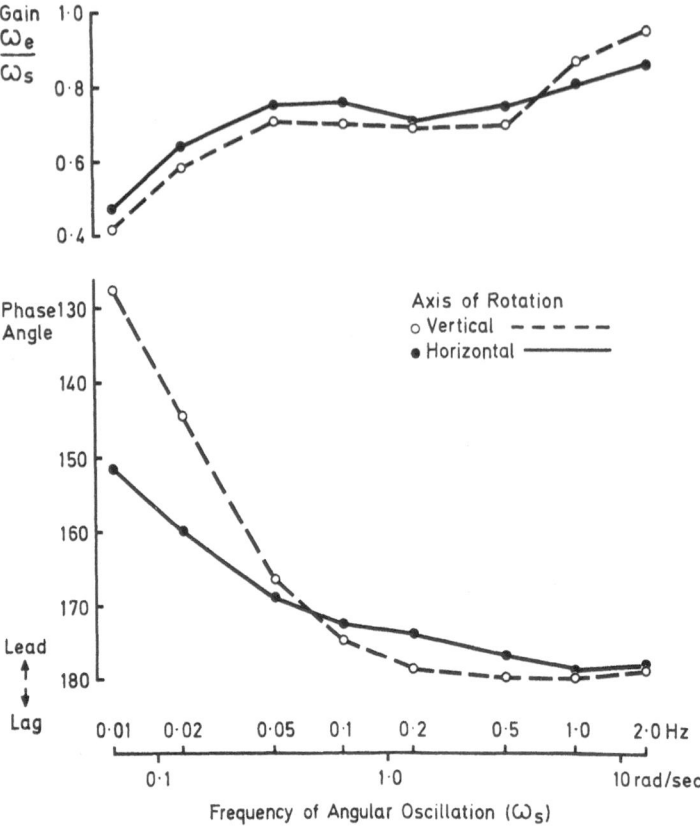

Fig. 8. Gain and phase plots obtained from measurement of lateral eye movements evoked by sinusoidal oscillation in yaw (rotation in longitudinal or z body axis) about earth vertical and horizontal axes. Peak angular velocity of the stimulus was ± 30 deg/sec at all test frequencies. Mean values from 9 subjects.

Unexpected features of responses recorded at the higher frequencies (1 Hz and 2 Hz) were the increase in gain and the absence of significant phase error. This finding was confirmed in an additional experiment carried out on six subjects who experienced sinusoidal oscillations in a frequency range 0.2 Hz to 5 Hz which were presented in a randomized order. The axis of rotation was vertical and, as before, the peak angular velocity of the stimulus was ± 30 deg/sec. Special attention was given to the fixation of the head by means of a dental bite, adjustable side plates and a brow strap. Figure 10 combines the vertical axis data from Figure 9 and the results obtained with the higher frequency stimuli. Despite the use of different subject groups, there was close agreement in the replicated measures of system gain and phase angle. At the higher frequencies, phase angle could not be measured with accuracy, principally because of the increase in signal-to-noise ratio, as the amplitude of stimulus and eye movement decreased with frequency. However, visual comparison of the records of eye and turntable position reveal that the compensatory eye movement was closely matched in phase to that of the stimulus over the frequency range 0.5 Hz to 5 Hz.

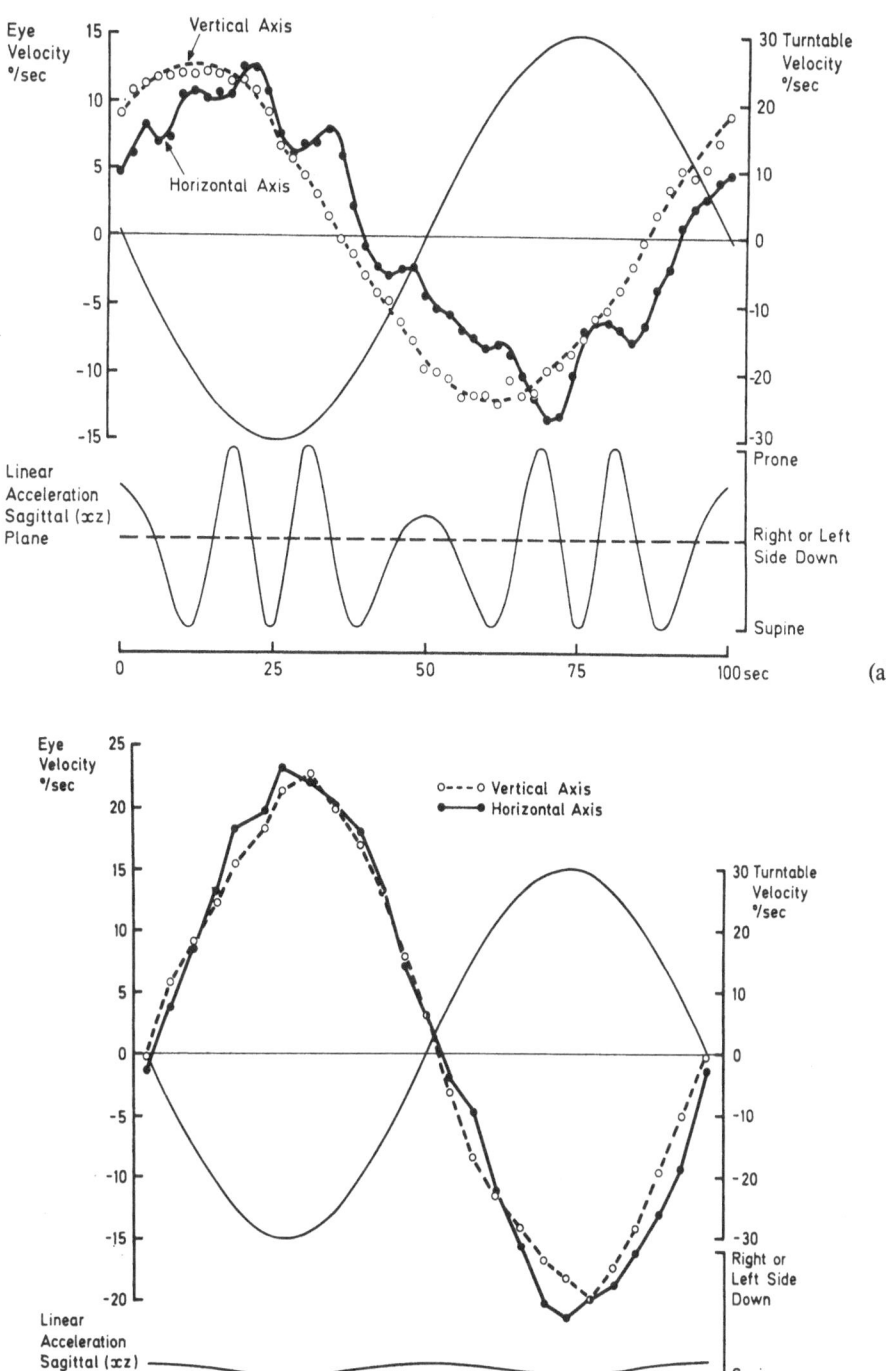

Fig. 9. Comparison of slow phase eye velocities during oscillation about vertical and horizontal axis at 0.01 Hz (a) and 0.2 Hz (b). Each point is the mean eye velocity during 2 cycles in (a) and 5 cycles in (b) from 3 subjects. The continuous lines show turntable velocity and the orientation of the subject to gravity during horizontal axis rotation.

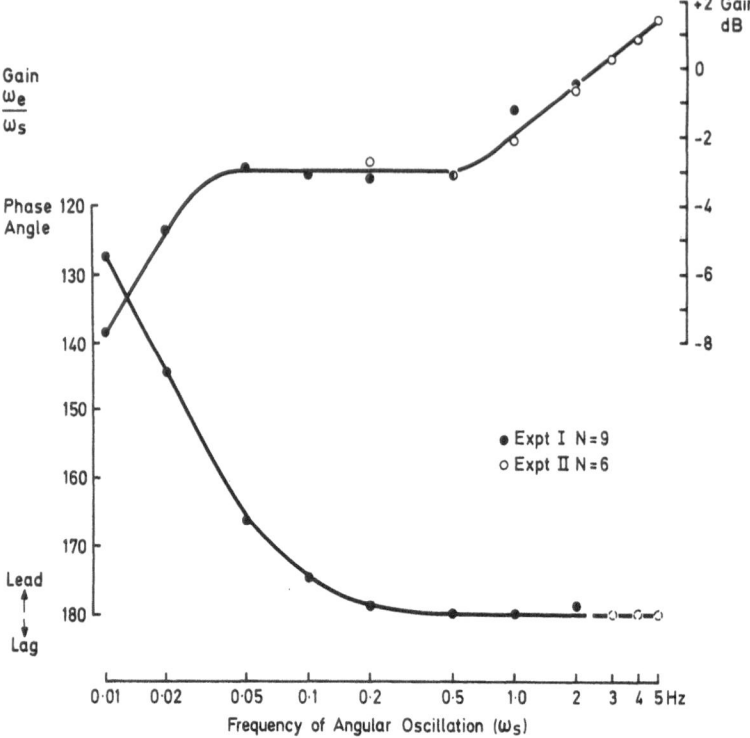

Fig. 10. Gain and phase plots of lateral eye movements evoked by sinusoidal oscillation in yaw about an earth vertical axis. Solid circles are from Figure 8 which cover the frequency range 0.01 Hz to 2.0 Hz. Open circles are mean values from a different group of 6 subjects who experienced oscillations in the frequency range 0.2 Hz to 5.0 Hz. Broken open circles show estimates of phase angle made from visual inspection of the electro-oculographic records.

The rising gain characteristic was consistently observed in all the experimental subjects. On average, the frequency at which the gain plot inflected was 0.5 Hz and the rate of increase gain with frequency was +5 dB per decade. The reason for this apparent departure of the response of the vestibulo-ocular reflex from that of a second order system which adequately describes its behaviour at frequencies below 0.5 Hz (Mayne, 1950; Hixon and Niven, 1961; Melvill Jones and Milsum, 1965; Meiry, 1966) must await further study. However, it is perhaps significant that the gain of the vestibulo-ocular reflex increases from 0.7 to 1.0 in that frequency band where the stabilization of eye position by the fixation reflex undergoes a rapid decrement.

References

Benson, A. J.: 1966, in *Proceedings Second Symposium on the Role of the Vestibular Organs in Space Exploration*, NASA-SP-115, National Aeronautics and Space Administration, Washington, D.C., pp. 119–213.

Benson, A. J.: 1967, in *Proceedings Third Symposium on the Role of the Vestibular Organs in Space Exploration*, NASA-SP-152, National Aeronautics and Space Administration, Washington, D.C., pp. 421–432.

Benson, A. J.: 1968, *J. Physiol.* **197**, 85P.

Benson, A. J. and Bodin, M. A.: 1965, *Acta Otolaryng.* **61**, 517.

Benson, A. J. and Bodin, M. A.: 1966a, *Aerospace Med.* **37**, 144.

Benson, A. J. and Bodin, M. A.: 1966b, *Aerospace Med.* **37**, 889.

Benson, A. J., Guedry, F. E., and Melvill Jones, G.: 1967, *J. Physiol.* **191**, 26P.

Collins, W. E.: 1968, *Aerospace Med.* **39**, 257.

Correia, M. J. and Money, K. E.: 1968, Rept. No. 728, D.R.E.T., Toronto, Canada.

Correia, M. J. and Guedry, F. E.: 1964, NAV-SAM-905, U.S. Naval Sch. Aviat. Med., Pensacola, Fla., U.S.A.

Fraser, T. M.: 1966, NASA-SP-102, National Aeronautics and Space Administration, Washington, D.C.

Guedry, F. E.: 1966, in *Proceedings Second Symposium on the Role of the Vestibular Organs in Space Exploration*, NASA-SP-115, National Aeronautics and Space Administration, Washington, D.C., pp. 185–198.

Head, H.: 1920, Med. Res. Council Special Rept. 53, H.M.S.O. London, U.K.

Hixon, W. C. and Niven, J. I.: 1961, NAV-SAM-57, U.S. Naval Sch. Aviat. Med., Pensacola, Fla., U.S.A.

Janeke, J. B.: 1968, *On Nystagmus and Otolith; A Vestibular Study on Responses as Provoked by a Cephalo-caudal Horizontal Axial Rotation*, Doctoral Thesis, University of Amsterdam, Amsterdam, The Netherlands.

Magnus, R.: 1926, *Lancet* **ii**, 531, 585.

Malcolm, R. and Melvill Jones, G.: 1969 (in preparation).

Mayne, R.: 1950, *J. Comp. Physiol. Psychol.* **43**, 309.

Meiry, J. L.: 1966, NASA-CR-628, National Aeronautics and Space Administration, Washington, D.C.

Melvill Jones, G. and Milsum, J. H.: 1965, *IEEE Trans. Biomed. Bioeng.* **12**, 54.

Niven, J. I., Hixon, W. C., and Correia, M. J.: 1965, NAV-SAM-953, U.S. Naval Sch. Aviat. Med., Pensacola, Fla., U.S.A.

Perry, D. H. and Naish, J. M.: 1964, *J. Roy. Aero. Soc.* **68**, 645.

Saito, I., Wada, H., Yagura, S., and Kato, N.: 1968, *Jap. J. Aerospace Med.* **6**, 6.

Steer, R. W.: 1967, *The Influence of Angular and Linear Acceleration and Thermal Stimulation on the Human Semicircular Canal*, Doctoral Thesis, Massachusetts Institute of Technology, Boston, Mass., U.S.A.

Young, L. R.: 1968, in *Symposium on Technical and Biological Problems in Cybernetics*, Yerivan, Armenia, U.S.S.R. *Automatica*, 1969, **5**, 369.

THE THRESHOLD VALUE FOR STIMULATION OF THE
HORIZONTAL SEMICIRCULAR CANALS

W. J. OOSTERVELD

Vestibular Department, Ear, Nose and Throat Clinic, Wilhelmina Hospital,
University of Amsterdam, Amsterdam, The Netherlands

1. Introduction

Vestibular threshold values are the smallest specific stimulations able to create a vestibular sensation or a vestibular reflex under certain, well defined conditions.

The threshold value for rotational nystagmus was defined in 1957 (Lachmann *et al.*, 1957) as the smallest rotational acceleration that can provoke an ocular nystagmus during the stimulation period. Groen and Jongkees (1948) defined the vestibular threshold for an angular acceleration as the value of the smallest angular acceleration which during the application of the stimulation causes either the sensation of a rotation or a nystagmus. It was pointed out theoretically in 1875 (Mach, 1875) that the smallest angular acceleration for a cupular reflex should be about 1 deg/sec². Fischer (1933) obtained the same result in his studies.

Table I points out the values reported by various other investigators. Notably, these limits range from 2.5 to 0.04 deg/sec².

The vestibular threshold is affected by the time of its measurement (Mittermaier, 1952), age and psychological factors (Haas and Eidebenz, 1967), stress and fatigue (Kornhuber, 1961), and drugs and alcohol (Aschan, 1956; Oosterveld, 1970). Differences are also apparent when subjects are studied in the sitting and vertical positions (Güttich and Hazeyama, 1967). Imposing a series of angular accelerations increases the vestibular threshold (adaptation, habituation) (Mittermaier and Rossberg, 1956). The different techniques used to determine this threshold may also be responsible for the wide range of reported values. These techniques have included electromyography of the neck muscles in pigeons (Van Eyck, 1953a, 1953b), electro- and photo-nystagmography, measurement of the sensation of rotation and observation of the oculogyral illusion.

The effect of gravity on the vestibular threshold for angular accelerations has been discussed by this investigator (Oosterveld and Laarse, 1968; Oosterveld, 1969). Lower values of gravity bring the threshold down; higher values increase it. So in weightlessness, cupular function is at its greatest sensitivity.

In 1905, Mulder explained variations in the threshold values for angular acceleration described by a number of authors who found varying values when the sensation of rotation was used as an indicator. Notably, when nystagmus was used as the parameter to measure the threshold of the vestibular organ, these variations were by no means smaller. Mulder showed that the product of time (T) and angular acceleration (α), required to reach the threshold of rotational sensation, as well as for nystagmus,

D. E. Busby (ed.), Recent Advances in Aerospace Medicine, 262–268. All Rights Reserved.
Copyright © 1970 by D. Reidel Publishing Company, Dordrecht - Holland.

TABLE I

Literature review of 25 publications concerning the determination of the threshold value of the vestibular organ for rotational accelerations in the horizontal plane. The minimum and maximum values, as well as the average value, described in these articles are indicated.

	Threshold for angular accelerations in deg/sec^2		
	Minimum	Maximum	Average-value
Mach (1875)	–	–	1.0
Mulder (1908)	–	–	2.0
van Wulfften Palthe (1922)	1.6	–	2.0
Fischer (1933)	–	–	1.0
Arslan (1934)	0.5	1.0	–
Mowrer (1935)	0.45	1.56	–
Buys and Rylant (1939)	–	–	0.8
Groen and Jongkees (1948)	0.5	–	–
Hulk and Jongkees (1948)	0.75	5.0	2.5
de Vries (1953)	0.38	–	–
Schierbeek (1953)	–	–	3.0
Aschan et al. (1952)	0.4	1.2	–
Hilding (1953)	0.25	3.0	0.75
van Eyck et al. (1956)	1.8	2.2	–
van Eyck et al. (1957)	1.5	–	–
Pfaltz (1957)	–	–	0.2
Ek et al. (1959)	0.04	–	–
Montandon et al. (1960)	0.6	1.07	0.8
Hennebert (1961)	0.4	1.0	–
Decher (1962)	0.2	0.8	0.37
Haas et al. (1965)	0.47	–	–
Bochenek and Gromowa (1967)	0.2	1.1	–
Haas and Eidebenz (1967)	0.43	0.6	–
Clark and Stewart (1969)	0.04	1.0	0.37

is constant within certain limits. The 'Law of Mulder' indicates that the beginning of the perception of angular acceleration is dependent on the product of acceleration and stimulus duration. This constant value of $\alpha \cdot T$, about 2.5 deg/sec, applies to stimulus durations from 0.5 to 6 sec (Van Egmond et al., 1943; Groen, 1956). Other authors (Löwenstein and Sand, 1940) proved that $\alpha \cdot T$ is less for shorter times of acceleration. The least value of T they used in experiments was 0.5 sec. For perception of an acceleration of 80 deg/sec^2, the duration has to be at least $\frac{1}{45}$ sec (Van Rossem, 1907). Thus the vestibular system is extremely sensitive to angular acceleration. The threshold value is so dependent on non-vestibular factors that the definition of this threshold depends largely on these factors.

Groen states in the discussion of a paper (Montandon et al., 1969) that the best way to define the vestibular threshold is to perform cupulometry where the wanted product is produced immediately, in contrast to the method which determines the minimum angular acceleration and omits the duration of its application. Before discussing the vestibular threshold more thoroughly one must define in a more detailed way, what is meant by this concept. Montandon and co-workers (1969) state that "the threshold of vestibular nystagmus is a frequency threshold which corresponds to the lowest grade of intensity of a continuous and constant stimulation which is able to provoke and to maintain until the end of the stimulating period a nystagmic reaction of a definite direction and of one beat per second". Experiments of others (Ek *et al.*, 1959) have shown that constant acceleration does not lead to such a pattern (adaptation), and the nystagmus threshold is not the same as the threshold of the vestibular system for rotatory stimulations. The most sensitive method to determine the threshold to angular acceleration in humans appears to be the oculogyral illusion (Roggeveen and Nijhoff, 1956). The lowest value reported utilizing this method was 0.04 deg/sec^2.

This investigator was interested in knowing at what angular accelerations people sitting in airplanes perceive the sensation of a turn. The perceptions of angular accelerations were investigated using blindfolded subjects in 1922 (Van Wulfften Palthe, 1922). In experiments using a small airplane, no sensation was experienced when angular accelerations had values below 1.6 deg/sec^2. It was stated that "an accurate enquiry in the case of the isolated semicircular-canal functions is only possible in an airplane and can never be realized with the spinning chair, as with the latter, influence of the superficial and the deeper sensibility can not be excluded".

When an airplane makes a turn in the horizontal plane, a short roll occurs, followed by a stationary position in which the airplane makes an angle with the horizontal plane, the inclination or banking angle being θ. In this stationary position, the airplane flies a pure circle. Around the yaw axis a short-lasting angular acceleration creates an angle speed in the horizontal plane. An angle speed will be perceived as an increase of gravity, for the angle speed provokes a centrifugal acceleration. In the stationary position the angular speed of the airplane is constant with regard to the center of the circle. The angular speed in combination with the inclination of the airplane increases the acceleration in the direction of the yaw axis, z (Figure 1). This acceleration presses the subject with mass m into his seat, and notwithstanding the inclination of the airplane, he remains directed perpendicularly to his seat. The resultant n_z of centrifugal acceleration and gravity (g) is equal to $mg/\cos\theta$ (Figure 2). Precise measurement of n_z will allow calculation of θ, since values of m and g are constant.

2. Stationary Turns

Perception of angular acceleration at the onset of turns was studied with 30 normal subjects, who were seated at the centers of gravity of DC 8 and DC 8-63 commercial jet airplanes of KLM Royal Dutch Airlines. The parameters used for identifying perception were nystagmography and the oculogyral illusion. Nystagmography was performed with a battery-fed Elema mingograph. The oculogyral illusion was created in a 4-ft long, dark-painted, wooden box, in which a luminous cube of metal wire was fixed.

The magnitude of angular acceleration at the onset of a turn can be determined

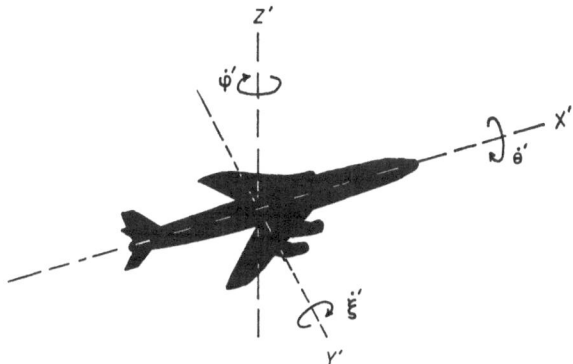

Fig. 1.   Schematic composition of the airplane flight axes in the three dimensions:
$X' = $ roll axis, $Y' = $ pitch axis, $Z' = $ yaw axis.

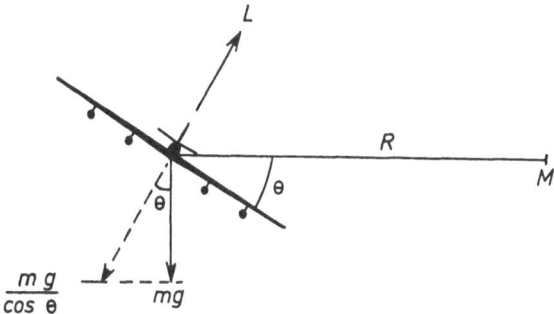

Fig. 2.   Position of an airplane making a turn. The inclination angle θ indicates the value of the acceleration, n_z, which is equal to $mg/\cos\theta$. The airlift L has the same size as the product of mass (m) and gravity (g). During turn, the value of n_z increases with the product of $1/\cos\theta$.

by the equation $\ddot{\varphi}' = \theta g/v \cos\theta$. As g (gravity) and v (speed) are non-variable factors, the angular acceleration depends on the banking angle θ of the airplane. Thus, as this angle is known, the angular acceleration can be calculated. In this study, it ranged from 0.3 to 2.0 deg/sec^2.

Electronystagmography did not show a clear nystagmus or other specific eye movement. The oculogyral illusion presented more information. Of the 30 subjects 25 were able to perceive the rotation around the yaw axis at an acceleration of 0.3 deg/sec^2; 28 perceived an acceleration of 0.5 deg/sec^2. All were sensitive to an acceleration of 1.0 deg/sec^2 (Table II).

One must keep in mind that this method of creating an angular acceleration also introduces a roll with an angular acceleration in the lateral vertical plane. These results seem to contradict the 1.6 deg/sec^2 threshold reported above. However, it should be noted that the observation of the oculogyral illusion in a modern jet plane is a much more sensitive method than the investigation of the sensation without the help of a light point in an older, vibrating, propeller-driven plane.

TABLE II

Thirty subjects were exposed to angular accelerations with a value of 1.0, 0.5 and
0.3 deg/sec². Observation of the oculogyral illusion proved that most of them were
sensitive to an acceleration of 0.3 deg/sec².

	Angular accelerations deg/sec²		
	1.0	0.5	0.3
Oculogyral illusion			
Right	30	28	25
Wrong	0	0	1
No response	0	2	4

3. Spiral Turn

Another point of interest in our experiments was the detection of the lowest value of
acceleration an individual could perceive. In order to produce a very small acceleration, a spiral turn (banking turn) was flown by the airplane (Figure 3). This means

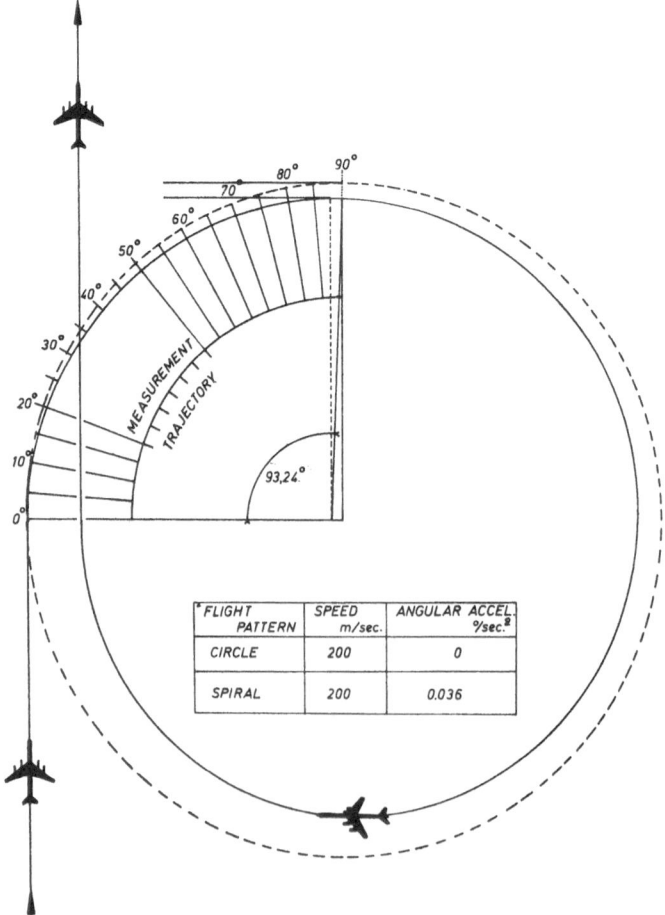

Fig. 3.   Flight pattern in the horizontal plane of an airplane performing a stationary (---) and a
spiral turn (——). A measurement trajectory of 10 sec is indicated.

that the flight path was like a segment of a spiral. The angular acceleration persists as long as the spiral is flown. It is nearly impossible for the flyer to make a pure flight pattern, but when he is flying spiral turns, he cannot avoid some segments with a very small acceleration. By asking the flyer to fly many turns it was possible to gain information from a few spiral turns with the desired magnitude of acceleration. The acceleration size was measured and calculated from exact observation of the increase of the bank angle θ, the changes of the compass bearing and the airspeed v, as well as from measurements of the resultant acceleration n_z using a very sensitive electric accelerometer (Figure 4). Since the acceleration n_z is equal to $mg/\cos\theta$, the inclination

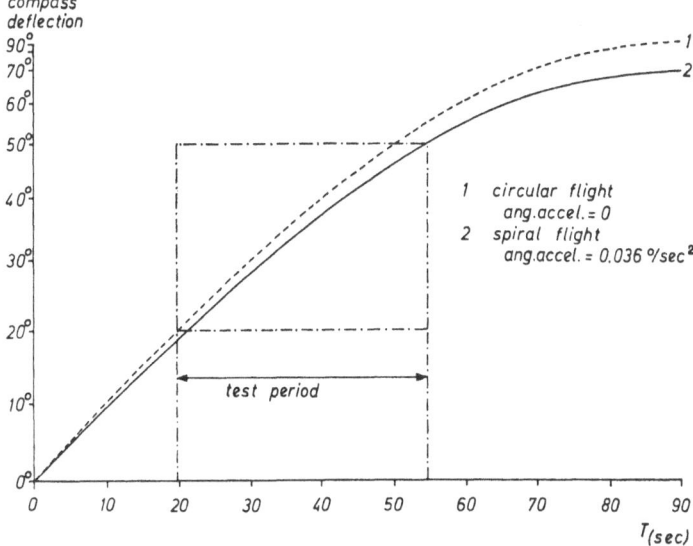

Fig. 4.   Changes in compass bearing during a stationary and a spiral turn. Following exact observation the angular acceleration can be calculated.

angle θ can be easily calculated. In a spiral turn, in contrast to a normal turn, the angle θ increases in a linear way. When the rate of increase of θ is known the acceleration can be calculated from the equation $\ddot{\varphi}' = \theta g/v \cos\theta$. Only spiral segments in the beginning of the turn were used in order to leave $\cos\theta$ close to unity. In 2 of the 5 subjects, an oculogyral illusion occurred during a 10-sec acceleration of 0.036 deg/sec² (Table III). In the 3 other subjects, no oculogyral illusion was elicited in angular accelerations of up to 0.041 deg/sec².

In earlier publications, this investigator (Oosterveld and Laarse, 1968; Oosterveld, 1969) described the effect of gravity on the threshold for angular accelerations. Since the resultant of centrifugal acceleration and gravity never exceeded 1.03 g in these studies, only a very small effect on the threshold value could be expected.

Thus one can state – as described in the past by various authors – that the threshold value of the horizontal semicircular canal depends upon a combination of factors. The lowest value measured during these experiments was 0.036 deg/sec². This is the lowest one ever described in humans.

TABLE III

Exposure of 5 subjects to small angular accelerations in the horizontal plane. Two of them were sensitive to an acceleration with a value of 0.036 deg/sec^2.

	Angular accelerations deg/sec^2					
Subject	0.025	0.032	0.036	0.038	0.040	0.041
L. de B.	–		+	+	+	
G. v. d. K.		–	+		+	+
E. W.			–			–
K. K.			–		–	–
S. P.				–	–	–

Bibliography

Arslan, M.: 1934, *Rev. Laryng.* **55**, 79.
Aschan, G.: 1956, *Acta Otolaryng.* Suppl. **129**.
Aschan, G., Nylen, C. O., Stahle, J., and Wersäll, R.: 1952, *Acta Otolaryng.* **6**, 451.
Bochenek, Z. and Gromowa, L.: 1967, *Pract. Otorhinolaryng.* **29**, 118.
Buys, E. and Rylant, P.: 1939, Arch. Int. Physiol. Biochem. **49**, 101.
Clark, B. and Stewart, J. D.: 1969, in *Preprints of Scientific Program* Annual Scientific Meeting, Aerospace Medical Association, San Francisco, Calif., U.S.A.
Decher, H.: 1962, *Z. Laryng. Rhinol.* **41**, 838.
De Vries, H.: 1953, *Acta Otorhinolaryng.* **15**, 87.
Ek, J., Jongkees, L. B. W. and Klijn, J. A. J.: 1959, *Acta Otolaryng.* **50**, 292.
Fischer, M. H.: 1933, *Klin. Wschv.* **12**, 1925.
Groen, J. J.: 1956, *Physics in Medicine and Biology* **6**, 37.
Groen, J. J. and Jongkees, L. B. W.: 1948, *J. Physiol.* **107**, 1.
Güttich, H. and Hazeyama, F.: 1967, *Z. Laryng. Rhinol.* **46**, 89.
Haas, E. and Eidebenz, H.: 1967, *Z. Laryng. Rhinol.* **46**, 96.
Haas, E., Kraenbring, C., and Pfänder, H.: 1965, *Z. Laryng. Rhinol.* **44**, 180.
Hennebert, P. E.: 1961, *Confin. Neurol.* **21**, 416.
Hilding, A. C.: 1953, *Ann. Otol.* **62**, 5.
Hulk, J. and Jongkees, L. B. W.: 1948, *J. Laryng.* **62**, 70.
Kornhuber, H. H.: 1961, *Acta Otolaryng.* Suppl. **159**, 113.
Lachmann, J., Bergmann, F., and Monnier, M.: 1957, *Helv. Physiol. Acta.* **15**, C5–C6
Löwenstein, O. and Sand, A.: 1940, *Proc. Royal Soc. Med.* **129**, 256.
Mach, E.: 1875, *Grundlinien der Lehre von den Bewegungsemfindungen.* W. Engelmann, _ ipzig.
Mittermaier, R.: 1952, *Z. Laryng. Rhinol.* **31**, 360.
Mittermaier, R. and Rossberg, G.: 1956, *Arch. Ohr.-, Nas.- u. Kehlk.-Heilk.* **168**, 313.
Montandon, A., Huguenin, S., Rohr, A. *et al.*: 1969, *Acta Otolaryng.* **67**, 293.
Montandon, A., Russbach, A., and Fumeaux, J.: 1960, *Confin. Neurol.* **20**, 253.
Mowrer, O. H.: 1935, *J. Comp. Physiol. Psychol.* **19**, 177.
Mulder, H.: 1908, Thesis. University of Utrecht, Utrecht, The Netherlands.
Oosterveld, W. J.: 1969, *Aerospace Med.* **40**, 382.
Oosterveld, W. J.: 1970, *Aerospace Med.* (in press).
Oosterveld, W. J. and Laarse, W. D. van der: 1968, *Ned. T. Geneesk.* **112**, 31.
Pfaltz, C. R.: 1957, *Arch. Ohr.-, Nas.- u. Kehlk.-Heilk.* **172**, 131.
Roggeveen, B. L. and Nijhoff, P.: 1956, *Acta Otolaryng.* **46**, 553.
Schierbeek, P.: 1953, *Pract. Otorhinolaryng.* **15**, 87.
Van Egmond, A. A. J., Groen, J. J., and Jongkees, L. B. W.: 1943, *Ned. T. Geneesk.* **87**, 1793.
Van Eyck, M.: 1953a, *Acta Otolaryng.* **48**, 306.
Van Eyck, M.: 1953b, Arch. Int. Physiol. Biochem. **61**, 113.
Van Eyck, M., Jongkees, L. B. W., and Klijn, J. A. J.: 1956, *Pract. Otorhinolaryng.* **18**, 282.
Van Eyck, M., Jongkees, L. B. W., and Klijn, J. A. J.: 1957, *Acta Otolaryng.* **47**, 402.
Van Rossem, A.: 1907, Thesis. University of Utrecht, Utrecht, The Netherlands.
Van Wulfften Palthe, P. M.: 1922, *Acta Otolaryng.* **4**, 415.

CENTRAL REGULATION OF VESTIBULAR FUNCTION

J. J. GROEN

Academic Hospital, Utrecht, The Netherlands

1. Introduction

The normal overall function of the vestibular system can be considered as the result of at least three interdependent activities:

(1) Afference generated in the peripheral organ by mechanical stimulation of the hair cells which activate the afferent neurons.

(2) Inhibition of the afference by efference generated in the central nervous system, to a degree depending upon the afference. The efference is transmitted along the Rasmussen bundle, terminating upon the hair cells of the peripheral organ, so reducing the transfer function between hair cell and neuron.

(3) Pattern center activity generated in the central nervous system when labyrinthine stimulation has a repetitive character.

2. Afference

In the laboratory, the isolated peripheral organ shows a resting activity measurable with an electrode as a constant stream of action potentials in the transsected vestibular nerve. When this isolated preparation is stimulated, as for example, on a torsion swing, the resting activity in the ampullar nerve of the lateral canal is modulated sinusoidally (Figure 1). The frequency of the action potentials rises and falls rhythmically with the movement of the swing. This response will stay the same for hours on end. There is neither adaptation nor fatigue (Groen *et al.*, 1952; Ledoux, 1958).

3. Inhibition

If the test animal is left intact and alive, adaptation of the peripheral organ to constant stimulation can be demonstrated (Figure 2). An electrode is brought into contact with the ampullar nerve from which the nerve sheath has been partially removed, saving the artery which serves the labyrinth. If lidocaine is applied to the nerve at a point between the electrode and the central nervous system, adaptation disappears and unbridled peripheral activity, as in an isolated preparation, will be recorded. As soon as the lidocaine blockade wears off, adaptation reappears, reducing activity to its former magnitude (Goetmakers, 1968). In the frog, this reduction is considerable; the normally adapted state has one-third of the maximum, unadapted sensitivity. Under constant stimulation, sensitivity is still further reduced within two minutes to even one-tenth of its maximum value. If left alone, this extra adaptation will return to its normal value in about 5 min (Figure 3). From this, it may be concluded that there

D. E. Busby (ed.), Recent Advances in Aerospace Medicine, 269–275. All Rights Reserved.
Copyright © 1970 by D. Reidel Publishing Company, Dordrecht-Holland.

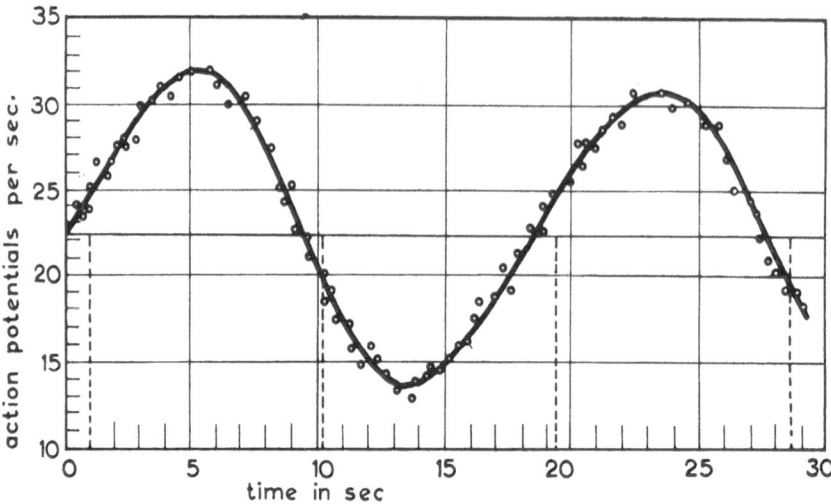

Fig. 1.   Frequency of the action potentials of a single nerve fiber preparation of the ampullar nerve of the lateral canal of a ray during a sinusoidal stimulation on a torsion swing with a period of 18.4 sec. The dotted lines represent the turning points of the swing.

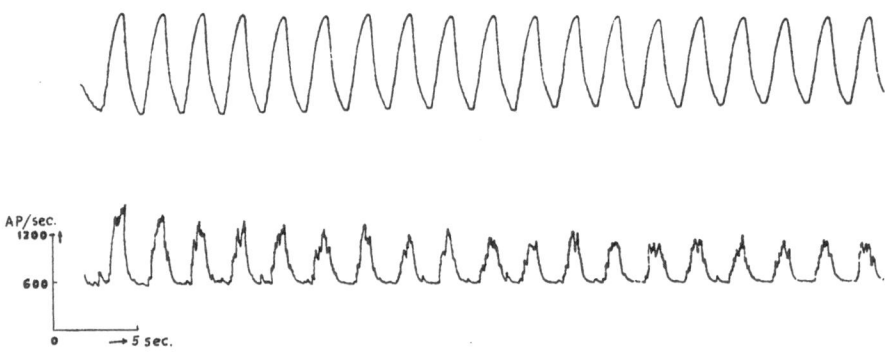

Fig. 2.   Adaptation phenomenon (lower trace) in the ampullar nerve of the lateral canal of a frog during sinusoidal stimulation on a torsion swing with a period of 2.5 sec (upper trace).

is an efference activity which inhibits the peripheral organ to a degree depending upon the intensity and duration of the stimulation.

Similar phenomena have been observed in the human test subject. The human appears to be in a constantly adapted state, the degree of adaptation among others depending upon previous vestibular experience (Figure 4). The inhibition responsible for this adaptation shows itself among others in shortening of duration of post-stimulatory phenomena such as nystagmus and sensation; the shorter they last the more adapted he is. Figure skaters, ballet dancers, fighter pilots and all those who submit themselves daily to intense rotational stimulation have attained the highest degree of adaptation (Figure 5). In contrast to the frog's recuperation time of 5 min, man needs days, even weeks, to regain the normal state of adaptation. This condition

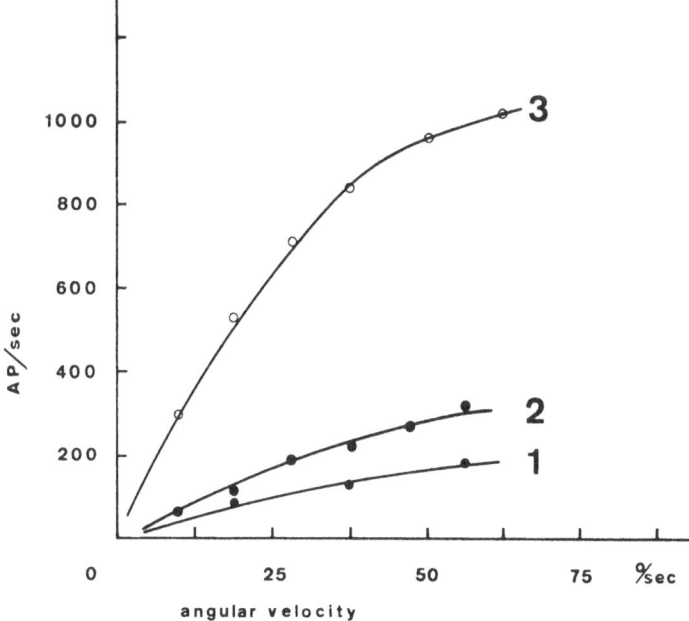

Fig. 3. Neural response (frequency of action potentials) of the ampullar nerve of the lateral canal of a frog during sinusoidal stimulation on a torsion swing (as in Figure 2), as a function of the magnitude of the stimulus (angular velocity) under different conditions. – (1) response after adaptation; (2) response before adaptation; (3) response after the animal had died. This shows a considerable amount of adaptation to exist in the condition before adaptation (graph 2).

of prolonged sensitivity reduction is called 'retention' (Krijger, 1954; Aschan, 1954; Hood and Pfaltz, 1954).

The loop consisting of the hair-cells with the afferent nerve, its central projection together with the efferent nerve returning to the hair-cells, forms a cybernetic system, the function of which is comparable to the automatic volume control circuit of a hearing aid. It is highly probable that this cybernetic loop is not the only one in the vestibular system.

4. Pattern Center

If man or animal is submitted to prolonged repetitive stimulation of his labyrinths, a copy of the motion pattern will be projected gradually in this pattern center, the location of which is unknown at the moment. It must be somewhere in the central nervous system, presumably in the reticular formation. This pattern center, by means of its copy activity and in collaboration with vestibular afference, keeps control of body balance and orientation; anticipation of body movement is taken care of and sensation is partly compensated. An example of pattern center activity is given by the passenger on ocean-going vessel. He will at first stumble around the ship, each movement taking him by surprise, even causing symptoms of sea sickness. After 3 days he will be used to the ship's heaving and rolling, he will no more notice the ever-changing balance demands; he will feel at ease, nauseating symptoms also having disappeared.

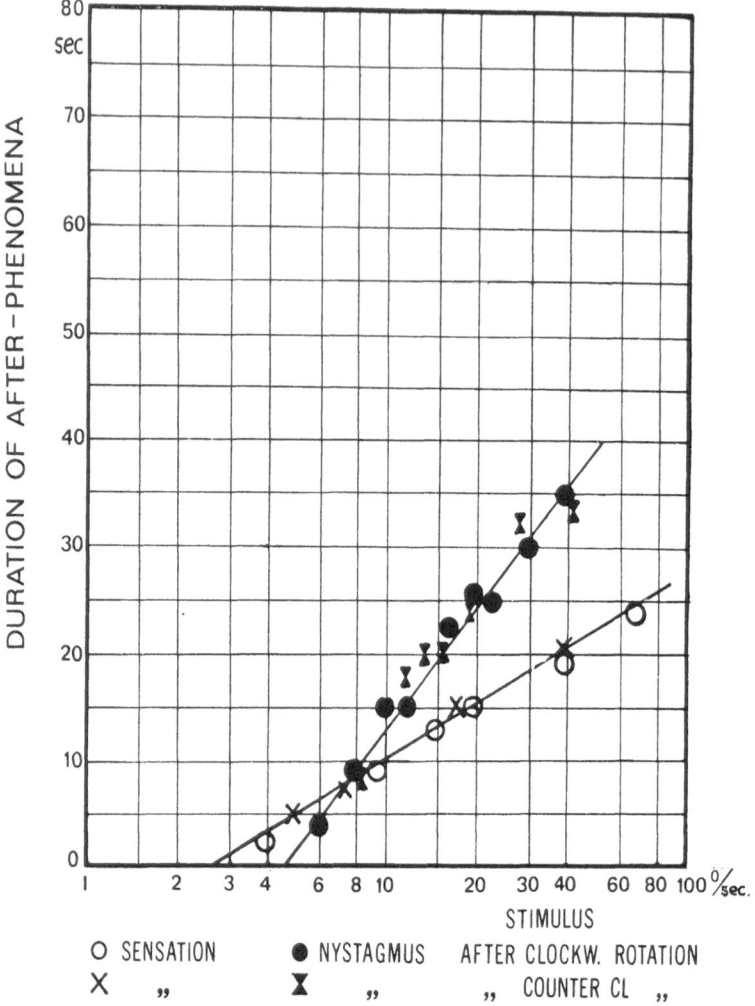

Fig. 4. Duration of after-phenomena with a normal human test subject on a turning chair as a function of the magnitude of the stimulus (angular velocity prior to the stopping). Sensation lasts shorter than nystagmus, the former being more inhibited than the latter.

As soon as he disembarks he will be unsteady on firm ground. When he walks in the vaguely lit corridor of his hotel, the walls will suddenly move over. In his bed he will go through all the ship's movements. Usually it will take 1 to 3 days to get rid of these after-phenomena, but in some cases these after-phenoma can last a month before the phantom ship definitely vanishes. These after-phenoma are due to his pattern center, where the copy of the ship's complicated movement was gradually built up, persisting after the cessation of the real movement (Groen, 1957). Comparable observations have been made with human test subjects in a rotating room (Guedry, 1965).

In a laboratory experiment on normal human test subjects, pattern center activity can be demonstrated within a quarter of an hour of uninterrupted periodic stimulation on a torsion swing (Clemens and Festen, 1969). Test subjects were selected for total

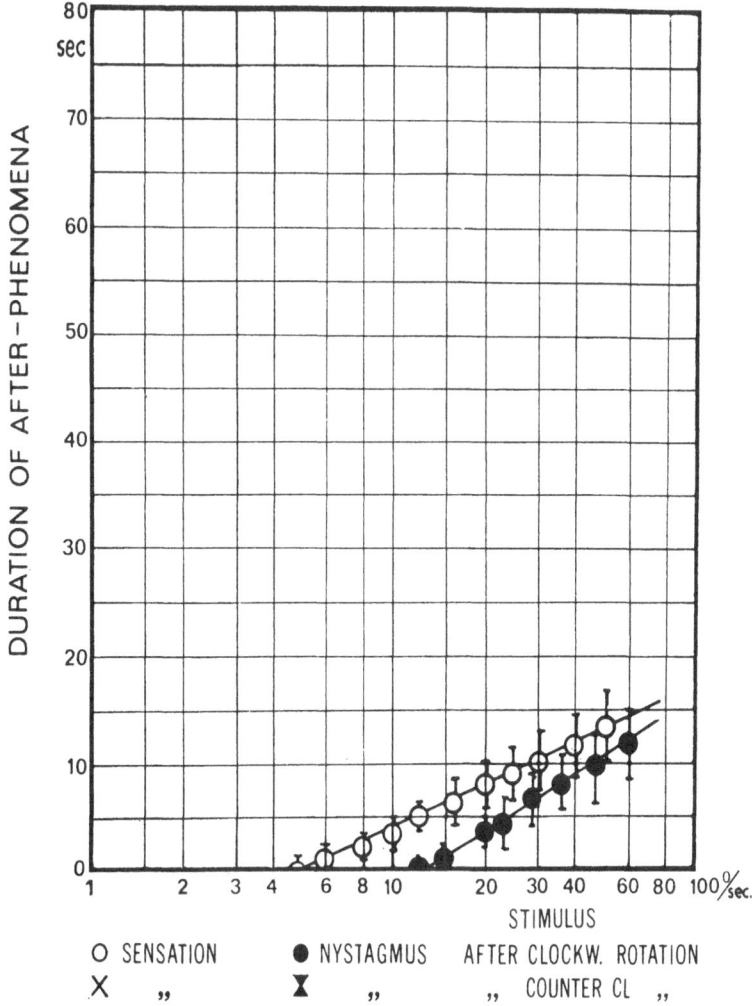

Fig. 5. The same data as in Figure 4 but now for fighter pilots who show far more inhibition of their vestibular responses, the durations of which are considerably reduced.

absence of latent nystagmus or spontaneous eye movements. The test was carried out in complete darkness. The stimulation lasted 15 min. Then the swing was stopped in an outward position, thus force-free, lest residual mechanical stimulation would occur. During and after the swinging, eye movements were continuously recorded in the usual way. Several phenomena could be observed.

(1) During the oscillatory period, eye movements are at first approximately sinusoidal on which nystagmus is superimposed.

(2) Gradually, inhibition will suppress nystagmus, but eye movements go on roughly sinusoidally.

(3) Eye movements then will also decrease gradually to reappear a few oscillations afterwards (Figure 6).

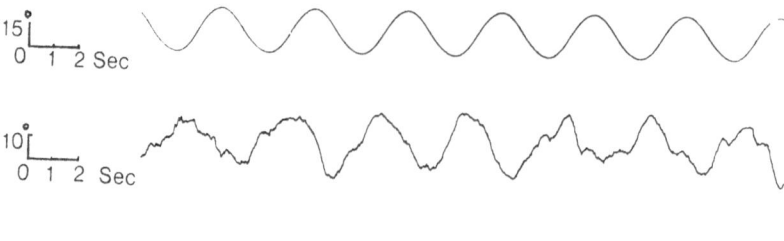

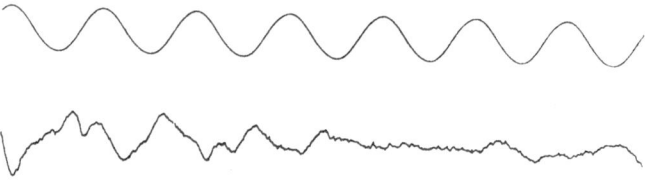

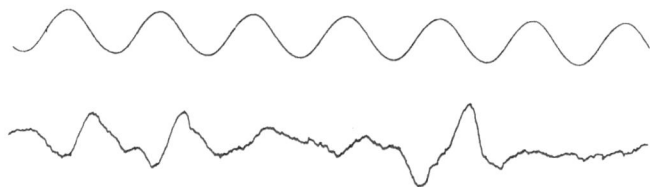

Fig. 6. Per-oscillatory eye movements (lower tracings) of a test subject on a torsion swing (upper tracings) submitted to sustained sinusoidal oscillation. The picture represents the recording during the tenth minute. Inhibition has reduced nystagmus almost completely whereas smooth eye movements persist. This one also declines to reappear after a few swingings with a changed phase difference in relation to the swing. The three pairs of tracings are reproductions of a continuous recording; beginnings and ends overlap.

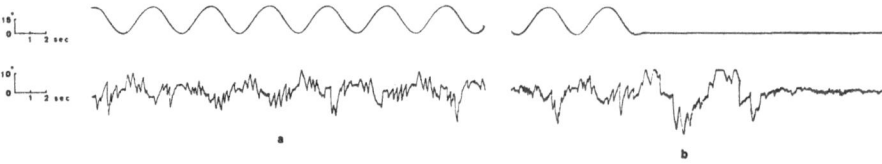

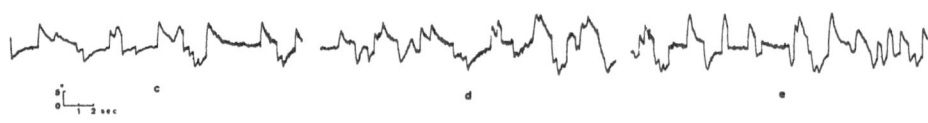

Fig. 7. Per- and post-oscillatory eye movements on torsion swing. – (a) upper trace: torsion swing (period 4.1 sec); lower trace: per-oscillatory eye movements; (b) upper trace: torsion swing stops; lower trace: eye movements go on after stopping; (c), (d), (e) post-oscillatory eye movements, 3.5, 5.5 and 10 min since stopping.

(4) This waning and waxing goes on while the swinging lasts.

(5) After the stopping of the swing, almost one-half of the test subjects demonstrated one or two complete eye oscillations with nystagmus superimposed, as if the swing had not stopped (Figure 7).

(6) During the post-oscillatory period, spontaneous eye oscillations will reappear in clusters every 5 min or thereabouts for one-half an hour or more.

(7) When the originally symptom-free test subjects are retested the next day, they will show spontaneous eye movements and nystagmus without any provocation.

From these observations, it may be concluded that a pattern center copy of sinusoidal character is developed during the 15 min oscillatory period. This copy interferes by beating with the afference of the vestibular organs. The copy persists on cessation of the swinging; this would explain the spontaneous extra eye oscillations afterwards and on the next day. It appears that only those who are able to develop a copy produce inhibition as well.

5. Conclusions

The central nervous system regulates the flow of vestibular messages in several interrelated ways, two of them having been discussed in detail – inhibition and copy formation. They show the complexity of so-called normal vestibular function.

References

Aschan, G.: 1954, *Acta Otolaryng. Suppl.* **116**, 24.

Clemens, A. and Festen, H.: 1969, *Acta Otorhinolaryng.* (in press).

Festen, H. and Clemens, A.: 1969, *Adv. Otorhinolaryng.* **17**, 101.

Goetmakers, R.: 1968, *Adaptatie van het evenwichtsorgaan*, Doctoral Thesis, University of Utrecht, The Netherlands.

Goetmakers, R.: 1970, *Adv. Otorhinolaryng.* **17**, 106.

Groen, J. J.: 1957, *Practica Otorhinolaryng.* **19**, 524.

Groen, J. J., Löwenstein, O., and Vendrik, A. J. H.: 1952, *J. Physiol.* **117**, 329.

Guedry, F. E.: 1965, *Psychophysiological Studies of Vestibular Function. Contributions to Sensory Physiology*, Vol. I, Academic Press, New York.

Hood, J. D. and Pfaltz, C. R.: 1954, *J. Physiol.* **124**, 130.

Krijger, M. W. W.: 1954, *De betekenis van het evenwichtsorgaan voor de vlieger*, Doctoral Thesis, University of Utrecht, Utrecht, The Netherlands.

Ledoux, A.: 1958, *Acta Otorhinolaryng.* **12**, 13.

TRACKING PERFORMANCE DURING SINUSOIDAL STIMULATION OF THE VERTICAL AND HORIZONTAL SEMICIRCULAR CANALS*

F. E. GUEDRY, JR.

U.S. Naval Aerospace Medical Institute, Pensacola, Fla., U.S.A.

and

A. J. BENSON

Royal Air Force Institute of Aviation Medicine, Farnborough, U.K.

1. Introduction

In the past, the greater part of the experimental investigation of the semicircular canals of man has involved stimulation of the horizontal canals by angular acceleration about an Earth-vertical axis. Typically, the vertical axis (z-axis) of the head has been approximately aligned with the axis of rotation which in turn has been aligned with gravity. However, in aerospace flight the vertical canals are frequently stimulated, and, of course, the axis of rotation is usually not aligned with gravity. Because of the complexities of linear and angular accelerations in flight, an understanding of the perceptual and reflex responses to vestibular stimulation in flight demands an understanding of how various sensory inputs from the canals, otoliths, eyes, and other systems are analyzed and stored by central processes.

The work described here deals directly with only one part of this over-all problem. The effects of vertical-canal stimulation will be compared with effects of horizontal-canal stimulation when the axis of rotation is aligned with gravity. Initially this line of investigation in our laboratory was prompted by a question from the National Aeronautics and Space Administration. It was anticipated that an emergency abort procedure during a particular stage of an Apollo flight would produce capsule rotation about the man's y-axis (an axis through the ears) at a rate of 200 deg/sec, persisting for as long as 12 sec, followed by deceleration to a stable attitude. The question was: To what extent would nystagmus and disorientation immediately after the rotation degrade an astronaut's ability to reposition the capsule into a safe re-entry attitude? It was anticipated that time, a matter of 20 or 30 sec, could be critical.

During investigations of the effect of y-axis rotation, Hixson and Niven (1964) discovered that visual acuity for observer-fixed eye charts after an angular impulse differed substantially, depending upon whether the stimulus produced upbeating or downbeating nystagmus. These findings have been confirmed in subsequent studies (Guedry, 1968a: Hixson and Niven, 1969). It is to be expected that comparable

* This study was supported by the U.S. Army Aeromedical Research Laboratory and the National Aeronautics and Space Administration.

D. E. Busby (ed.), Recent Advances in Aerospace Medicine, 276–288. All Rights Reserved.
Copyright © 1970 by D. Reidel Publishing Company, Dordrecht-Holland.

rotational stimuli in the flight environment would impair visibility of cockpit instruments and hence the ability of the pilot to fly by instruments with accuracy (Guedry,
1968b; Jones, 1965). The experiment reported here examines the effect of vestibular
stimulation on an extrapolation of the instrument flying task, viz. compensatory
tracking during various conditions of display luminance.

2. Procedure

The test situations are illustrated in Figure 1. Throughout most of the experiments,
the stimulus to the semicircular canals was a sinusoidal oscillation about an Earth-
vertical axis with a period of 25 sec. The subject was positioned with head on center in
one of two positions: upright, so that rotation was about his z-axis, or left side down,
so that rotation was about his y-axis.

The visual display, tracking equipment, and recording setup are illustrated sche-
matically in Figure 2. The visual display was a cross-pointer indicator usually referred
to as a glide-slope meter; it is commonly used in aircraft for instrument landing
approaches. This was illuminated by a projector fitted with neutral-density filters,
which gave instrument-pointer luminances of 0.01, 0.1, 1.0, and 10.0 ft-lambert. The
forcing function for the display was a continuous, unpredictable signal made of five
independent sinewaves in the frequency band 0.01 to 0.25 Hz.

The subject's task was to keep the vertical needle of the display centered in null
position. A voltage proportional to deviation from the null position was recorded, and

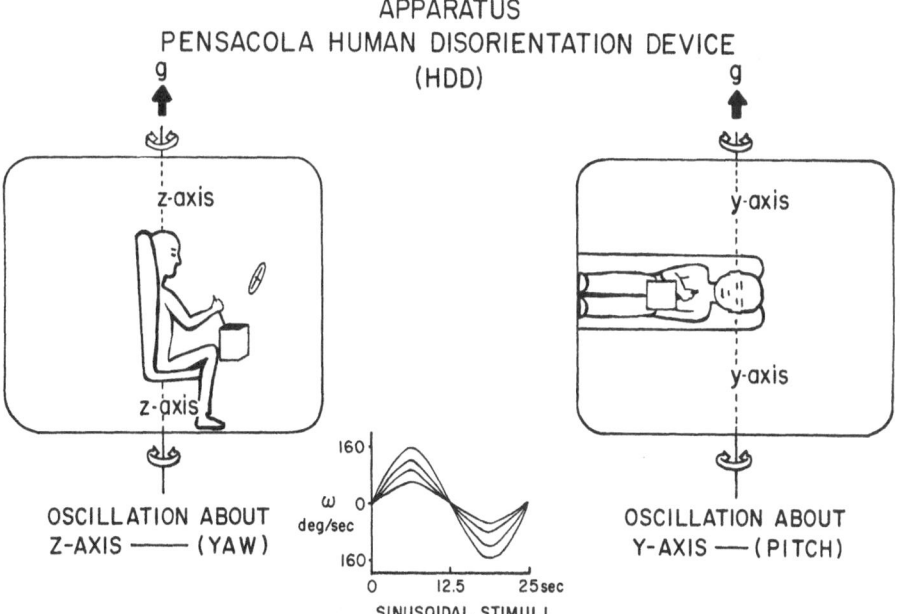

Fig. 1.   Positions used for stimulating the horizontal semicircular canals (picture on left) and the
vertical semicircular canals (picture on right) on the HDD.

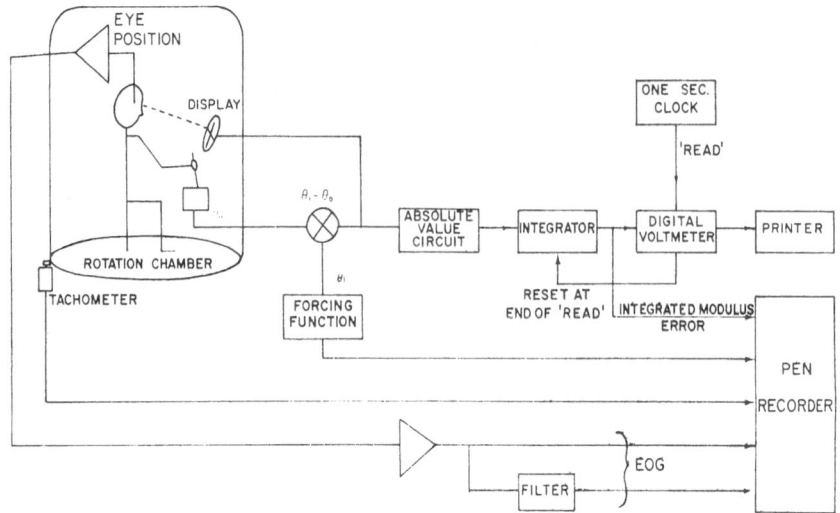

Fig. 2.   Schematic illustration of data processing and recording system.

its absolute value over successive 1-sec periods provided error scores that were used as measures of performance. Lateral and vertical eye movements were recorded by the conventional oculographic technique. A sample record is shown in Figure 3. A more complete description of the apparatus and procedure has been presented in a separate report (Gilson *et al.*, 1969).

Subjects were young men from the laboratory staff and from the Naval Aviation Schools Command, Pensacola, Fla. From 5 to 20 subjects participated in each of a series of experiments; 47 subjects in all were tested.

3. Results

Figure 4 summarizes two experiments in which the effect of display luminance on performance and on nystagmus was recorded. The left half of Figure 4 refers to results obtained during sinusoidal oscillation about the z-axis (yaw axis), and the right half refers to results obtained during sinusoidal oscillation about the y-axis (pitch axis). In both cases the axis of rotation was aligned with gravity, and the stimulus velocity was varied sinusoidally with a frequency of 0.04 Hz and maxima of 159 deg/sec.

Performance decrement during the course of each stimulus cycle was biphasic, with the peak decrements occurring just after the two stimulus-velocity maxima. It is apparent that luminance level of the instrument face was an important determinant of performance, especially between 0.01 and 1.0 ft-lambert. Increase in luminance from 1.0 to 10.0 ft-lambert yielded only slight additional improvement. Because these luminance values are within a range recommended for aircraft instrument lighting (Morgan *et al.*, 1963), the demonstrated effects of luminance on tracking performance during dynamic vestibular stimulation would seem to have practical implications for

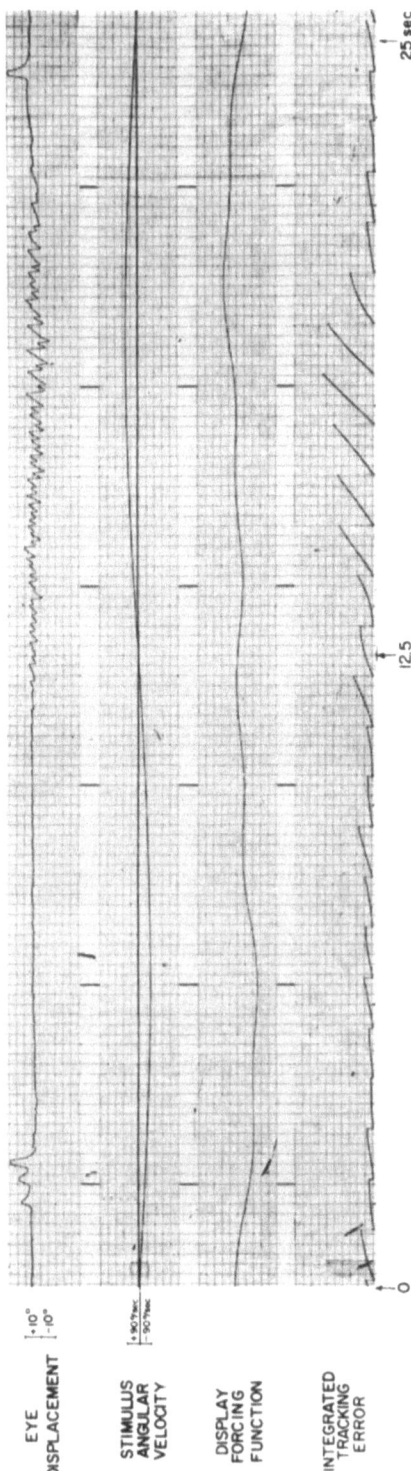

Fig. 3. Polygraph record of the stimulus and response data. This record is from sinusoidal oscillation about the subject's *y*-axis when instrument luminance was 0.1 ft-lambert. Note the absence of nystagmus (upper tracing) and good performance (bottom tracing) during backward pitch (0–12.5 sec) and the strong nystagmus and poor performance during forward pitch (12.5–25 sec).

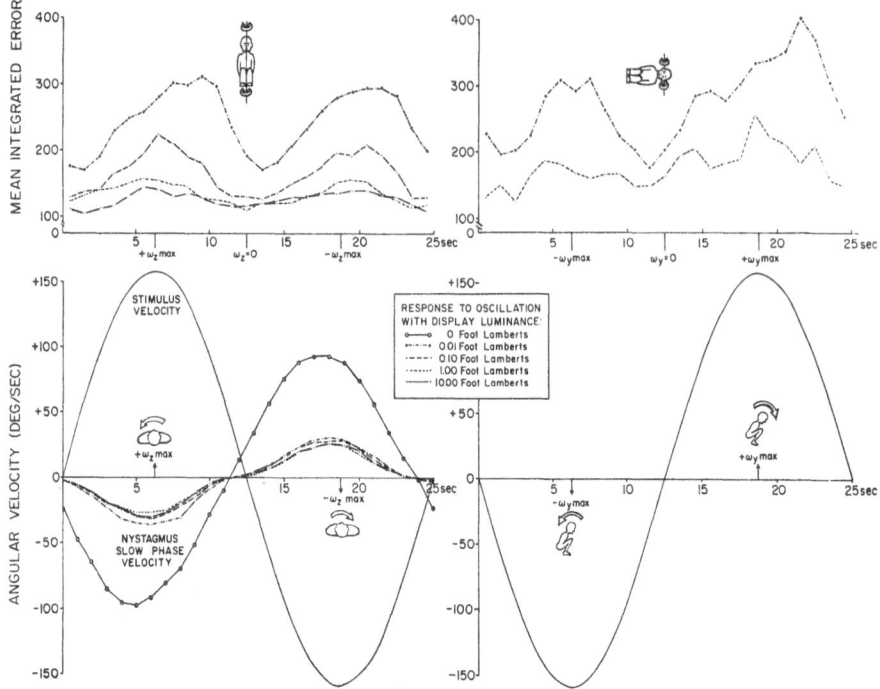

Fig. 4. Effect of luminance on tracking performance (upper graphs) and on nystagmus (lower left graph) during sinusoidal oscillation about the z-axis (graphs on the left) and during sinusoidal oscillation about the y-axis (graphs on the right). Solid curves in lower graphs depict stimulus velocity with respect to time. In upper left figure, $N = 20$ subjects × 10 cycles; nystagmus was recorded from 5 of these 20 so that $N = 5$ subjects × 10 cycles in the lower left figure. In the upper right figure, $N = 6$ subjects × 5 cycles. Although 15 subjects were tested, 9 were eliminated because of sickness. Vertical nystagmus was not successfully recorded with this stimulus, and thus no plots of vertical nystagmus are presented in the lower right graph.

cockpit lighting. Comparison of the nystagmus in the dark (0 ft-lambert in Figure 4) and when the display was illuminated revealed that even at the lowest level of display luminance (0.01 ft-lambert), nystagmus slow-phase velocity was reduced to about one third of that obtained in the dark. However, somewhat to our surprise, increasing display luminance from 0.01 to 10.0 ft-lambert, a one thousandfold increase in brightness, gave little additional suppression of nystagmus. Thus it may be concluded that a given level of nystagmus degrades tracking performance, and the amount of degradation depends upon the luminance level of the instrument.

Noteworthy are the differences in effects of luminance level on task performance when stimuli produced nystagmus of different directions. During stimuli directed to produce leftbeating and rightbeating nystagmus (oscillation in 'yaw'), performance was about the same for these two directions; but during forward pitch it was inferior to performance during backward pitch. Unfortunately, an adequate comparison of directional effects was complicated by two problems. First, under these test conditions (oscillation 'in pitch', 0.04 Hz, 159 deg/sec maximum velocity), the quality of recordings of vertical nystagmus was very poor, especially when fast phase was down. This was probably due, at least in part, to eyelid artifacts (Ford, 1959; Jones *et al.*, 1964). Second, because of motion sickness only 6 of 15 subjects were able to complete a test session, even though the length of the test session was reduced by eliminating two of the luminance levels and by reducing the number of 'steady-state' cycles per run. Thus the directional effects revealed by the performance measures could not be evaluated in detail.

In another experiment, however, the magnitude of canal stimulation was reduced (Figure 5). Under these circumstances adequate records of vertical nystagmus were obtained, and also the incidence of sickness was substantially reduced. Thus responses in yaw and in pitch from one set of subjects could be compared. In this experiment instrument luminance was maintained at 0.1 ft-lambert.

It was found that nystagmus slow phase velocity and performance decrements were greater during 'pitch forward' than during the other stimulus conditions. Figure 5 also illustrates differences in phase relations of vertical and horizontal nystagmus to the stimulus. Measurement of the point of reversal of the mean slow-phase velocity revealed that phase advance of compensatory vertical nystagmus was about 30 to 40 deg, whereas for the horizontal nystagmus it was about 15 deg.

In an earlier paper (Guedry, 1968a), it was concluded that the differences in vertical nystagmus (up vs. down) were attributable to differences in visual suppression of these two reactions. This conclusion was based on results indicating that the upbeating

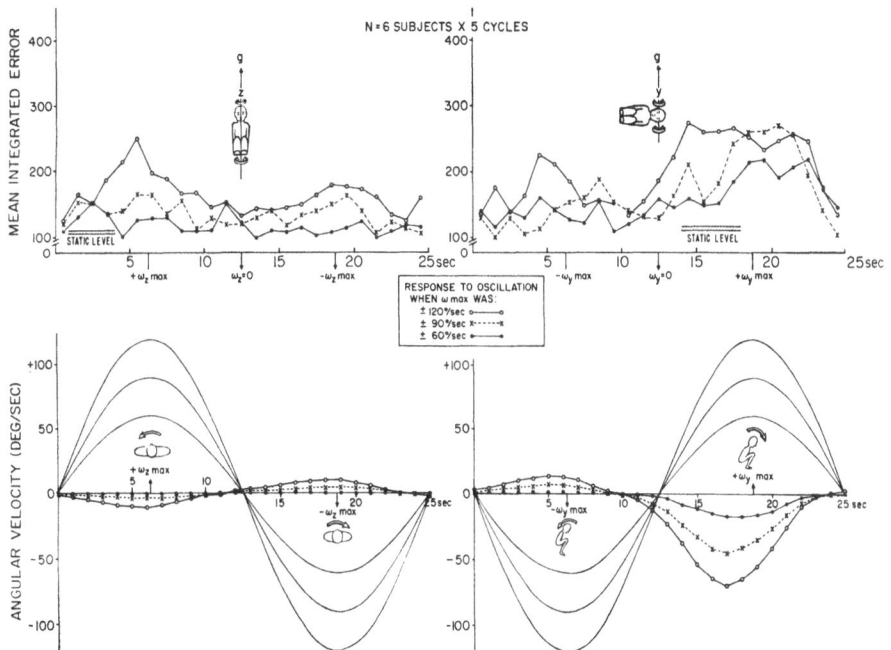

Fig. 5. Effect of peak stimulus velocity on performance (upper graphs) and nystagmus (lower graphs) during sinusoidal oscillation about the *z*-axis (graphs on the left) and about the *y*-axis (graphs on the right). Luminance level of the instrument was 0.1 ft-lambert. Each of 6 subjects participated in all conditions of this experiment.

and downbeating nystagmus are equal in magnitude when elicited in darkness, but unequal when elicited during visual stimulation. Results in the present series of experiments, however, were not entirely consistent with this finding. When a sinusoidal stimulus with a peak-to-peak velocity change of ±90 deg/sec was used, vertical nystagmus in the dark was slightly greater in the fast-phase down direction, as shown in Figure 6. During tracking, with either the 0.01 or the 1.0 ft-lambert luminance level, the difference in the two directions of nystagmus was accentuated apparently due to differential visual suppression of the reactions. Following this, when subjects were again tested in the dark, there was a much more pronounced difference between downbeating nystagmus and upbeating nystagmus. In other words, there was a response decline in nystagmus in the dark from the beginning to the end of the session, and the decline in upbeating nystagmus was greater than the decline in downbeating nystagmus. Only 6 subjects participated in this experiment, but there was a similar

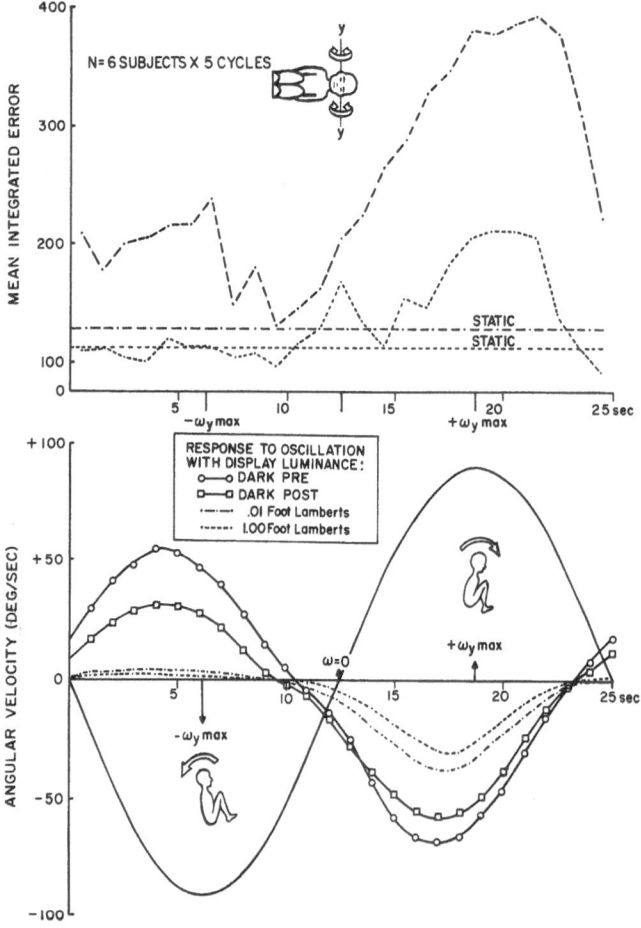

Fig. 6.   Effect of luminance on performance (upper graph) and on nystagmus (lower graph) during sinusoidal oscillation about the *y*-axis when the peak stimulus velocity was ±90 deg/sec. Each of 6 subjects participated in all conditions of this experiment.

difference in response decline in all 6, suggesting that this effect was probably not attributable to chance (sign test: $P=0.016$). Thus a minor difference in slow-phase velocity in the dark was accentuated in the light, and the direction of the reaction most affected by the light also showed the greater response decline from the beginning to the end of the test session.

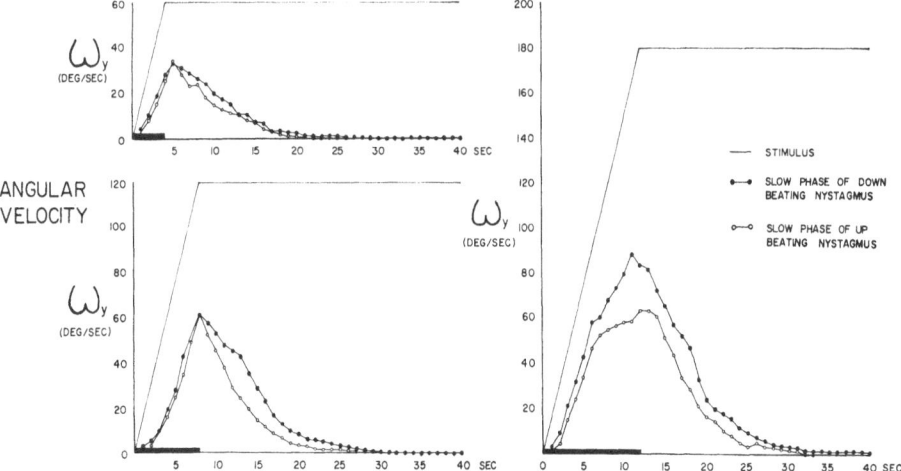

Fig. 7.   Comparison of mean slow-phase velocity of upbeating nystagmus and downbeating nystagmus produced by 15 deg/sec² accelerations maintained for 4, 8, and 12 sec. Nystagmus was recorded in darkness from 8 subjects.

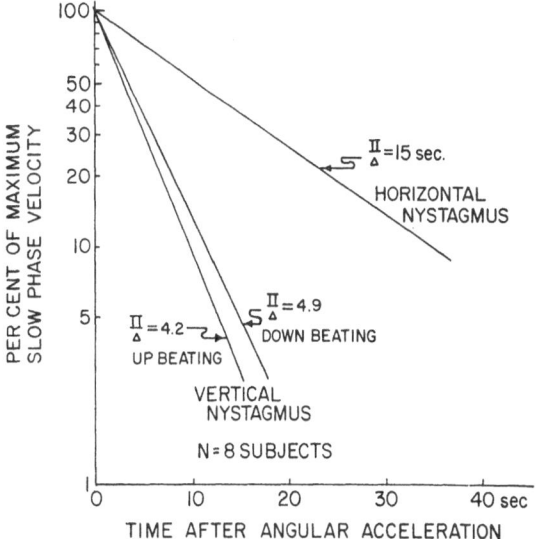

Fig. 8.   Comparing mean slopes of nystagmus decay curves following angular impulses. Slopes were obtained by least-squares fit through paired values of nystagmus velocity and time. The ordinate scale is logarithmic.

To investigate further the differences between the two vertical nystagmus reactions in the dark, another group of 8 subjects were tested by a series of 'ramp' stimuli that involved the following changes in angular velocity: 60-deg/sec change, 120-deg/sec change, and 180-deg/sec change. The mean results shown in Figure 7 indicate that maximum slow-phase velocities of the two reactions in darkness are approximately equal for the 60-deg/sec change and for the 120-deg/sec change, but the mean reactions appear to be unequal with the 180-deg/sec change.

The rate of decay of vertical nystagmus in the dark after each of the ramp stimuli was about the same for the two directions of response: but in either direction, the rate of decay was very fast as compared with that of horizontal nystagmus under similar circumstances, as shown in Figure 8. These linear plots represent the mean slopes of the best-fitting straight lines, as determined by the method of least squares, through plots of paired values of $\log_e$ of slow-phase velocity and time. According to the terminology introduced by Van Egmond *et al.* (1949) and Groen (1960), Π/Δ represents the time constant of the cupula restoration as inferred from the decline of responses such as nystagmus, and it is calculated from the reciprocal of the slopes of curves such as those in Figure 8. The difference in Π/Δ between vertical and horizontal nystagmus is statistically reliable (cf. Jones, 1965; Benson and Bodin, 1966), and it is consistent with the differences in phase relations apparent in Figures 4, 5, and 6 above. The small difference in Π/Δ between downbeating and upbeating nystagmus may be attributable to chance.

There were also characteristic differences between upbeating and downbeating nystagmus in regard to beat frequency (Figure 9). During sinusoidal oscillation about the y-axis ($\omega_y[\max] = \pm 90$ deg/sec, 0.04 Hz), downbeating nystagmus had a higher frequency than upbeating nystagmus in the dark (sign test: $P = 0.016$). Illumination.

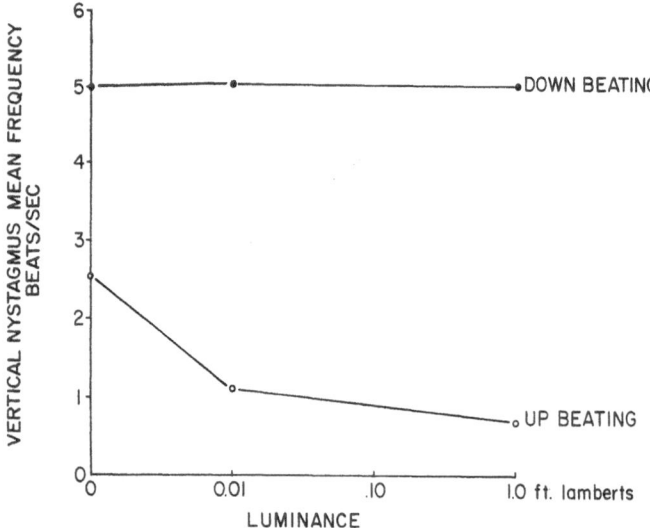

Fig. 9.   Effect of luminance on mean number of nystagmus beats per second during a 3-sec interval encompassing the point of maximum slow-phase velocity. Stimulus was oscillation about the y-axis at 0.04 Hz, with peak velocity of 90 deg/sec. $N = 6$ subjects $\times$ 5 cycles.

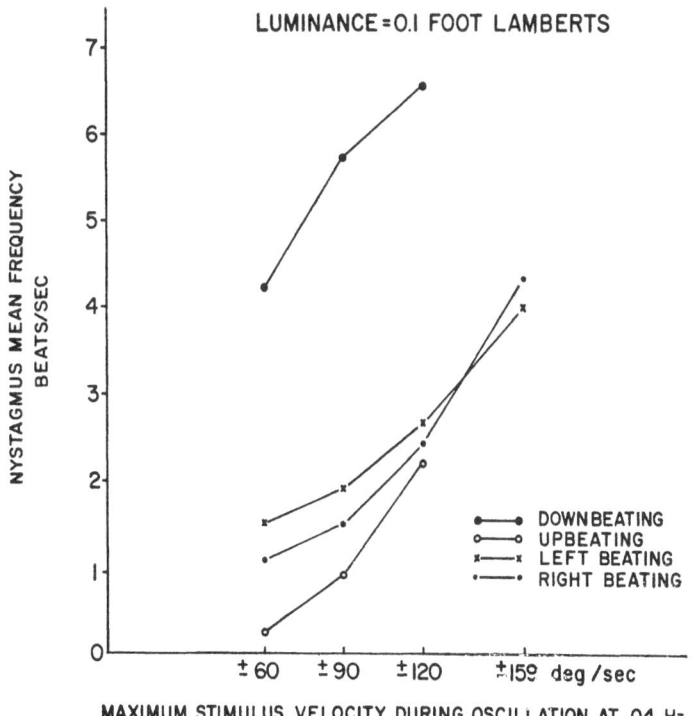

Fig. 10. Effect of peak stimulus velocity on mean nystagmus beat frequency (during 3-sec interval of maximum slow phase velocity) for different nystagmus directions. The luminance level was 0.1 ft·lambert and the oscillation frequency was 0.04 Hz. Mean ordinate values for 60, 90, and 120 deg/sec points on the axis of abscissa are based on one group of 6 subjects × 5 cycles. Mean ordinate values for the 159-deg/sec abscissa point are based on another group of 5 subjects × 10 cycles.

irrespective of luminance level, did not influence the frequency of downbeating nystagmus, whereas it reduced the frequency of the upbeating nystagmus. Hence, the directional difference in frequency manifested in the dark was accentuated by the introduction of light.

Further evidence of the difference between upbeating and downbeating nystagmus was afforded in experiments in which the display luminance was constant (0.1 ft-lambert), but the magnitude of sinusoidal stimulus was altered (Figure 10). Again it was found that downbeating nystagmus had a higher frequency than upbeating nystagmus. The frequency of horizontal nystagmus (right-or leftbeating) was more akin to the upbeating vertical nystagmus than to the downbeating vertical nystagmus. This impression of a similarity between rightbeating, leftbeating, and upbeating nystagmus is supported by comparison of the slow-phase velocity of nystagmus presented in Figure 5 above, but it is not supported by the relative decay rates illustrated in Figure 8.

4. Summary and Conclusions

Visual tracking performance comparable to that involved in instrument flight can be disrupted by strong semicircular canal stimulation. The amount of performance degradation depends upon the luminance level of instruments; this is true within a range of luminance levels recommended for cockpit lighting. Increasing the luminance level from 0.01 ft-lambert to 1.0 ft-lambert substantially improves the tracking of instruments during vestibular nystagmus. Increasing luminance from 1.0 to 10.0 ft-lambert provides only a slight additional improvement in performance. It should be noted that whereas sustained sinusoidal oscillations like those in the present experiments are not likely to be duplicated in conventional aircraft, rotational stimuli can attain magnitudes sufficient to degrade visual performance in flight (Jones, 1965), and individuals differ significantly in their ability to see under these circumstances (Guedry, 1968a, b).

The direction of the semicircular canal stimulus relative to the man also controls the amount of degradation in performance. Stimuli producing vertical nystagmus with fast phase down produce much stronger nystagmus and much greater performance degradation than stimuli producing vertical nystagmus with fast phase up or horizontal nystagmus of either direction.

In the present experiments, two kinds of directional effects were noted in regard to vestibular reactions. One was the difference between nystagmus up and nystagmus down with stimuli of equal magnitude but opposite directions about the man's y-axis. The other was the difference between horizontal nystagmus and vertical nystagmus produced by stimuli about the z and y-axes, respectively.

The difference in the rates of decay of horizontal and vertical nystagmus after an angular impulse and the difference in the stimulus-response phase relations during sinusoidal stimulation suggest that the time constant of the vertical canals is considerably shorter than the time constant of the horizontal canals (Jones et al., 1964). However, central mechanisms may also be involved. During natural movement, stimulation of the vertical canals by rotation about the y-axis almost always involves a change in orientation relative to gravity, because the axis of rotation is not vertical. It has been clearly demonstrated that nystagmus is influenced by changes in orientation relative to gravity, probably as a result of a central interplay of otolith and canal information (Benson, 1966; Guedry, 1966; Guedry, 1969). The otoliths are believed to be a faster responding system than the canals (Jongkees and Groen, 1946; de Vries, 1950). The continual natural interplay between vertical canals and otoliths in controlling eye movements may result in a central processing of peripheral information which is more rapid for the information supplied by the vertical than that supplied by the horizontal semicircular canals. In other words, some of the differences in response to vertical- and horizontal-canal stimulation may be a result of central rather than peripheral factors.

In regard to the differences in upbeating and downbeating nystagmus, it seems unlikely that this can be attributed to differences in the dynamics of the particular semicircular canals involved because the same canals were involved in both reactions. The visual system may account for some of the differences noted. Downbeating nystagmus in the dark is stronger than upbeating nystagmus with intense canal stimuli, and there is evidence (Benson and Guedry, 1969) which suggests that the same kind of difference exists when moving visual targets elicit a visual-tracking response in the absence of vestibular stimulation. This implies a bias in the oculomotor system in favor of downbeating nystagmus, irrespective of whether the vestibular or visual system initiates the eye movement. With vestibular stimuli which produce equal slow-phase velocities, however, downbeating vestibular nystagmus is much less suppressed by the introduction of vision than is upbeating nystagmus. 'Retinal smear' seems to be a less effective error signal in one direction than another, either due to some curious visual effect or due to oculomotor responses which have a directional bias. Whatever the reasons, downbeating nystagmus was less affected by vision than upbeating, leftbeating, or rightbeating nystagmus.

Finally, let us consider some speculations about functional aspects of these responses. Typically, locomotion is forward as opposed to lateral or backward. During rapid forward movement it is necessary to attend briefly to an array of visual stimuli at or below eye level while maintaining clear vision of more distant objects. This ability to suppress optokinetic stimuli from important visual detail below eye level may account for some of the differences between upbeating and downbeating nystagmus. Also, the most likely consequence of faulty locomotion is a forward tumble; consequently, reactions to correct for forward tumble may be faster than other reactions. Probably the first emergency visual action during forward tumble is a rapid downward glance. The utricular and saccular otolith surfaces are curved such that the frontal and horizontal head planes are well supplied with otolith-bearing sensory epithelia. This structural characteristic may be a significant factor in correcting head position and eye position during forward pitch. Further evidence indicative of an emergency reaction during forward pitch may be adduced from the 'Coriolis vestibular reaction'. During clockwise rotation about an Earth-vertical axis, a right lateral head tilt produces an experience of backward pitch, while the return head movement to upright produces an experience of forward pitch. Even when the two head movements are controlled to deliver angular impulses of equal magnitude to the semicircular canals, subjects typically report displeasure and fear reactions during the perception of forward pitch which are much greater than the effects reported during backward pitch (Guedry and Montague, 1961). This may be related to the differences between upbeating and downbeating nystagmus in the present experiments.

To develop an understanding of man's reactions during aerospace operations, a necessary starting point is a clear understanding of the physics of motion and its relation to the mechanics of the vestibular receptors. But this is only a starting point. Perceptions and reactions during the complex angular and linear accelerations in aerospace operations are also influenced by the central processing of sensory inputs from the vestibular, visual, and somatosensory systems. This central processing is undoubtedly conditioned by past experience of the individual in his natural environment and in his flight environment. When the flight environment introduces unnatural combinations of sensory inputs, the past flight experience of the individual is especially important in determining his reactions.

References

Benson, A. J.: 1966, in *The Role of the Vestibular Organs in Space Exploration*, NASA SP-115, National Aeronautics and Space Administration, Washington, D.C., p. 199.

Benson, A. J. and Bodin, M. A.: 1966, *Aerospace Med.* **37**, 889.

Benson, A. J. and Guedry, F. E.: 1969 (in preparation).

Egmond, A. A. J. van, Groen, J. J., and Jongkees, L. B. W : 1949, *J. Physiol.* **110**, 1.

Ford, A.: 1959, *Arch. Ophthal.* **61**, 899.

Gilson, R. D., Benson, A. J., and Guedry, F. E.: 1969 (in preparation).

Groen, J. J.: 1960, *Acta Otolaryng., Suppl.* **163**, 59.

Guedry, F. E.: 1966, in *The Role of the Vestibular Organs in Space Exploration*, NASA SP-115, National Aeronautics and Space Administration, Washington, D.C., p. 185.

Guedry, F. E.: 1968a, Wenner-Gren Center International Symposium Series.

Guedry, F. E.: 1968b, *Aerospace Med.* **39**, 570.

Guedry, F. E.: 1969, Presented to *International Congress of Oto-Rhino-Laryngology*, Mexico City, Mexico.

Guedry, F. E. and Montague, E. K.: 1961, *Aerospace Med.* **32**, 487.

Hixson, W. C. and Niven, J. I.: 1964, Letter report to NASA Manned Spacecraft Center, Houston, Tex., U.S.A.

Hixson, W. C. and Niven, J. I.: 1969, NAMI-1079, Naval Aerospace Medical Institute, Pensacola, Fla, U.S.A.

Jones, G. Melvill: 1965, *Aerospace Med.* **36**, 976.

Jones, G. Melvill, Barry, W., and Kowalsky, N.: 1964, *Aerospace Med.* **35**, 984.

Jongkees, L. B. W. and Groen, J. J.: 1946, *J. Laryngol.* **61**, 529.

Morgan, C. T., Cook, J. S., Chapanis, A., and Lund, M. W.: 1963, *Human Engineering Guide to Equipment Design*, McGraw-Hill, New York, N.Y., U.S.A.

Vries, H. L. de: 1950, *Acta Otolaryng.* **38**, 262.

UN NOUVEAU TEST DE DÉSORIENTATION SPATIALE AVEC QUELQUES RÉSULTATS CONCERNANT LE RÔLE DES OTOLITHES DANS LE MÉCANISME DE RÉORIENTATION

U. BRANDT

Medical Department, Swedish Air Force, Stockholm, Sweden

1. Introduction

L'appareil vestibulaire contient deux systèmes de récepteurs sensoriels: les canaux semicirculaires, influencés par des impulsions d'ordre cinétique; les otolithes, mis en jeu par des excitants d'ordre statique. Il faut y adjoindre un troisième mode de stimulation, dont l'action se manifeste à la fois sur les cupules et sur les otolithes: celui de déplacement rectiligne le long d'un axe horizontal (mouvement de translation) ou d'un axe vertical (mouvement d'ascenseur). L'appareil vestibulaire est étroitement intégré dans le mécanisme de l'équilibration, qui fait encore appel, surtout chez l'homme à toutes sortes d'autres afférences: de la vision, de la sensibilité profonde et superficielle.

Le rôle du système vestibulaire dans l'équilibration demeure mal défini: il est sujet à une continuelle ré-évaluation. Le maintien ou le rétablissement de l'équilibre spatial n'est pas non plus lié nécessairement au fonctionnement de cet appareil.

Les importantes informations que nous ont fourni empiriquement les expériences de ces dernières années où une cinquantaine d'êtres humains ont pu opérer dans un milieu de sous- ou zérogravité pendant des durées allant à plusieurs jours, semblent démontrer nettement que ces états n'auraient qu'une influence facilement surmontable sur les récepteurs vestibulaires et sur les répercussions que cette influence pourrait avoir sur l'organisme en général.

Il est cependant bien connu que ces sujets avaient été soumis après sélectionnement à un entraînement spécial. L'homme semble toutefois avoir la faculté de fonctionner 'vestibulairement' d'une façon satisfaisante dans un milieu où la gravitation n'existe plus ou serait sensiblement réduite.

Dans notre milieu terrestre avec sa gravitation constante, dans l'activité du vol conventionnel, le rôle joué par l'appareil vestibulaire dans l'orientation spatiale, l'interaction entre otolithes, canaux semicirculaires, vision et proprioception soulève toujours des problèmes. Cette méconnaissance provient en large partie du manque de signaux objectifs pouvant être de manière incontestable attribués spécifiquement ou bien aux otolithes ou bien aux canaux semicirculaires.

J'ai l'intention ici d'apporter une contribution à cette question de sélectionnement de signes otolithiques en fondant ma démonstration sur une série d'expériences effectuées dans la centrifugeuse humaine. Ce travail a fait l'objet d'une thèse, dont je donne ici la raison et quelques résultats qui me semblent particulièrement intéressants. J'ai posé la question de la façon suivante: des méthodes d'investigation visant à stimuler spécifiquement l'appareil otolithique, celles qui usent de la centrifugeuse ou de la chaise tournante à position eccentrique, sont particulièrement dignes d'intérêt puisqu'on peut y produire des forces centrifugales, donc des accélérations linéaires, bien définies quant à leur quantité et leur direction par rapport aux macules.

Les réponses classiques sont, ou bien la contre-rotation du globe oculaire, signe objectif, ou bien le changement de position dans l'espace (fictif), connu sous le nom d'illusion optogravique. Graybiel (1953) s'est particulièrement intéressé à ce signe subjectif, sans toutefois apporter des preuves irréfutables en faveur d'un rapport direct entre cet effet et l'appareil otolithique. Le mécanisme de la réorientation spatiale me semble trop complexe pour être ainsi simplifié.

Ma question a donc été: est-il possible d'obtenir ces deux réponses simultanément en les référant à un même excitant statique? En ce qui concerne le comportement de l'œil et ses changements de position, existerait-il, outre la contre-rotation d'autres-variations de position de l'œil pouvant être mises en relation directe avec non seulement la direction mais aussi avec la grandeur de l'excitant statique en puissance?

Inutile de souligner l'importance capitale de la deuxième partie de la question. Si en effet l'œil accuse des redressements compensateurs non seulement autour de l'axe visuel (axe Z) mais aussi suivant les deux autres axes (axes Y et Z), si l'on peut montrer que ces changements sont fonction de l'excitant statique en puissance et reviennent régulièrement de sujet à sujet, on pourrait en conclure que l'œil serait cet accéléromètre physiologique observable ouvrant des horizons nouveaux à l'investigation de la fonction otolithique.

2. Méthode

Pour obtenir simultanément ces deux réponses, j'ai procédé comme suit: corps et tête immobilisés, le sujet, privé de toutes références visuelles, est placé en position assise dans une cage située à une distance connue du centre de rotation (Figure 1). Un dispositif optique projète sur un écran représenté par une demi-sphère dont le centre coïncide avec le milieu de la tête du sujet, un objet visuel, en l'occurrence une croix faiblement lumineuse, qui par manipulation, peut être actionnée suivant les trois axes X, Y et Z, soit par le sujet, soit à l'insu de celui-ci, par l'expérimentateur.

L'objet visuel projeté sur l'écran est produit par un petit projecteur situé au-dessus de la tête du sujet (Figure 2).

Occupant la position variable, qui lui est imposée au départ, le sujet est incité à rapporter tout déplacement apparent de l'objet visuel. Il indique ainsi, non seulement son horizontale apparente, mais aussi les déplacements latéraux et ceux qui se produisent dans le sens de la hauteur, en ramenant l'indicateur à la position initiale ('centrifugeuse arrêtée'). Il est ainsi obtenu trois valeurs angulaires – une pour chaque axe – exprimant quantitativement la réponse du sujet à un excitant statique donné, cet excitant pouvant être calculé dans chaque cas.

La méthode ne visant qu'à interroger les gravicepteurs, l'accélération angulaire (passage d'une vitesse à une autre) est réduite à des valeurs sousliminales ($<0.5°/sec^2$).

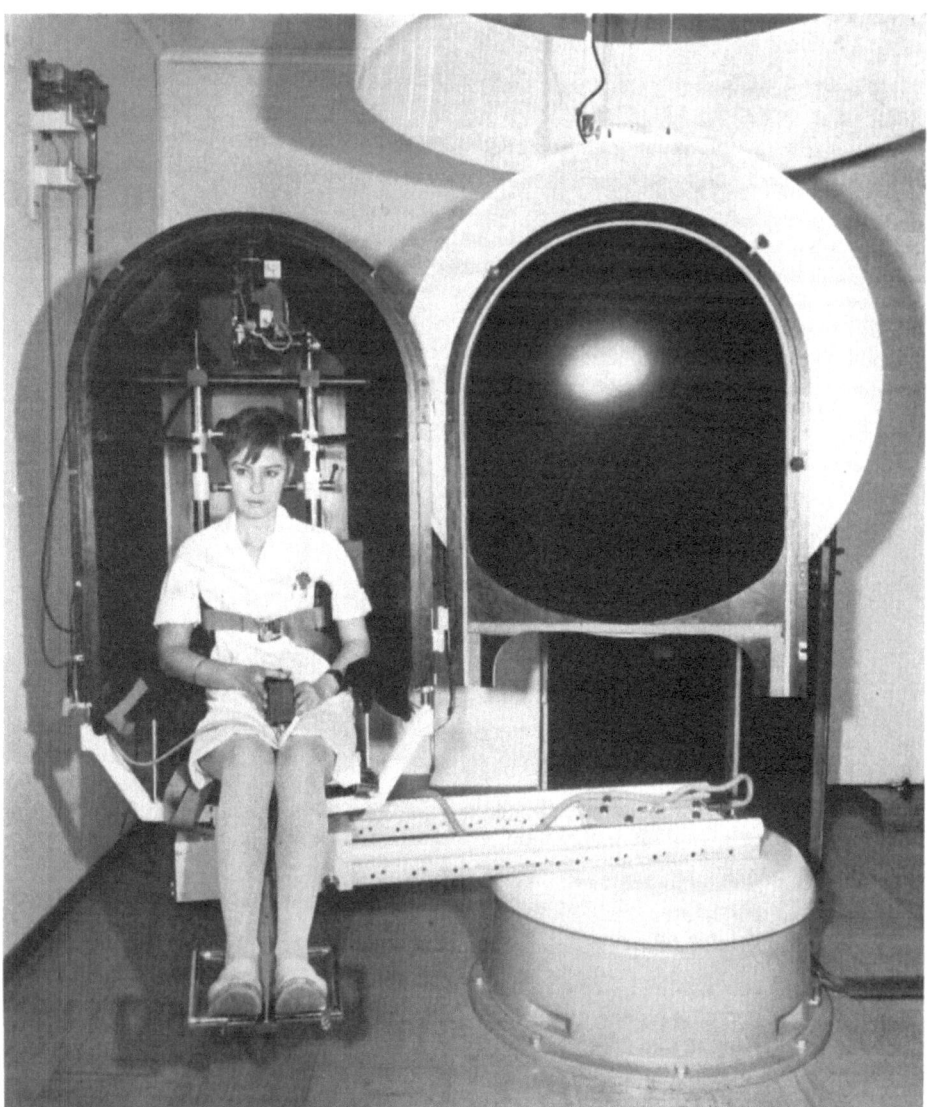

Fig. 1.   Le sujet est placé, tête et corps immobilisés, privé de toutes références visuelles, dans une cage située à une distance connue du centre de la centrifugeuse. Il a devant lui un écran à forme de demi-sphère sur lequel est projeté l'objet visuel émis par le projecteur placé au-dessus de lui et qu'il peut actionner suivant les trois axes par manipulation à distance. La caméra n'est pas représentée sur l'illustration.

Toutes les manœuvres sont dirigées à partir d'une unité de contrôle (Figure 3), qui emmagasine également toutes les valeurs obtenues pour permettre ensuite leur traitement par ordinateur.

Pour obtenir une réponse à la deuxième partie de ma question, concernant les redressements compensateurs de l'œil, j'ai eu recours au filmage à l'infrarouge,

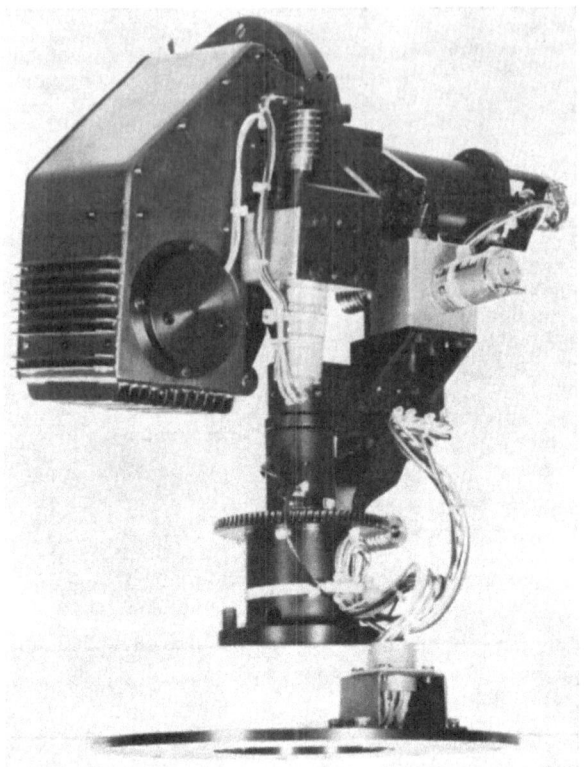

Fig. 2.   Vue de l'appareillage optique. Les déplacements de l'objet visuel peuvent être enregistrés triorthogonalement par un dispositif spécial.

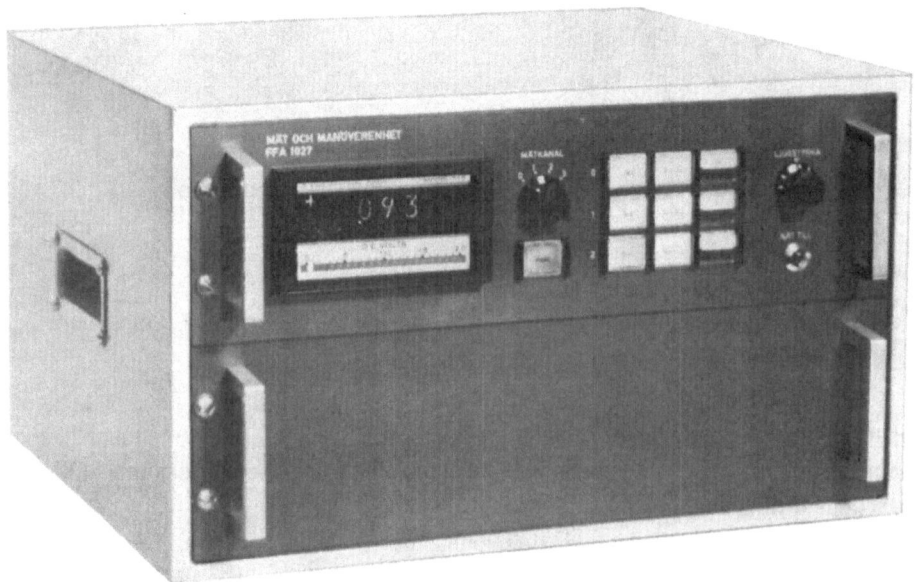

Fig. 3.   Unité de manœuvre et d'enregistrement. Les valeurs enregistrées sont traitées par ordinateur.

puisque toutes les opérations doivent se faire dans le noir absolu. Préalablement à la réponse subjective et à chaque échelon d'excitant statique un très court métrage de film (Kodak Infra High Speed 16 mm) est enregistré par une camera placée devant l'œil du sujet. A cet effet des radiations infrarouges émises par un projecteur muni d'un filtre (Kodak Wratten Infrafilter No. 87) entrent en action. Pendant cette opération de filmage, le dispositif indicateur de position est éteint tandis que le sujet est incité à fixer avec l'œil filmé un point phosphorescent situé sur le bord de l'objectif.

Une image-étalon 'centrifugeuse à la vitesse zéro') pour chaque sujet et position de sujet est comparée avec deux images obtenues à chaque échelon, par superposition, dans un liseur qui sert à agrandir les microphotographies de journaux. J'ai donc eu la ressource de travailler sur des agrandissements de la taille d'une page de journal et de mesurer avec très grande précision les changements de position, les déplacements, les torsions etc., en me servant des détails de la pupille, de l'iris et en me référant à deux points fixes indépendant des mouvements oculaires.

Toutes les valeurs obtenues ont été converties en valeurs angulaires et il m'a ensuite été possible d'intégrer les réponses subjectives et objectives dans une même représentation graphique en y faisant également figurer l'excitant statique (vecteur G).

Inutile de souligner que toutes ces opérations furent extrêmement laborieuses puisqu'elles se firent en grande partie manuellement. Plus de mille photographies furent ainsi évaluées.

Les résultats sont néanmoins d'une valeur incontestable, puisque les conclusions que j'ai cru pouvoir tirer de cette étude semblent démontrer que l'œil, dans les conditions expérimentales appliquées, par son comportement, dessine l'existence d'une mécanisme s'opérant au niveau de l'organe statique qui serait une preuve physiologique de l'hypothèse de polarisation de Spoendlin (1966).

3. Résultats

De façon générale il a pu être montré que tous redressements compensateurs de l'œil qui se produisent autour de l'axe visuel (axe Z) ou suivant les deux autres axes (axes Y et X) se font en sens inverse des déplacements de l'objet visuel. Elles leur sont quantitativement très inférieures. Dans certains cas et pour certaines positions des sujets, il existe un rapport net entre la quantité de l'excitant statique en puissance et les valeurs angulaires des torsions oculaires quel que soit l'axe autour duquel se font celles-ci. Il y a également une certaine proportionnalité entre réponses subjectives et grandeur de vecteur G.

Il ne sera donné ici que les principales représentations graphiques où figurent les deux réponses en fonction de l'excitant statique.

A. SUJETS TOURNÉS DANS LE SENS DE LA ROTATION ('HEADING FORWARD')

Dans cette série, l'excitant statique agit dans le plan frontal. Les informations obtenues en huit étapes consécutives, se renouvelant de sujet à sujet et correspondant à une augmentation de 10° de l'inclinaison du vecteur G proviennent de trois séances: sujets assis droit, inclinés 50° vers l'intérieur, inclinés 50° vers l'extérieur.

La Figure 4 illustre le développement des deux réponses autour de l'axe Z. Les Figures 5 et 6 donnent les deux réponses pour les axes Y et X. La Figure 7 donne une idée d'ensemble, où le comportement de l'œil pour les trois axes est représenté pour les trois séances de la série.

B. SUJETS FACE AU CENTRE DE ROTATION ('HEADING CENTRIPETAL')

Dans cette série, l'excitant statique agit dans le plan sagittal. Les sujets sont examinés, d'abord en position assise droite, puis inclinés vers l'extérieur, l'axe longitudinal du corps formant un angle de 50° avec la verticale. Ne sont donnés que les résultats concernant l'axe Y (Figure 8).

4. Discussion

L'investigation de l'appareil otolithique est rendue singulièrement ardue par le manque de signes objectifs pouvant être liées directement avec son fonctionnement. Dans mon expérimentation, j'ai essayé d'évaluer ces signes tels qu'ils ont été obtenus par une méthode spéciale usant de la centrifugeuse humaine. J'ai cru devoir insister sur la nature de l'excitant: les conditions expérimentales permettent de faire abstraction de la composante susceptible de stimuler les canaux semicirculaires.

Dans mon introduction, je n'ai pas cru devoir me rallier à l'opinion suivant laquelle la sensation d'un changement de position dans l'espace puisse exprimer, à l'exclusion d'afférences provenant d'autres systèmes sensoriels, un effet purement otolithique. La réponse subjective, qui exprime la réorientation spatiale du sujet, est en effet le résultat final d'un mécanisme d'équilibration extrêmement complexe, mettant en jeu des réflexes fondamentaux où le rôle de l'appareil vestibulaire apparaît comme très mal défini.

La réponse objective – les redressements compensateurs de l'œil en fonction du vecteur G – me semble en tant qu'expression otolithique plus intéressante. Il a pu être montré, en effet, que ces redressements ne se font pas seulement autour de l'axe Z (contrerotation) mais, pour certaines positions, également et d'une façon régulière, suivant les deux autres axes (axes Y et X). Une fixation volontaire de l'œil n'empêche pas celui-ci d'opérer de très petites révolutions de quelques degrés autour des trois axes possibles. Il existe de plus un rapport incontestable entres ces redressements et la direction – dans certains cas la grandeur – du champs de force imposé.

Il a pu être montré également l'existence d'un rapport entre les deux réponses, celles-ci se dirigeant en principe en sens contraire, la réponse objective demeurant quantitativement très inférieure à la réponse subjective. Il y a très souvent une dis-

→

Fig. 4.   Réponses objectives et subjectives pour dix sujets soumis au vecteur G agissant dans le plan frontal. Résultats concernant l'axe Z pour les trois positions: inclinaison vers l'extérieur, droite et inclinaison vers l'intérieur. La représentation graphique permet une comparaison entre les deux réponses.

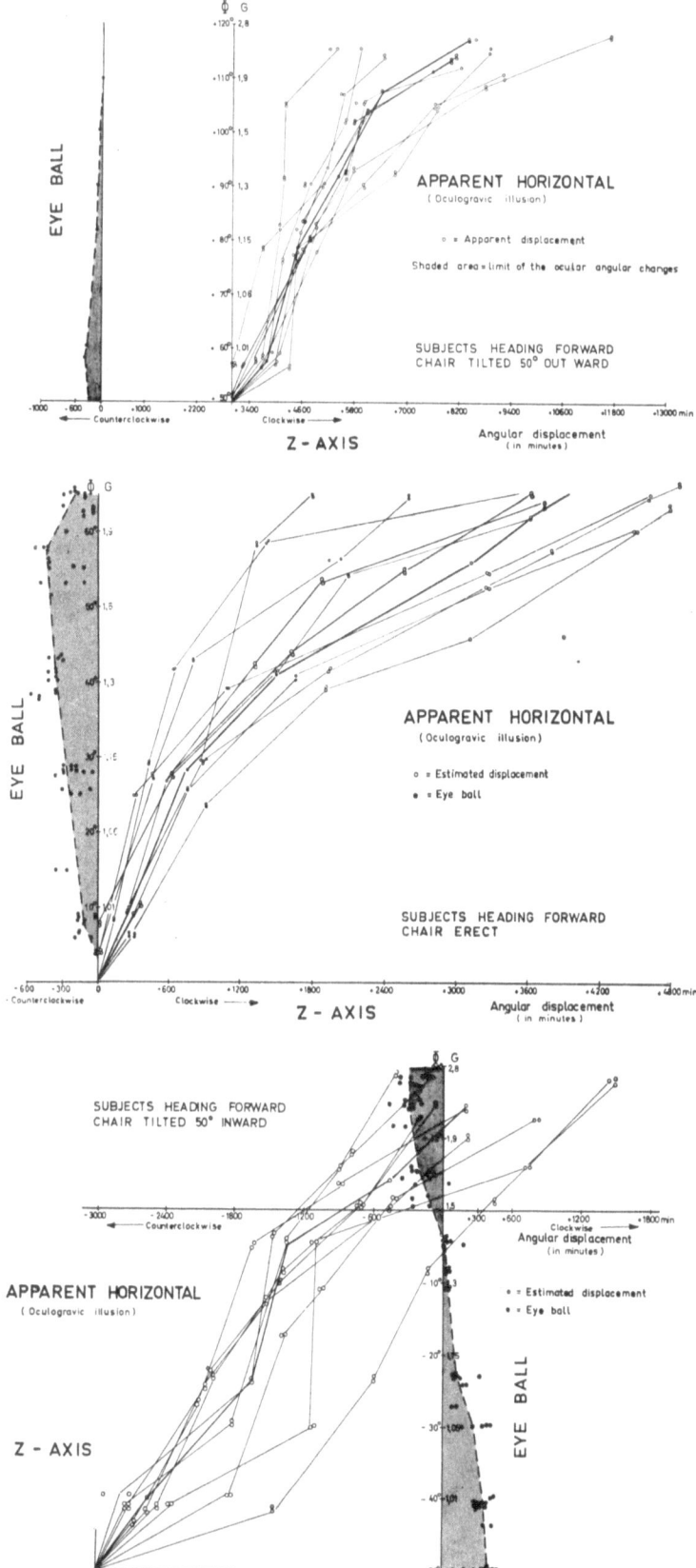

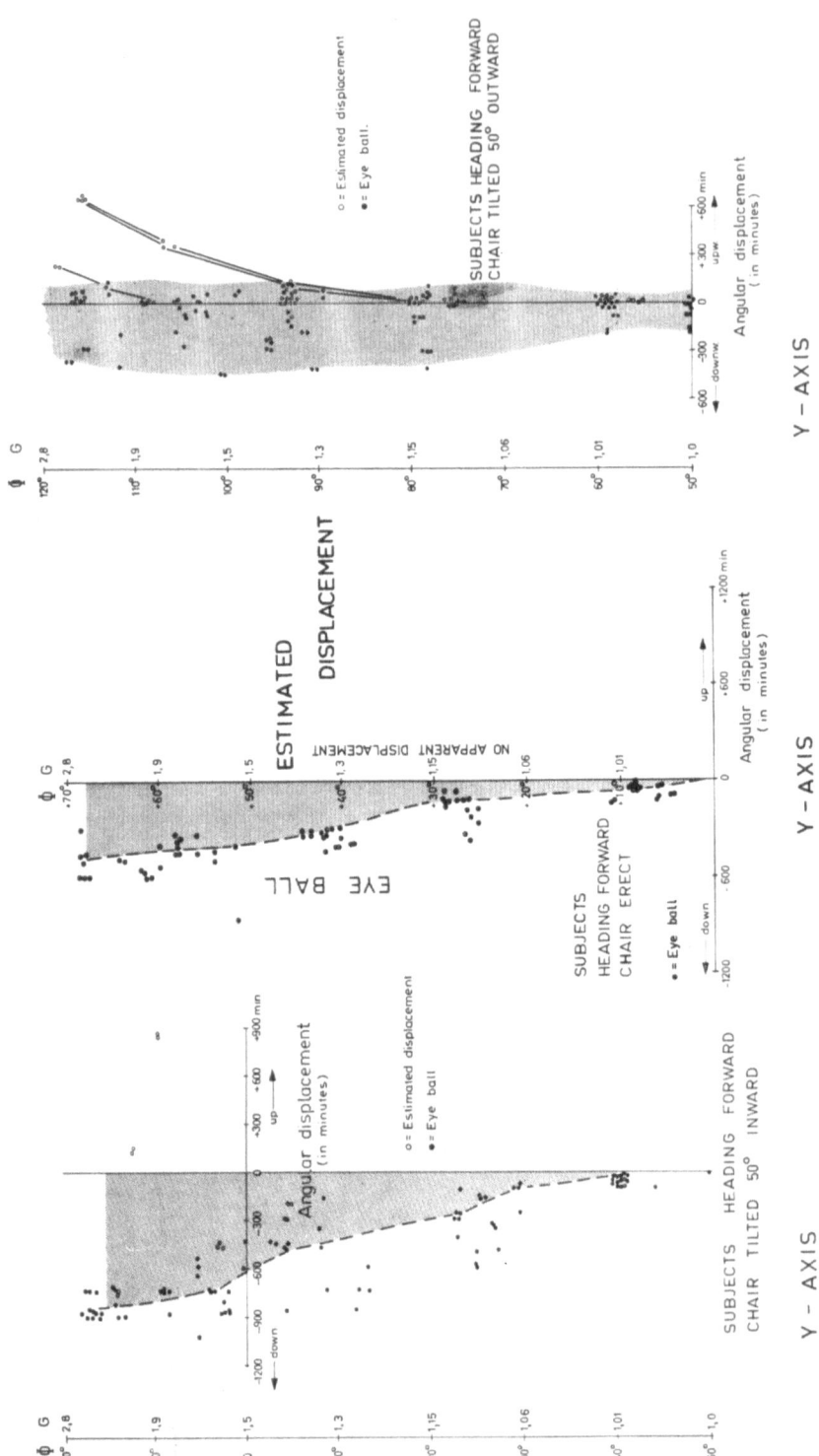

Fig. 5.　Mêmes réponses concernant l'axe *Y* pour les mêmes sujets. La réponse subjective est pratiquement inexistante tandis que l'œil se déplace régulièrement vers le bas pour les positions 'tilted inward' et 'erect' mais d'une manière indécise pour la position 'tilted outward'.

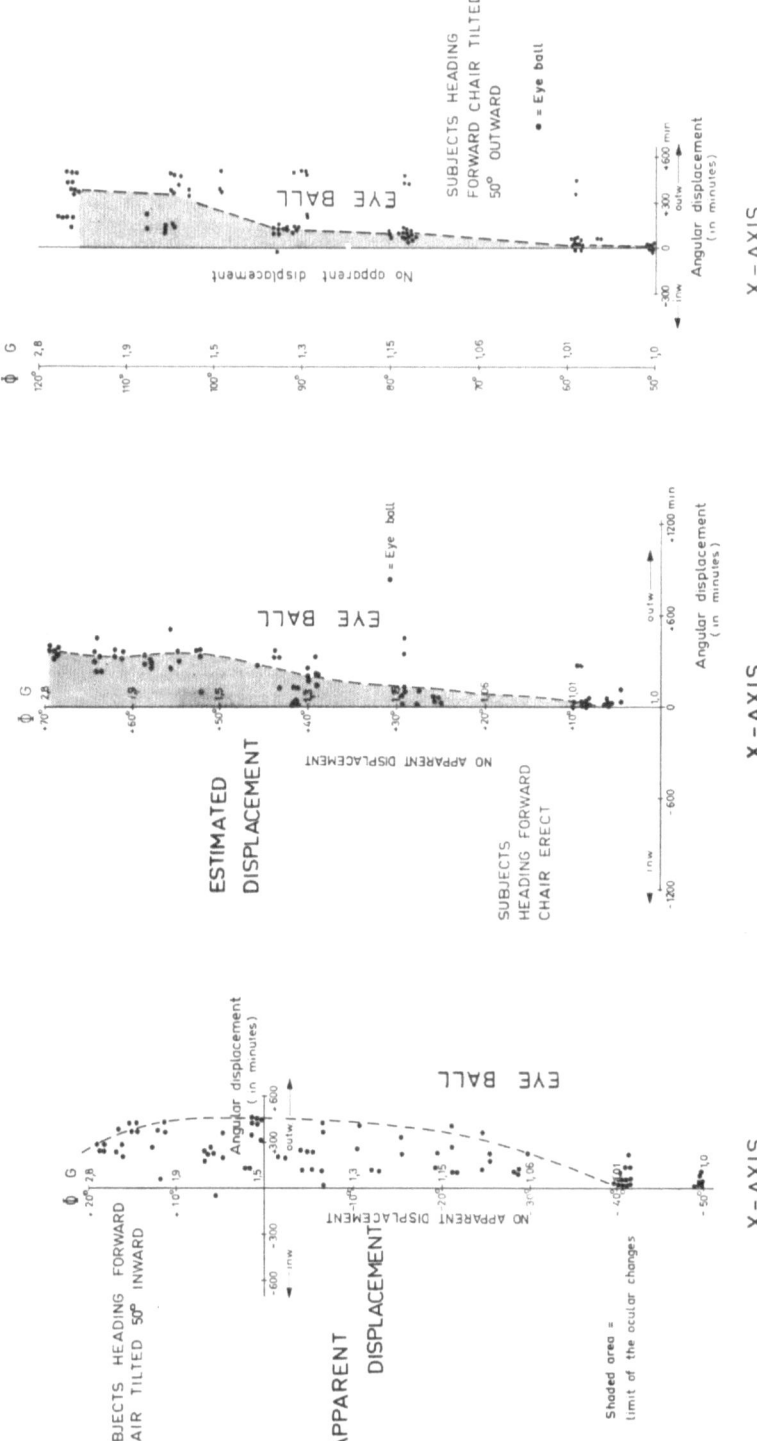

Fig. 6.   Mêmes réponses concernant l'axe *X*. Il n'y a pas de réponse subjective. L'œil accuse de très petites torsions vers l'extérieur.

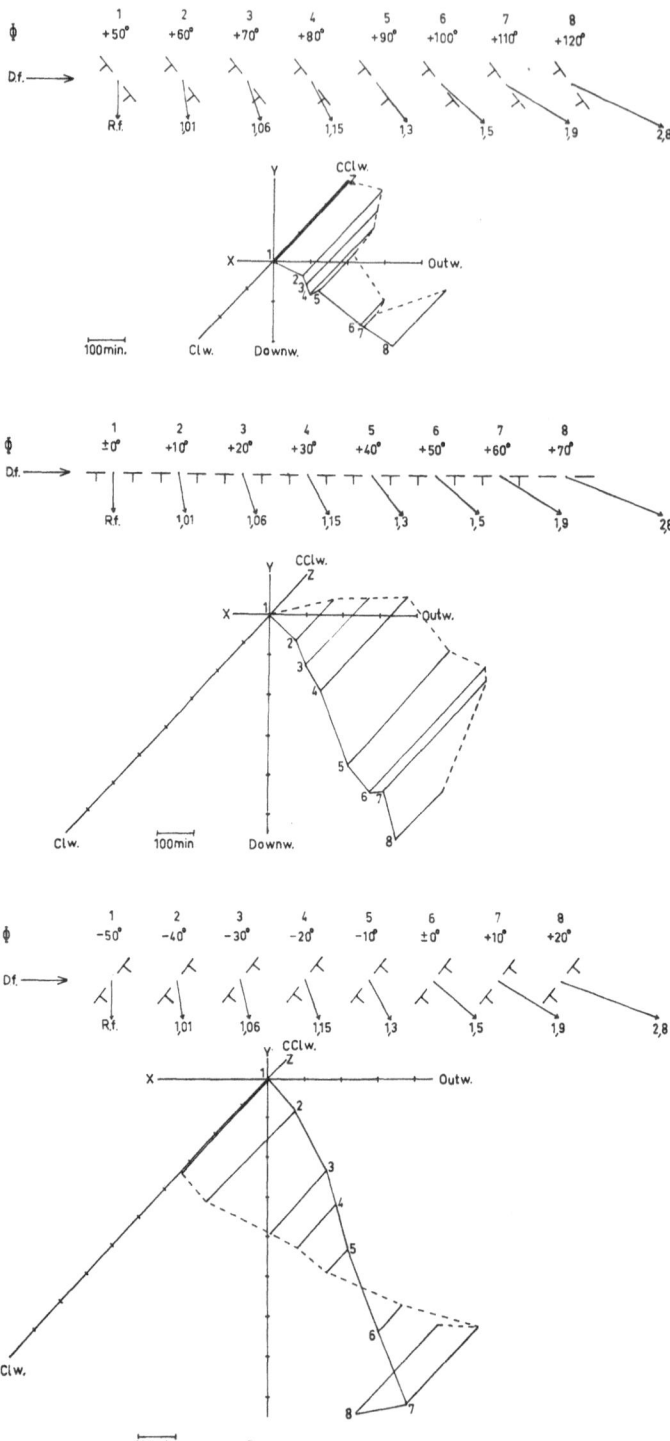

Fig. 7.   Comportement de l'œil pour les trois axes (représentation triorthogonale) pendant la même expérience. La direction du vecteur G (D.f.) par rapport aux otolithes et sa grandeur (calculée) est indiquée pour les huit échelons.

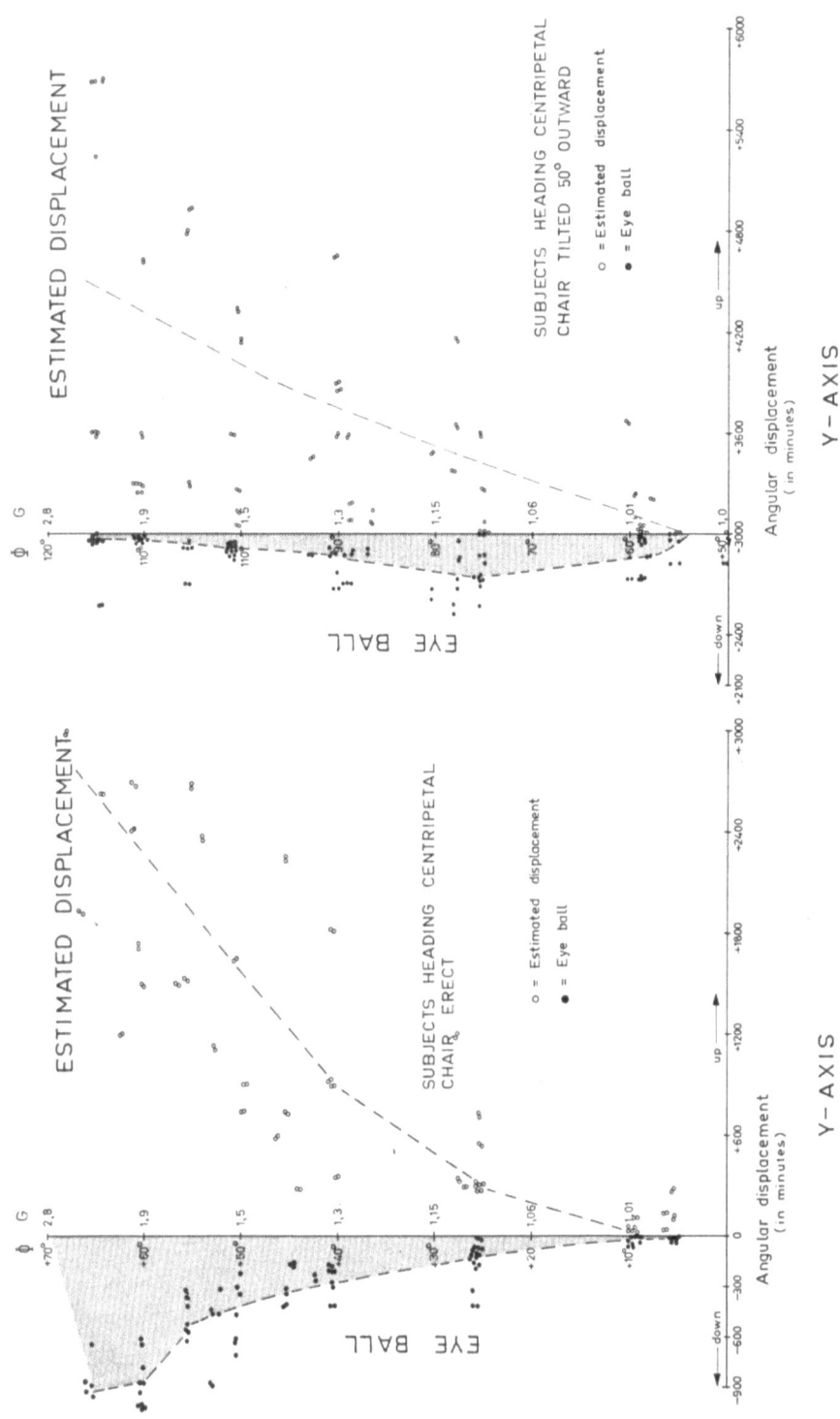

Fig. 8. Réponses objectives et subjectives pour huit sujets, soumis au vecteur *G* agissant dans le plan sagittal. Résultats concernant l'axe *Y* pour deux positions : droite et inclinée vers l'extérieur. La comparaison entre les deux positions permet de situer un rapport entre la réponse subjective et la grandeur du vecteur *G*, apparaissant moins nettement pour la position inclinée. Il faut observer le comportement de l'œil pour cette même position, celui-ci revenant à sa position initiale malgré l'augmentation de l'incidence relative du vecteur *G* et surtout de grandeur.

sociation entre le développement des deux réponses suggérant l'existence de mécanismes sensoriels différents à la base de celles-ci.

J'ai examiné d'autre part si ces comportements de l'œil n'étaient pas tout simplement des artéfacts – les preuves n'apparaissent pas dans ce court exposé, mais je considère que cette éventualité, envisagée dans ma thése, ne peut pas exister. Il m'a semblé intéressant de comparer les relations possibles entre d'une part les mouvements oculaires en fonction des directions du vecteur G, de l'autre, l'effet de ces mouvements en supposant que ceux-ci initiés par une action de ce même vecteur sur les macules. J'ai pensé, en effet, qu'un déplacement des otolithes par le fait d'un excitant statique aurait un effet spécifique sur certains muscles oculaires qui seraient à leur tour activés par les sections polarisées de la saccule et l'utricule (hypothèse de Spoendlin, 1966).

En analysant, par rapport à la direction relative du stimulus statique, ces redressements, j'ai trouvé en général une identification entre les effets escomptés et enregistrés, ce qui permettrait de lier les zones polarisées des macules avec l'action sur des muscles oculaires bien définis.

5. Conclusion

Dans ces conditions expérimentales (noir absolu, accélérations linéaires variables par leur direction et par leur grandeur, composante angulaire sous-liminaire etc.) le comportement de l'œil semble dessiner un mécanisme sensoriel au niveau des otolithes. La principale conclusion serait donc que l'œil, considéré comme indicateur objectif multidimensionnel de la fonction otolithique, peut servir comme instrument d'investigation de cette fonction. Ces expériences semblent en outre apporter une preuve physiologique de l'hypothèse de polarisation de Spoendlin (1966).

6. Références

Graybiel, A.: 1953, *Arch. Ophthal.* **24**, 249.
Spoendlin, H.: 1966, in *The Vestibular System and Its Diseases* (ed. by R. J. Wolfson), University of Pennsylvania Press, pp. 39–68.

IMPORTANCE OF LABYRINTHINE AND OTHER SENSORY INFORMATION FOR NORMAL DRIVING

N. G. HENRIKSSON and A. NILSSON

Ear, Nose and Throat Department, University of Lund, Lund, Sweden

1. Introduction

The mechano-receptors in the labyrinths are stimulated during normal traffic driving at levels of motion well above the minimum perceptible. However, little is known about to what extent this information is exploited for normal driving. This initiated a study exploring how variations in peripheral sensory information might influence normal driving. This study was carried out in six consecutive steps:

(1) An analysis was made of the driver as a receptor of physical impulses.

(2) A car simulator was designed and constructed.

(3) Driving students were tested in the car simulator.

(4) Normal subjects were tested when exposed to combinations of impaired visual, vestibular and proprioceptive inputs.

(5) Driving ability was studied as a function of age.

(6) The driving ability of patients with various lesions of the vestibular system was assessed.

2. The Driver as a Receptor of Physical Impulses

Physiological experiments have determined the smallest accelerations – angular or rectilinear – necessary to stimulate the vestibular and the proprioceptive systems. Thus it is possible by physical calculations to determine the traffic situations that present threshold values for these systems (Table I).

TABLE I

Traffic situations which reach threshold values required to stimulate non-visual sensory organs (superficial and deep sensitivity, and the vestibular organ)

Sensory organ	Threshold values	Corresponding traffic situation
Semicircular canal system	5 deg/sec^2 for 1 sec	A skidding movement giving a deviation of the car of 2.5 deg after 1 sec
Otoliths and proprioceptive system	1 deg backwards or forwards	Acceleration from 0 to 6 km/hr in 10 sec
Otoliths and proprioceptive system	3 deg towards the side	Driving around a curve with a radius of 50 m at a speed of 18 km/hr

It is evident that quite ordinary traffic situations will provide stimuli reaching or exceeding the thresholds for the vestibular and the extero- and proprioceptive systems (Henriksson *et al.* 1965).

3. Car Simulator Device

In order to reproduce the sensory information one receives during driving more adequately, it is necessary to expose the test subject to various kinds of movements which stimulate not only the visual system, but also the proprioceptive system and the vestibular apparatus. As shown in Figure 1, a dentist's chair with an adjustable back and arm rests was mounted on ball-bearings in such a way that it could be easily rotated. By turning a steering wheel, as in a car, the test subject could control the rotatory movements of the device. The chair made rotatory accelerations clockwise when the steering wheel was turned clockwise, and counter-clockwise when it was turned counter-clockwise.

There was no 'zero position' of the steering wheel; thus it was impossible to bring the chair to a steady standstill. The chair could be brought to a quick stop easily, but would immediately begin to accelerate in either direction, depending on the position of the wheel. The smallest acceleration was available at the 'zero position' of the wheel, being 6 deg/sec in either the clockwise or counter-clockwise directions. For example, turning the steering wheel clockwise through 45 deg, when the chair was stationary, gave the chair an angular acceleration of 18 deg/sec^2. Therefore, the angular velocity

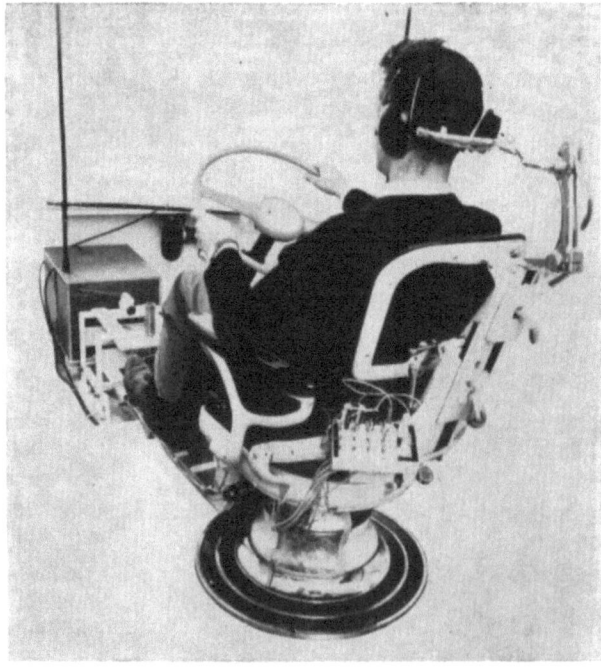

Fig. 1.   The car simulator.

after 1 sec of turn was 18 deg/sec. If the wheel was then turned very quickly counter-clockwise through 45 deg, the velocity diminished (deceleration) at a deceleration of 18 deg/sec^2 to a stand-still at the end of the next second; the chair then would imme-diately begin to accelerate counter-clockwise at an acceleration of 18 deg/sec^2.

The total angular deviation of the chair during a pre-test period was determined by an electronic device and used as a measure of driving ability. The smaller the total deviation, the better the driver could command his 'vehicle'.

The technician operating the test could apply rotatory accelerations of 65 deg/sec^2 for 2 sec, imitating skidding movements which a test-subject could counteract with the steering wheel (Henriksson *et al.*, 1965).

4. Tests of Driving Students in Car Simulator

Thirty-six driving students from five different driver education programs were studied. During a period of one month, the instructors in these programs selected one group (A) of 15 good and rapid learners, and another group (B) of 21 slow learners from a

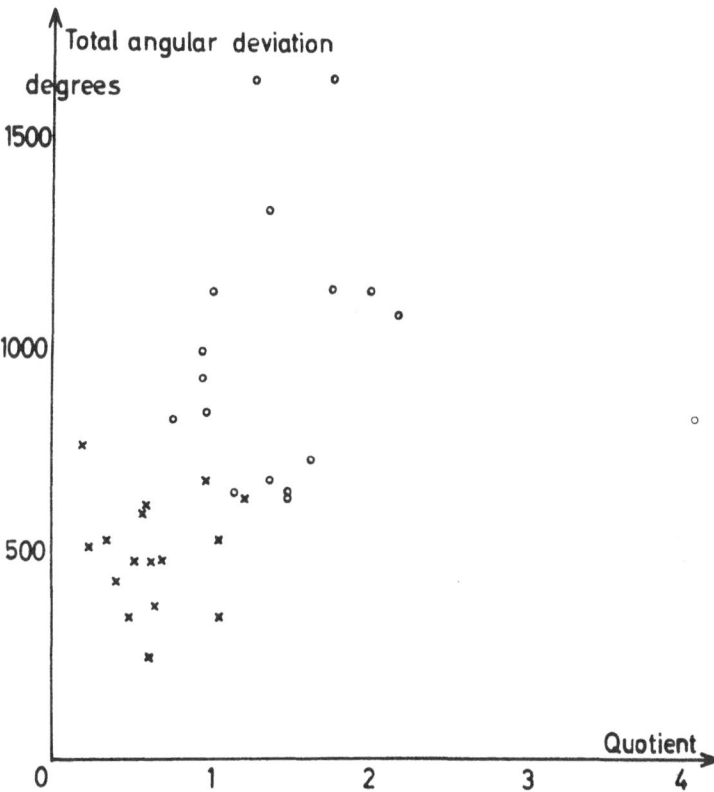

Fig. 2.   Total angular deviation in simulated driving tests with skids plotted against corresponding learning quotient at the Driver Education Institute. (Learning quotient = the number of lessons taken at the institute/number of parts of the training program the students had completed. A high quotient thus indicates a slow learning.)

group of about 800 students available at that time. The test subjects were selected and tested in the simulator after they had commenced training, but before their final examination for the driver's licence.

As shown in Figure 2, the total angular deviation of the simulator was to a high degree a function of the time necessary to learn how to drive in the driver education institute. From this and other similar experiments, it is quite clear that a student's driving ability in the car simulator very much reflected at least the ability to learn in a short time how to drive a car (Henriksson *et al.*, 1965).

5. Tests with Impaired Visual, Vestibular and Proprioceptive Inputs

Thirty subjects were exposed to a driving test under the conditions shown in Figure 3. The proprioceptive inputs were impaired by sitting on cushions. The vestibular information was disturbed by rotation (a deceleration from 120 deg/sec to standstill in 2 sec prior to test). Visual inputs were diminished by having the subjects drive in complete darkness except for one small orientating visual target of light. In the sequence of tests with impaired sensory information reference periods of driving with optimal conditions were put in. In this way the effect of a continuous improvement in driving ability during the test was eliminated. The decrease in performance caused by the loss of each specific sensory input or combinations of these inputs could thus be calculated as a difference between the test and the preceding reference test.

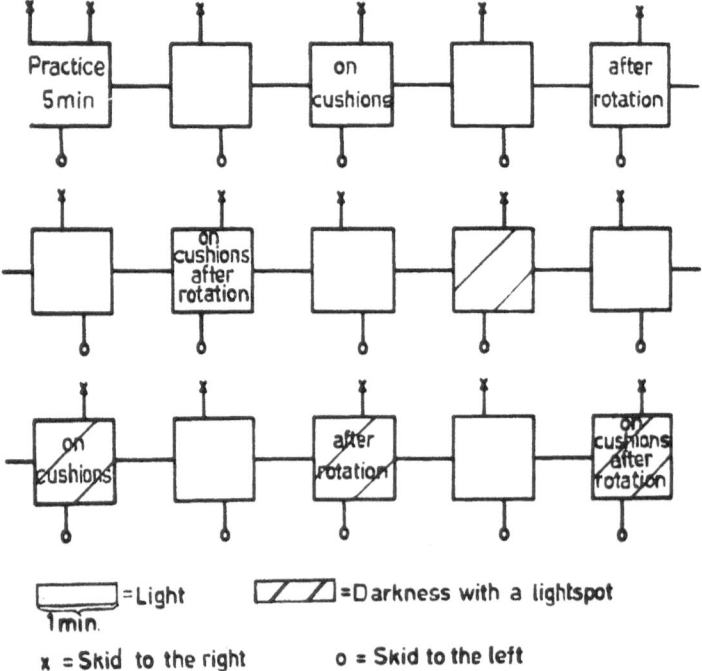

Fig. 3. Performance of the test. The white squares correspond to driving in optimal conditions exposed to one skid to the right and one to the left.

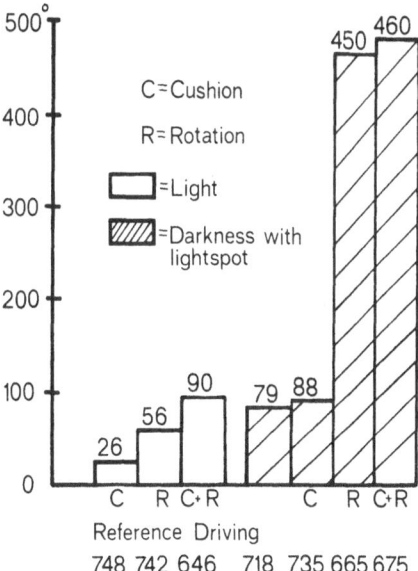

Fig. 4.   Effect on driving ability of (a) sitting on cushions, (b) driving immediately after rotation, (c) driving in darkness (except for one spot of light for orientation), and effects of combinations of altered sensory inputs during driving.

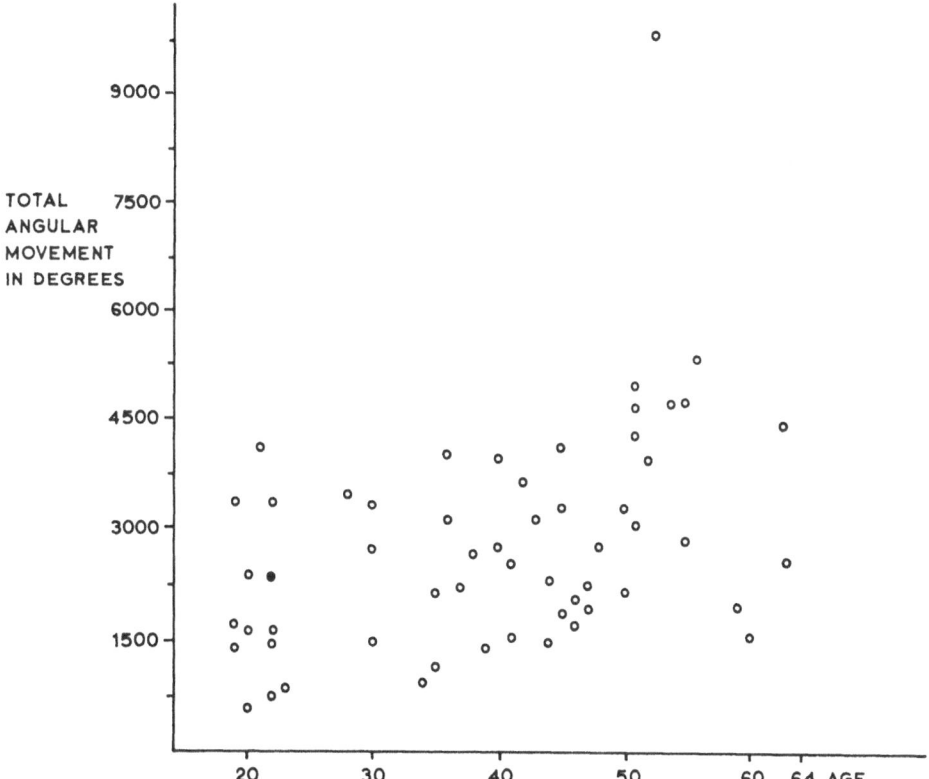

Fig. 5.   Total angular deviation of car simulator as a function of test subject age.

As shown in Figure 4, the decrease of sensory inputs during driving had only a minor effect upon driving ability. Post-rotatory stimulation influenced normal driving to a moderate degree. Combinations of proprioceptive and vestibular defects in orienting information did not affect driving ability to a great degree. Extremely reduced visual inputs did not decrease one's ability to handle the car simulator seriously. In fact, not until the test subject was exposed to both post-rotatory stimulation and a decrease in visual inputs was there a pronounced decrease in the normal handling of the traffic simulator.

These findings indicate that drivers who tend to have acute attacks of vertigo might be in a better position to compensate for their vertigo when driving under optimum lighting conditions. Therefore, there is good reason to advise patients with a tendency for attacks of vertigo to avoid driving in darkness.

6. Relationship of Driving Ability and Age

Figure 5 presents data on the total angular deviation of the car simulator for subjects of various ages. These data indicate that there was an inverse relationship between

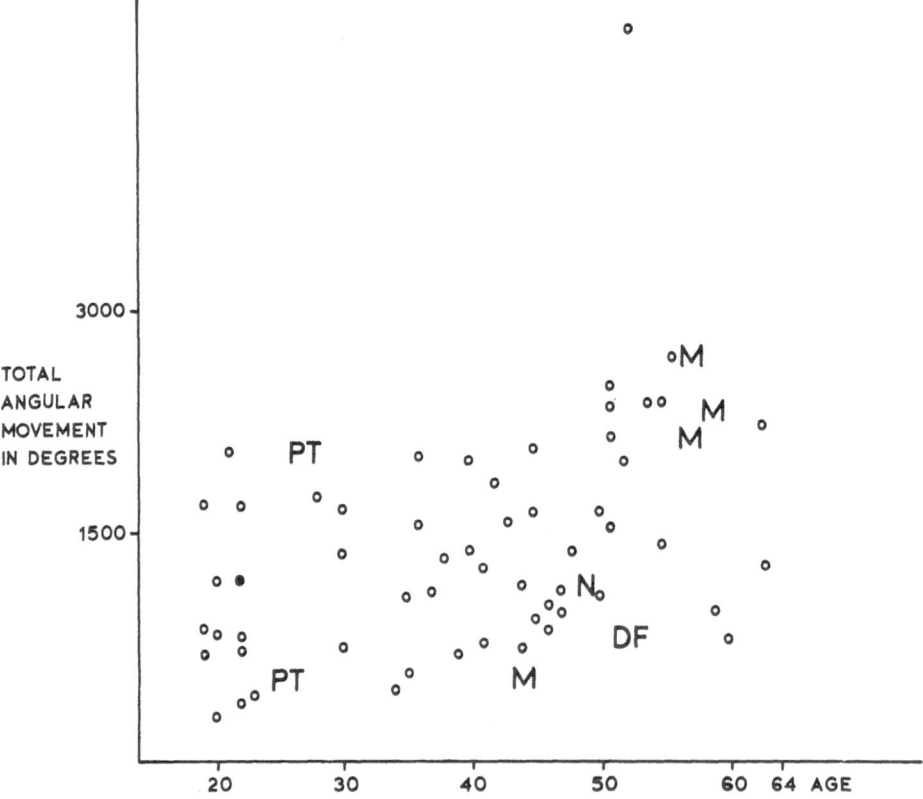

Fig. 6.   Total angular deviations of normal individuals in the car simulator as a function of age together with corresponding values of 4 patients with Menière's disease (M), two post-traumatic cases (PT), one deaf-mute (DF) and one case with acute neuronitis (N).

increasing age and the ability to handle the car simulator. It is apparent that young drivers are more apt to learn how to handle the car simulator more rapidly than elderly drivers. For this reason a study of how various disorders might affect the driving ability must take into account also the age of the patient.

7. Effect of Vestibular Disorders on Driving Ability

To a diagram representing the driving ability of normal individuals as a function of age was added data on the driving ability of several patients with various disorders of the vestibular system (Figure 6). These patients were tested in darkness with adequate proprioceptive information, but with visual information reduced to one single target of light in an otherwise dark room. As shown in this figure, subjects suffering from post-traumatic vertigo, neuronitis, congenital deafness, and Menière's disease did not control the simulator significantly different from that expected of normal individuals of the same age. Even immediately after labyrinth destruction by surgery, two cases of Menière's disease reached normal scores. There was even no difference between pre- and post-operative scores in these tests (Figure 7).

The two cases with labyrinth destruction were tested less than 24 hr post-operatively, and yet a normal driving ability was found. This finding contrasts with the observation that subjects under post-rotatory conditions were not at all able to drive in a normal or nearly normal way. The explanation for this difference might perhaps

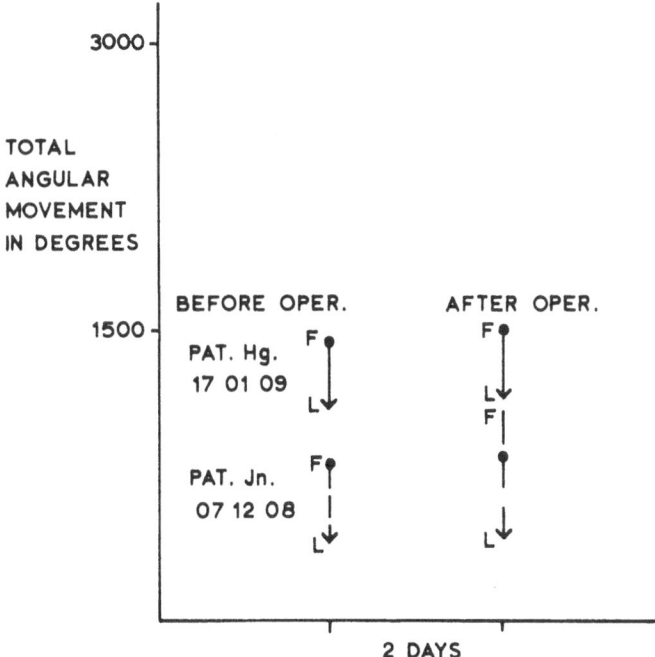

Fig. 7. Total angular deviation in the simulator of two Menière's disease cases before and after labyrinth destruction.

be that enough compensation takes place during the first 24 hr after labyrinth destruction to allow the patient enough orientation for normal driving, while such a compensation would not take place in the post-rotatory situation. Another explanation for this difference would be that in the post-rotatory situation, both labyrinths give inadequate information, while in the cases with labyrinth destruction, only one labyrinth was defective.

8. Comparison of Driving Ability of Accident-Prone and Accident-Free Drivers

As vestibular disease had very little effect on ability to handle the car simulator, an attempt was made to study the ability of accident-prone young drivers to handle the car simulator. The results were compared with those from drivers never involved in accidents, but with otherwise identical driving backgrounds. No difference was found in the way these groups handled in the simulator. On the other hand, significant differences were found between the groups in their personality profiles, as studied by a psychological test battery (Andersson *et al.*, 1970).

9. Conclusions

Inputs from the visual, proprioceptive and vestibular systems are utilized in driving. Extensive loss or defects in information provided by any one of these systems did not produce a pronounced loss in driving ability in a car simulator. When exposed to both post-rotatory stimulation and reduced visual inputs, driving ability is markedly reduced.

Patients with vestibular disorders, even after acute labyrinthectomy, do not show a significant loss of driving ability, probably due to rapid compensation allowing almost normal orientation while driving. Individuals who suffer acute attacks of vertigo should be advised not to drive in darkness. A comparison of accident-prone and accident-free, young car drivers showed personality, but no driving ability differences.

References

Andersson, A. L., Nilsson, A., and Henriksson, N. G.: 1970, *Brit. J. Psychol.* (in press).
Henriksson, N. G., Nilsson, A., and Andersson, A.: 1965, *International Road Safety and Traffic Review* 13 (3).
Henriksson, N. G., Prytz, S., Andersson, A., and Nilsson, A.: 1965, *International Road Safety and Traffic Review* 13 (4).
Henriksson, N. G., Turesson, A., Nilsson, A., and Andersson, A.: 1965 *International Road Safety and Traffic Review* 14 (1).

STUDIES OF EFFECTS OF VARIATIONS IN THE DIRECTION AND MAGNITUDE OF THE GRAVITATIONAL-INERTIAL FORCE ENVIRONMENT ON THE CARDIOVASCULAR AND RESPIRATORY SYSTEMS

E. H. WOOD

Department of Physiology, Mayo Clinic and Mayo Foundation, Rochester, Minn., U.S.A.

1. Electronic Data Processing and Computer Analysis of Multiple Continuously Recorded Cardiovascular and Respiratory Variables During Changes in the Force Environment Produced on a Centrifuge

The cardiorespiratory effects of changes in the direction and magnitude of the gravitational-inertial force environment in man, chimpanzees and dogs have been studied over a number of years in this laboratory to determine the role of gravity in normal cardiopulmonary physiology (Banchero *et al.*, 1967; Coulam *et al.*, 1970a, b; Reed and Wood, 1970; Rutishauser *et al.*, 1967; Vandenberg *et al.*, 1968). Typically, intravascular and respiratory pressures and other variables from catheter strain-gauge manometer systems and other types of transducers are continuously recorded on paper photokymographs and magnetic tape throughout each centrifuge run. However, pressures cannot be read directly from these recordings for several reasons:

(1) Manometer baselines shift during the centrifuge run due to the effect of acceleration on the transducers and the fluid-filled catheter systems.

(2) The position of the animal and the heart and lungs within the thorax change, relative to the manometers, due to the increase in weight produced by the acceleration.

(3) Extravascular pressures recorded from fluid-filled catheters (*e.g.*, pleural and esophageal pressures) must be corrected for the vertical distance between the catheter tips and the zero pressure reference.

When these pressures must be measured from the paper recordings and corrected by hand, the data reduction problem is formidable. Programs have been written for processing these data more efficiently on the CDC 3200, both on-line for monitoring purposes and subsequent to the experimental procedure for more detailed analysis and study. These programs have been described in previous reports, and more recently, have been refined to simplify their use (Coulam *et al.*, 1970a). Briefly, consecutive ten-second intervals of the pressure data initially recorded on digital tape are analyzed, the appropriate corrections applied, and the results for each interval printed in alphanumeric characters. Approximately 30 such sets are printed for the usual centrifuge exposure of 60 sec at the plateau level of acceleration. Each set required approximately 15 sec of computer time, or roughly 7 to 8 min computer time for the complete run. At least one day would be required for hand analysis of each run, and then only a fraction of the run would be analyzed, possibly with less accuracy. Since there are typically 10 to 15 centrifuge runs performed in each study, the savings in time compared with hand methods of data reduction is very large.

Separate programs have been developed to simplify data reduction further and to verify the accuracy of the data reduction system. With the use of the computer, a continuous analog tape recording can be produced from the original digital tape, with all pressure corrections applied, and a continuous photokymographic record made of all the computer-corrected variables. In effect, use of the computer in this manner converts the photokymographic recording assembly into a multichannel, very high-speed *x-y* plotter. Unlike the original uncorrected photokymographic recording obtained in real time during the centrifuge exposures, real data can be quickly read directly from the computer-processed recordings. Furthermore, in the latter, the individual tracings can be more uniformly spaced, and overlapping greatly reduced so that visualization and interpretation of changes in each variable are facilitated. Continuous photokymographic recordings of this type have proved very valuable since they provide a quick visual check of the probable validity of the results being produced by the complete multi-channel analog-to-digital conversion – digital computer – digital-to-analog conversion data processing and computing assembly. All of the corrected 14 channels of continuous analog data obtained in each exposure can be conveniently displayed in a readily interpretable form by this technic and possible large errors in the data processing procedure, such as dropouts and transient channel overloads, which can readily escape detection when only sets of alphanumeric results are obtained, become immediately apparent. Detection of less obvious data processing, computing, and other types of errors is greatly facilitated when the results are converted back to complete continuous analog records which can be readily compared with the original unprocessed recordings of the same data, so that discrepancies between the two data sets and discontinuities in the processed data are apparent.

2. Gravity-Dependent Regional Differences in Intrathoracic Pressures and Pulmonary Arterial-Venous Shunts

Vertical gradients in pleural pressure and alveolar size in transverse and head-up positions plus 100% arterial-venous shunts in the most dependent regions of the lungs suggest atelectasis at these sites. Failure to find a gradient in alveolar size in the head-down position prompted study of intrapleural, intraesophageal, intrapericardial, right and left atrial pressures, total and regional pulmonary blood flow in anesthetized dogs studied without thoracotomy when head-up and head-down. Pleural and intrapericardial pressures were recorded at multiple sites between apex and base when head-up and head-down.

The computer is used in this project for real time calculation of cardiac output using the indicator-dilution curve method plus pressure data correction and display. The correction of pleural pressures yields pressure data which are corrected to some absolute body position (*e.g.*, sixth thoracic vertebra or to a mid-lung location). The computer programs are used to determine pleural pressures at desired phases in the respiratory cycle on a breath-to-breath basis.

Pleural and pericardial pressures were similar at the same vertical height in the thorax and negativity always increased with increased height. Average pleural gradients from apex to base were 0.7 and 0.8 ± 0.05 cm H_2O/cm and regional gradients smaller cephaled in the thorax when head-up and head-down, respectively. Average pericardial pressures near heart apex and base were -3 and -10 cm H_2O (head-up) and -10 and -2 ± 0.5 (head-down). Average vertical gradients were 1.0 ± 0.04 cm H_2O/cm, so transmural atrial pressures were independent of vertical height in the thorax, and cardiac outputs of 2.0 and 1.9 ± 0.2 l/min were similar when head-up and head-down. The discrepancy between the vertical pleural pressure gradient and the zero intra-alveolar pressure gradient renders lung function very susceptible to changes in direction and magnitude of the gravitational-inertial force environment, while elimination of regional differences in transmural pressures by compensated hydrostatic counter-pressures in the pericardium minimizes cardiac effects.

Simultaneous determinations of oxygen saturation of blood being withdrawn continuously via cuvette oximeters from left and right pulmonary veins, aorta, and pulmonary artery demonstrated regional differences in oxygenation of pulmonary venous blood in 10 anesthetized dogs studied without thoracotomy when in supine, left, and right decubitus positions. During air-breathing, the oxygen saturation of blood from the more dependent pulmonary venous catheter was lower than systemic arterial and pulmonary venous blood from the more superior pulmonary vein. A correlation was demonstrated between the vertical distance separating the pulmonary venous catheter tips and the difference in oxygen saturation of blood withdrawn from the two sites when in the supine and left decubitus positions. This correlation was of borderline significance in the right decubitus position. Desaturation of dependent pulmonary venous blood occurred when breathing 99.6% oxygen, indicating a large anatomic shunt. Deficient oxygenation of blood traversing dependent regions of the lung disappeared in less than 1 min following a change in body position placing the affected region in a superior region of the thorax. The P_{CO_2} of dependent pulmonary venous blood was uniformly higher than that from a superior vein and from the aorta, indicating regional difference in the ventilation-perfusion ratio. These results are believed related to effects of gravity on thoracic contents which produce pleural pressures at or near zero at the most dependent surfaces of the lung simultaneously with highly negative values at superior surfaces, resulting in a vertical gradient in size of the terminal airways and alveoli which apparently can extend to complete collapse in the most dependent regions of the lung.

3. Spatial Distribution of Pulmonary Blood Flow in Chimpanzees by Computer-Controlled External Scintiscanning and Display

Six chimpanzees have been studied. The animals were maintained in either the right or the left-lateral position in specially-molded half-body casts and fastened to the cockpit of the Mayo centrifuge. Control recordings, including isotope tagged micro-sphere injections for indicating pulmonary blood flow distributions, oxygen saturations, cardiac output measurements, and circulatory pressures were completed. The cen-trifuge was then engaged and repeat measurements were made on the chimpanzee at the 5.8 G_y level. Biplane X-rays were taken at 1 G_y and 5.8 G_y, which allowed for all pressure recordings to be subsequently corrected to mid-lung levels. The chimpanzee was then moved to the opposite right or left lateral position, and 1 G_y and 5.8 G_y measurements repeated. Following the centrifugation, the chimpanzee was positioned first in supine and then in prone half-body casts, and the regional distribution of pulmonary blood flow for all G_y conditions simultaneously determined, using the scintiscanning procedure.

Computer-produced oscilloscopic displays utilizing three-dimensional surface maps and contour plots in conjunction with images of the shape and volume of the excised lung and its interlobar fissures have been developed for study of the spatial distribution of isotope tagged 35 μ microsphere emboli in the lung from scintiscan data following their injection into the outflow tract of the right ventricle. Data indicate that the distribution of these emboli in different regions of the lung is proportional to the blood flow to these regions at the time of the injection.

Visualization of the surfaces representing count rates as a function of two spatial coordinates of various planes through the count matrix was achieved by a shading technic which creates the illusion of three dimensions on a photographic image of the display.

Isocount contour maps of transverse sections of excised lungs obtained following fixation by air drying while inflated to 30 cm H_2O were displayed and their spatial orientations indicated in images of the lungs and their component lobes generated from data fed into the computer by cursor tracing of the external lung borders and its interlobar fissures from each of the 1 cm slices into which the lungs were sectioned.

Determinations of the fractions of cardiac output traversing the two lungs and their component lobes and the rate of perfusion (blood flow per unit volume) of different regions in the lung are calculated from the scan matrix and these anatomical meas-urements.

If uniform microsphere tagging of the blood is achieved, the sectional contour maps, together with the anatomic data and three-dimensional count surface displays, provide the facility for display and study of complete information concerning the spatial distribution of pulmonary blood flow at the time of injection of the microspheres.

Figure 1 shows the three-dimensional regional distributions of radioactive micro-spheres, as determined from the scintiscan procedure and as processed by the digital computer. The larger the blood flow fraction is to one lung, the greater are the radio-active count values for that particular part of the anatomy, resulting in a 'peaked or mountain-like' three-dimensional effect. Increased inertial and gravitational forces are seen to alter the regional pulmonary flow patterns.

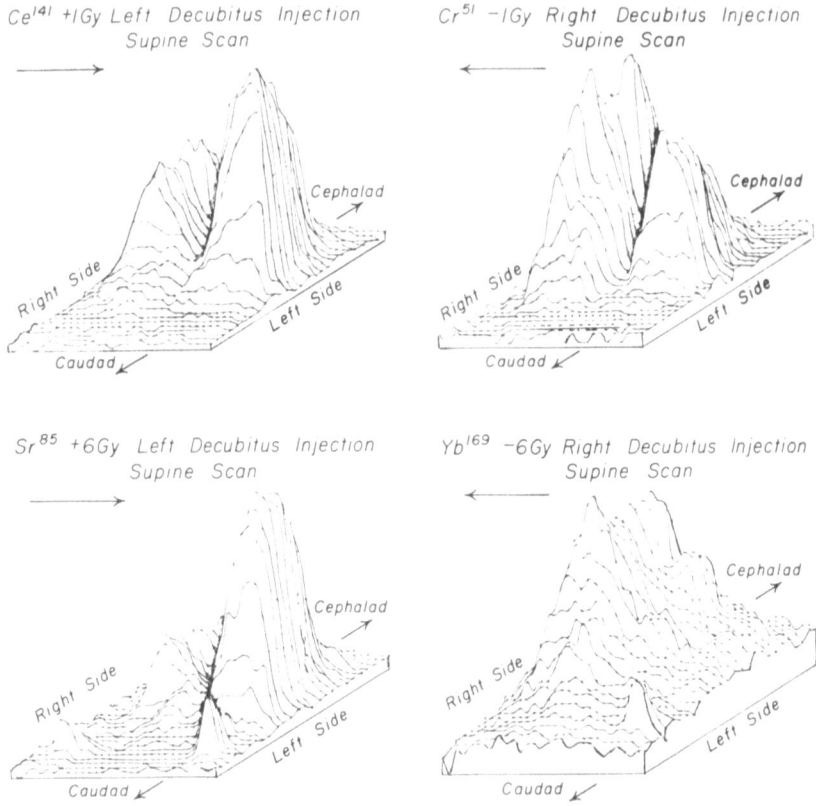

Fig. 1. Comparative three-dimensional views of the regional isotopic distributions which are believed to be related to regional pulmonary blood flow distributions. In all cases, the data are displayed as viewed by an observer looking towards the head from the left caudad side of the animal. The vertical height of any peak is proportional to the regional flow distribution at that point. All data were recorded simultaneously during a scintiscan of the ventral surface of the thorax, using isotopic, energy-discrimination technics. The data were scaled so that the peak activity of all curves was identical. Comparisons may be made, therefore, with respect to form only in this format. The arrow above each distribution indicates the direction of the inertial force environment. For this chimpanzee, increased G conditions tend to displace regional pulmonary blood flow toward the dependent direction. Other chimpanzees, during exposure to 6 G_y have shown redistribution of blood flows towards the midthoracic region where hydrostatic effects of the increased force environment would be expected to be minimal.

Acknowledgements

This study was supported in part by research grants NsG-327 from the National Aeronautics and Space Administration; AF F41609-68-C-0022 from the United States Air Force, Brooks Air Force Base; AHA CI 10 from the American Heart Association, FR7, and H-3532 from the National Institutes of Health, United States Public Health Service.

References

Banchero, N., Rutishauser, W. J., Tsakiris, A. G., and Wood, E. H.: 1967, *Circ. Res.* **20**, 65.

Coulam, C. M., Dunnette, W., Greenleaf, J. F., *et al.:* 1970a, Technical Report SAM-TR-70-6 U.S. Air Force, U.S. Sch. Aerospace Med., Brooks, AFB, Texas.

Coulam, C. M., Dunnette, W., and Wood, E. H.: 1970b, *Computers in Medicine* (in press).

Reed, J. H., Jr. and Wood, E. H.: 1970, *J. Appl. Physiol.* **28**, 303.

Rutishauser, W. J., Banchero, N., Tsakiris, A. G., and Wood, E. H.: 1967, *J. Appl. Physiol.* **22**, 1041.

Vandenberg, R. A., Nolan, A. C., Reed, J. H., Jr. and Wood, E. H.: 1968, *J. Appl. Physiol.* **25**, 516.

EFFETS DES ACCÉLÉRATIONS POSITIVES PROLONGÉES (+3 G$_z$) SUR LES VARIATIONS DU DÉBIT CARDIAQUE HUMAIN

Mesure par pléthysmographie électrique aortique transthoracique: influence du vêtement anti-G)

J. M. R. DEMANGE

Laboratoire de Médecine Aérospatiale du Centre d'Essais en Vol, 91 – Brétigny-sur-Orge, France

1. Introduction

La centrifugeuse humaine du Centre d'Essais en Vol de Brétigny a été utilisée pour déplacer des corps étrangers intraoculaires ou intrarachidiens ou pour le traitement des décollements de rétine. Les accélérations utilisées restaient inférieures à 3 G$_z$ mais pendant 20 à 30 min.

Ces accélérations de longue durée nous ont alors amenés à étudier les réactions circulatoires de sujets humains soumis à +3 G$_z$ pendant 20 à 120 min avec ou sans vêtement anti-G.

2. Technique de mesure

Un appareil de plethysmographie électrique (à 4 électrodes) permet de mesurer les variations du volume d'éjection systolique (stroke volume); comme Kubicek *et al.* (1966) et Coleman *et al.* (1966), nous plaçons les 2 électrodes d'injection respectivement autour du cou et à la partie inférieure du thorax, mais les 2 électrodes de recueils sont collés sur le thorax, devant l'image radiologique de l'aorte montante (Figure 1).

Le dépouillement graphique proposé par Kubicek *et al.* (1966) est utilisé et permet la mesure du volume d'éjection systolique. Les comparaisons avec des mesures de débit cardiaque par dilution de cardiogreen montrent une très bonne corrélation dans la majorité des cas, et une corrélation moins bonne avec des sujets très brévilignes dont l'image radiologique de l'aorte est courte, mais les variations du volume systolique restent proportionnelles.

La mesure de la pression artérielle est effectuée par enregistrement des bruits de Korotkoff et de la pression dans un brassard pneumatique brachial.

3. Expérimentation

Sur une centrifugeuse humaine, 5 sujets assis sur un siège Martin-Baker ont subis une accélération longitudinale de +3 G$_z$ pendant des durées variables (3 sujets ont présenté des malaises généraux à 20, 40 et 45 min), (2 sujets n'ont présenté aucun malaise et l'épreuve a été arrêtée à 70 et 120 min). Cinq autres sujets ont subis + 3 G$_z$ pendant 15 min, à ce moment un vêtement (anti-G suit) a été gonflé pendant 10 min et enfin dégonflé avant l'arrêt de l'expérience.

D. E. Busby (ed.), Recent Advances in Aerospace Medicine, 315–318. All Rights Reserved.
Copyright © 1970 by D. Reidel Publishing Company, Dordrecht-Holland.

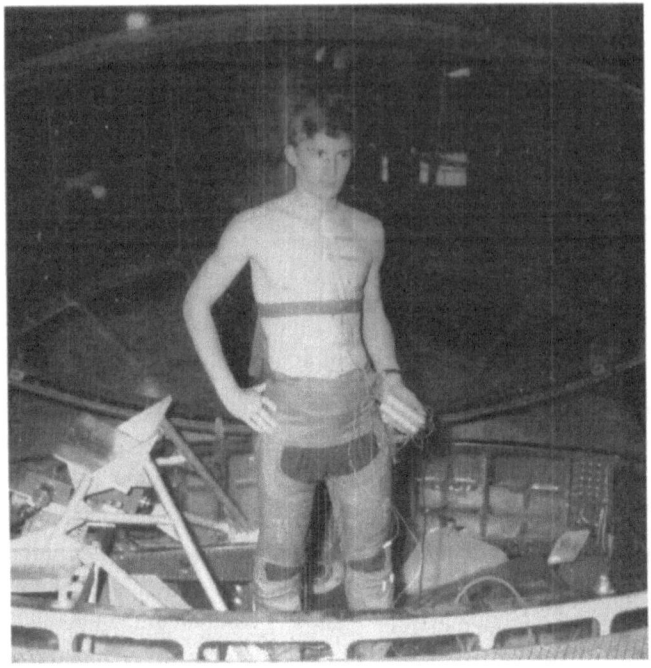

Fig. 1.　Sujet porteur des 4 électrodes du pléthysmographe électrique et du vêtement anti-*G*.

TABLEAU I

Sujets	A	B	C	D	E
PA (mm Hg)					
Avant départ	16/12	15/10	15/11	14/8	14,5/10
+ 3 G_z avant gonflage	18,5/14	17/14,5	19/15	17/12	19,5/10
+ 3 G_z gonflage	20/15	20/17	20/14	23/14	23/11
+ 3 G_z dégonflage	18/14	17/15	17/14*	15/12*	17/11
SV					
Avant départ	100%	100%	100%	100%	100%
+ 3 G_z avant gonflage	76%	80%	87%	68%	87%
+ 3 G_z gonflage	96%	90%	136%	150%	106%
+ 3 G_z dégonflage	73%	80%	81%*	89%*	82%
$\dot{Q}$					
Avant départ	100%	100%	100%	100%	100%
+ 3 G_z avant gonflage	100%	126%	108%	101%	94%
+ 3 G_z gonflage	126%	134%	156%	159%	105%
+ 3 G_z dégonflage	94%	116%	100%	127%	106%
f (coup par min)					
Avant départ	75	70	88	80	70
+ 3 G_z avant gonflage	100	110	110	120	75
+ 3 G_z gonflage	100	100	100	85	70
+ 3 G_z dégonflage	100	100	110	135	95

* Voile gris.

4. Résultats

Le départ de la centrifugeuse entraine une augmentation de la fréquence cardiaque f et de la pression artérielle (PA) et même du volume systolique (stroke volume – SV) et du débit cardiaque (cardiac output, $\dot{Q}$) (Tableau I). Après 2 à 3 min environ, les sujets se stabilisent, avec un SV diminué de 13 à 32%. Mais l'augmentation de f permet à $\dot{Q}$ de rester sensiblement normale. Les 3 sujets qui ont subis des malaises généraux

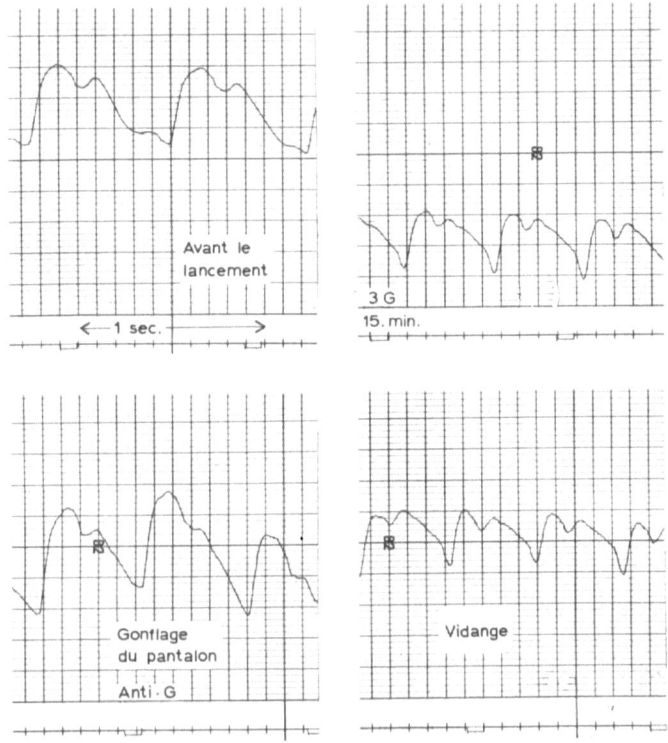

Fig. 2. Pléthysmographe électrique aortique transthoracique: à $+1\,G_z$, puis à $+3\,G_z$, puis avec gonflage et dégonflage du vêtement anti-G.

ont présenté brusquement une baisse nette de SV (jusqu'à 40%) et de PA. L'arrêt immédiat de la centrifugeuse a permis une récupération très rapide. Pour les 5 autres sujets, le gonflage du vêtement anti-G après 15 min entraîne une augmentation de PA, de SV et de $\dot{Q}$.

Après 10 min, le dégonflage entraîne une baisse de SV, mais l'accroissement de f permet de garder $\dot{Q}$ à environ 100% de la valeur avant le départ (Figure 2). Deux sujets ont présenté une baisse nette de PA et ont alors annoncé l'apparition d'un voile gris (gray-out). Des travaux en cours sur des sujets subissant $+5\,G_z$ montrent une accentuation de ces phénomènes.

5. Conclusions

La mesure du débit cardiaque par plethysmographie électrique permet de suivre en continu les variations circulatoires sous l'influence des accélérations G_z et présente un intérêt certain à l'entraînement et à la sélection du personnel navigant et au cours des longues utilisations thérapeutiques de la centrifugeuse.

Bibliographie

Coleman, B., Hertzman, A., D'Agrosa, L., et Flath, F.: 1966, AMRL-TR-66-65, Aeromedical Research Laboratories, Wright-Patterson AFB, Ohio, U.S.A.
Demange, J., Colin, J., et Boutelier, C.: 1968, *J. Physiol. (France)* **60**, Suppl. 2, 429.
Kubicek, W. G., Karnegis, J. N., Patterson, R. P., *et al.*: 1966, *Aerospace Med.* **37**, 1208.

RÉSISTANCE DU CORPS HUMAIN AUX ACCÉLÉRATIONS ÉLEVÉES DE COURTE DURÉE: EFFETS MÉCANIQUES ET HEMO-DYNAMIQUES

R. AUFFRET, H. SERIS, J. DEMANGE et R. P. DELAHAYE

Laboratoire de Médecine Aérospatiale du Centre d'Essais en Vol, 91 – Brétigny-sur-Orge, France

1. Introduction

En médecine aéronautique, il est classique de séparer par leurs effets physiologiques, les accélérations de courte durée (siège éjectable par exemple), des accélérations de durée plus longue (virage serré par exemple). Les accélérations de courte durée, d'une durée inférieure à la seconde, provoquent des effets mécaniques s'apparentant à la résistance des matériaux.

La résistance du squelette est alors fonction de l'amplitude de l'accélération, se son sens, de sa rapidité d'installation. L'abandon de bord d'un avion par siège éjectable provoque une accélération type courte durée. Les sièges éjectables actuels (cartouche à poudre) produisent une accélération suivant le grand axe du corps ($+G_z$) de l'ordre de 15 g pendant une durée de 0.2 sec, accélération atteinte en 0.05 sec environ. Pour les sièges à fusées, les chiffres temps d'établissement et amplitude de l'accélération sont à peu près les mêmes, mais la durée du plateau d'accélération est d'environ 0.4 sec. Dans ces conditions, avec des accélérations de ces durées, il n'y a jamais de modification de l'équilibre circulatoire. Le sang n'a pas le temps de s'accumuler en quelques dixièmes de seconde dans les parties basses du corps. La pleine conscience du sujet est conservée pendant l'éjection, mais cette accélération de 15g pendant quelques dixièmes de seconde peut produire des dégats osseux, plus particulièrement des lésions de la colonne vertébrale allant jusqu'à la fracture d'une ou plusieurs vertèbres. Ces dommages surviennent principalement lorsqu'au moment de l'éjection existent des accélérations complexes sur plusieurs axes liées à une perte de contrôle avion, ou si la position de sujet sur le siège est mauvaise (baquet siège trop bas, sangles mal serrées). Cette traumatologie vertébrale liée à l'éjection est décrite dans de nombreux travaux français et étrangers (cf. bibliographie).

Récemment, pour augmenter la sécurité du sauvetage dans des éjections à basse altitude, les constructeurs songèrent à augmenter la durée de combustion de la fusée. Ainsi dans les éjections vers le haut, en augmentant l'apogée de trajectoire du siège, on améliore la réussité de l'éjection près du sol, ou sur un avion avec une vitesse descentionnelle importante. L'accélération est alors de 15 g pendant 0.8 sec environ.

Ces nouveaux paramètres sont à l'intérieur du domaine de tolérance (Beckman, 1954) néanmoins ils s'approchent du domaine où se produisent les phénomènes hémo-dynamiques. Pour apprécier la tolérance physiologique à ces accélérations une expérience a été réalisée en centrifugeuse.

D. E. Busby (ed.), Recent Advances in Aerospace Medicine, 319–322. All Rights Reserved.
Copyright © 1970 by D. Reidel Publishing Company, Dordrecht-Holland.

2. Installation et protocole d'essais

En centrifugeuse, grâce au lancement par catapulte, il est possible d'approcher le profil d'accélération de l'éjection. Pour la centrifugeuse du Centre d'Essais en Vol de Brétigny avec la grande nacelle, 13.5 g seront obtenus en 1 sec, temps plus long que l'éjection réelle mais la durée 0.8 sec du plateau à 13.5 g suivi d'un freinage en 1 sec donne des renseignements voisins d'une éjection.

Pour que la forte accélération centripète produite par la centrifugeuse soit dirigée selon le grand axe du corps il faut que le sujet soit placé sensiblement horizontalement, la tête dirigée vers l'axe de rotation. Le temps très bref de lancement ne permet pas d'utiliser une nacelle 'libre' s'inclinant selon sa propre inertie et nécessité, avant le lancement, un basculement manuel de la nacelle qui amènera le grand axe du corps dans le prolongement de l'axe du bras portant la nacelle de la centrifugeuse. Cette position inconfortable rend difficile la mise en place correcte du dos, de l'expérimentateur sur le siège Martin-Baker MK 4 utilisé.

La surveillance du sujet était assurée par télévision. Deux caméras 16 mm noir et blanc ont enregistré les déplacements de la tête du sujet de face et de profil. Les films couleur n'ont pu être utilisés à cause du bourrage des caméras.

L'accélération sur l'axe Z, l'électrocardiogramme et la rhéographie de la base du crâne ont été enregistrés à chaque essai réalisé aux amplitudes d'accélération progressive: 6.5, 9, 11.5, et 13.5 g.

3. Enregistrements physiologiques

A. RHÉO-ENCÉPHALOGRAPHIE

Cette technique relativement récente d'exploration par voie externe du système circulatoire cérébral était utilisée. La méthode est basée sur l'enregistrement des variations d'impédance électrique craniennes, variations provoquées essentiellement par les modifications de la circulation cérébrale:

soit modifications du volume général (donc essentiellement veineux) entraînant des variations plus ou moins lentes de l'impédance de base.

soit modification plus faibles dues aux pulsations artérielles.

Une exploitation graphique de l'enregistrement des pulsations artérielles a été proposée par Demange (1967a, b). Elle est dérivée de celle mise au point par Nyboer pour la circulation périphérique et a permis par exemple de suivre l'évolution classique du débit sanguin cérébral sous l'influence de l'inhalation de CO_2 et de constater la faible influence du scalp dans la technique utilisée.

La technique dite à 2 électrodes est préférée à celle à 4 électrodes pour des raisons pratiqués, la deuxième n'étant d'ailleurs pas supérieure à la première pour l'étude de la circulation cérébrale globale ce qui n'est pas le cas pour l'étude de la circulation cérébrale locale, ou des circulations périphériques et thoraciques. Ces mesures rhéographiques cérébrales ont été pratiquées sur des sujets humains placés en centrifugeuse grâce à l'adaptation du matériel; elles ont permis de suivre les altérations pulsatiles cérébrales et l'effet protecteur des vêtements anti-*G* au cours d'accélérations de moyenne intensité.

Les fortes accélérations de courte durée décrites ci-dessus ne permettent guère une étude des pulsations artérielles (du fait des vibrations, en particulier) par contre, l'enregistrement de la variation de l'impédance de base a montré une baisse rapide mais relativement faible, traduisant probablement une certaine vidange rapide veineuse, mais aussi une récupération immédiate au cours de la décélération (des études statistiques sur sujets placés la tête en bas, puis en haut, avaient montré des variations d'impédance de base qui pourraient s'expliquer surtout par des variations du volume sanguin cérébral capillaire et veineux).

La récupération rapide semble suggérer que le siphon liquidien constitué par les gros vaisseaux cérébraux et les coeurs droit et gauche ne s'est pas désamorcé et donc que le cœur droit est resté suffisamment alimenté, probablement par le sang veineux issu de la partie supérieure du corps. Cette constatation viendrait à l'appui des travaux attribuant au débit cardiaque un rôle essentiel dans l'irrigation des gros vaisseaux cérébraux, irrigation persistant par effet siphon malgré un effondrement de la pression artérielle.

B. ÉLECTROCARDIOGRAPHIE

Malgré les difficultés d'enregistrement l'E.C.G. ne montre pas d'altération du rythme ou de l'amplitude des contractions cardiaques.

4. Résultats des essais

A. *Essais à 6.5 et 9 g*

Aucun trouble subjectif n'a été signalé par les expérimentateurs, ni perte de conscience, ni baisse de vision. Il faut néanmoins noter l'apparition de quelques algies de la région dorsale après des essais répétés.

B. *Essais à 11.5 g*

L'accélération commence à être durement ressentie par le sujet. Ni perte de conscience, ni voile, mais les douleurs vertébrales sont la règle.

C. *Essais à 13.5 g*

Un seul essai a été réalisé. Il n'y a eu ni trouble visuel, ni perte de connaissance. Le tassement du sujet, visible sur les films a été très important de l'ordre d'une quinzaine de centimètres. L'expérimentateur a ressenti une douleur assez intense au niveau des dernières vertèbres cervicales qui a persisté, s'est transformée en névralgie cervicale et brachiale avec altération radiologique d'un disque intervertébral et condensation de plateaux vertébraux.

5. Conclusions

Ces essais ont montré l'absence de trouble de la vision périphérique ou centrale ou à plus forte raison de perte de connaissance pour les niveaux d'accélérations cités.

Les syndromes douloureux vertébraux avec altérations radiologiques ont vraisemblablement pour origine la combinaison des accélérations sur les axes Z (longitudinal) et X transverse au moment du lancement et de l'arrêt de la centrifugeuse. Ils s'apparentent à ce que l'on rencontre lors d'éjections compliquées avec mauvaise position du corps au départ du siège. Ces phénomènes douloureux apparaissent d'autant plus rapidement que les trous de conjugaison présentent une petite taille.

Bibliographie

Beckman, E. L.: 1954, *J. Aviat. Med.* **25**, 50.
Demange, J.: 1967a, *Rev. Méd. Aérospatiale* **6**, 5.
Demange, J.: 1967b, *Rev. Méd. Aérospatiale* **7**, 162.

THE EFFECT OF SUPERSONIC FLYING ON THE URINARY CATECHOLAMINE EXCRETION IN PILOTS

R. DEBIJADJI. L. PEROVIĆ, and V. VARAGIĆ

Institute of Aviation Medicine, Zemun, Yugoslavia

1. Introduction

The quantitative evaluation of reactions to stress has attracted increasing interest in recent years not only from the point of view of obtaining information on the bodily changes occurring under stress situations, but also with respect to the necessity of selecting personnel suitable for special tasks and missions. It is widely believed that flying acts as a general stressor, inducing changes in neuroendocrine and metabolic functions. This concept has been tested in a variety of flying circumstances (Balke *et al.*, 1957; Debijadji, 1967; Euler, 1964; Frankenhaeuser, 1962; Hale *et al.*, 1965).

In conditions of supersonic flying, several factors, such as emotional tension, accelerations, vibrations, noise and fatigue, act on the human organism. All these factors might produce an activation of the sympatho-adrenal system. Therefore, it seemed of interest to investigate stress during flight at high altitude and at high speed by determining the urinary excretion of catecholamines.

In this study, the effects of piloting supersonic aircraft on urinary catecholamine output was investigated. This is particular interest to aviation medicine since the metabolism of these substances can be altered by emotional and other types of stress associated with flying (Bloom *et al.*, 1963; Demos *et al.*, 1969; Euler and Lundberg, 1954; Euler, 1964; Hale, 1962; Klepping, 1963; Ulvedal *et al.*, 1963).

2. Method

The supersonic pilots were divided in three groups: A, B and C. The pilots, ages 22 to 24 years, had very little flying experience in supersonic aircraft.

There were 16 pilots in group A. They flew at an altitude of 6000 m, at a speed of 750 to 850 km/hr. The 15 pilots in group B flew at an altitude of 13 000 m at a speed of 2100 km/hr. The 7 pilots in group C flew at the altitude of 18 500 m at a speed of 1850 km/hr. These pilots were group B pilots who flew about 2 hr after their first mission. The duration of each flight was 45 min. The pilots wore a partial pressure suit. All flying time was in the forenoon.

Urine samples were taken 45 min before flight and 45 min after landing. Adrenaline and noradrenaline were estimated according to the method of Euler and Lishajko (1959, 1961), using an Amince-Bowman spectrophotofluorometer.

Control data were obtained from 6 members of the laboratory staff (administrators and technicians). Urine samples were collected at the same time of day as those from the pilots. The average age of this group was the same as the pilot groups.

D. E. Busby (ed.), Recent Advances in Aerospace Medicine, 323–327. All Rights Reserved.
Copyright © 1970 by D. Reidel Publishing Company, Dordrecht-Holland.

3. Results

The influence of various types of flying on the urinary catecholamine excretion are presented in Table I. This table shows values obtained from the flyers before and after flight. In order to test the effect of flight, the urinary data were compared statistically with those obtained before flight.

For Group A, Table I and Figure 1 show that the post-flight excretion of adrenaline was increased in comparison with the values obtained before flight ($p < 0.001$). The

TABLE I

Urinary catecholamine excretion (ng/min), supersonic pilots

Group	Adrenaline (A)		Noradrenaline (N)		A + N	
	Before flight	During flight	Before flight	During flight	Before flight	During flight
A	10.5 ± 1.17 [a]	27.6 ± 2.36	23.2 ± 2.45	28.9 ± 1.53	33.7 ± 3.00	56.6 ± 3.01
		$p < 0.001$		$p < 0.05$		$p < 0.001$
B	13.1 ± 2.05	26.8 ± 2.25	23.2 ± 1.55	30.1 ± 1.89	36.0 ± 2.75	56.9 ± 3.36
		$p < 0.001$		$p < 0.01$		$p < 0.001$
C	12.3 ± 2.45	18.1 ± 1.97	23.3 ± 3.01	35.0 ± 2.60	35.6 ± 4.42	53.1 ± 4.03
		$p < 0.10$		$p < 0.02$		$p < 0.02$

[a] Numbers shown are mean $\pm$ SE. The p value is significant at the 0.05 level.

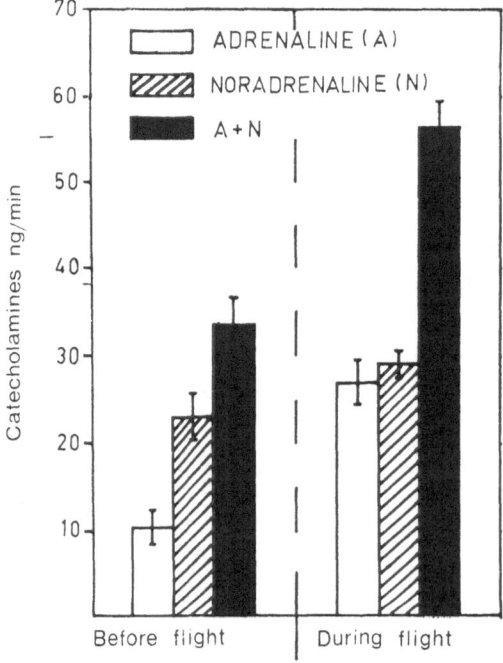

Fig. 1. Urinary output of catecholamines in group A (Mean $\pm$ SE).

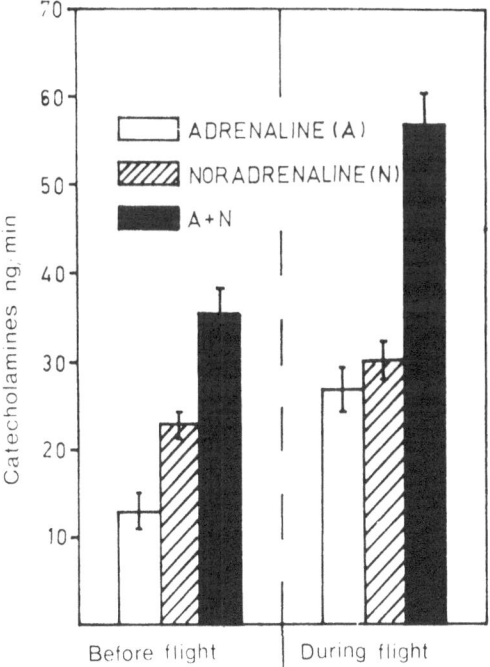

Fig. 2.   Urinary output of catecholamines in group B (Mean + SE).

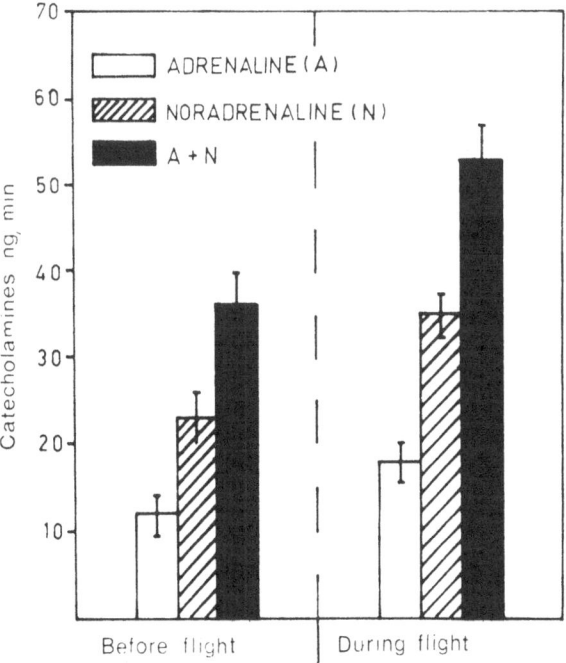

Fig. 3.   Urinary output of catecholamines in group C (Mean ± SE).

excretion of noradrenaline was also increased, but not to the same degree as was adrenaline ($p < 0.05$). For Group B, Table I and Figure 2 demonstrate that a significant increase occurred not only in the adrenaline output ($p < 0.001$) during flight, but also in the noradrenaline excretion ($p < 0.01$). As shown in Table I and Figure 3, no statistically significant variation was found in the catecholamine excretion of Group C pilots. It should be pointed out again that this flight was performed by pilots from group B, about 2 hr after their first flight.

Data in Table II represent the values for catecholamines in the nonflyer group and the supersonic pilots before the flight. It was found that the values for adrenaline and noradrenaline in flyers were significantly increased in comparision with those in the control group. It can be supposed that these increased values were connected with anticipation stress during flight preparation.

TABLE II

Anticipatory stress in pilots

Urinary variable ng/min	Nonflyers (6)[a]	Supersonic pilots (15)
Adrenaline (A)	5.6 ± 1.03[b] $\quad p < 0.001$	13.1 ± 2.05
Noradrenaline (N)	18.23 ± 2.10 $\quad p < 0.05$	23.2 ± 1.55
A + N	23.83 1.42 $\quad p < 0.001$	3.60 ± 2.75

[a] Number in parentheses is the number of cases.
[b] Numbers shown are Mean ± SE.

4. Discussion

Endocrine-metabolic analysis suggests that it was possible to appraise the effects of flight sensitivity on sympatho-adrenal, adrenocortical and metabolic activities. These observations also suggest that stress reactions to flight conform to the general adaptation syndrome pattern (Euler, 1964; Hale et al., 1959; Hale et al., 1965; Marchbanks, 1960).

In this experiment, an attempt has been made to evaluate quantitatively flight situations by urinary catecholamine analysis. The results indicate an increase in activity of the sympatho-adrenal system in pilots in groups A and B. In both groups, a significant increase in the adrenaline output occurred during flight. If the excreted adrenaline is presumed to be a reflection of the emotional state, then the pilots in groups A and B reacted in the same manner by the 'all or nothing' law. The higher excretion of noradrenaline in group B pilots is probably the consequence of the influence of physical factors of the flight on the organism encountered at the higher altitude and speed. It is possible that this increased excretion of catecholamines is at least in part due to low flying experience of the pilots. It has already been shown that the excretion of catecholamines and corticosteroids during flight can be related to the aircraft characteristics, weather conditions and flying experience (Demos *et al.*, 1969; Kramer *et al.*, 1966; Marchbanks *et al.*, 1963; Ulvedal *et al.*, 1963).

No significant difference in the pre-flight and in-flight catecholamine outputs was found in group C pilots. One would expect these pilots to have higher outputs than those of the other groups, since they flew at the highest altitude and speed. However this group was made up of group B pilots, who had flown previously on the same day. Therefore, it appears that stressors, when acting for the first time, induce adreno-cortical responses of fairly large magnitude. However, with continued or repeated stimulations, these responses diminish in magnitude (Marchbanks *et al.*, 1963). The values for adrenaline and noradrenaline outputs in group C are not the consequence of exhaustion of the sympatho-adrenal system, but of the adaptation of this system to the flying situation. Measuring of the urinary output of adrenaline and noradrenaline thus represents a sensitive parameter of the sympatho-adrenal medullary activity during flight performance.

5. Conclusion

The adrenaline and noradrenaline output was determined in supersonic pilots before and during flight at various altitudes and speeds. The significantly increased excretion of adrenaline during flight is most probably due to the emotional state of the pilots. The excreted amount of adrenaline during flying stress suggests that the pilots in groups A and B reacted by the 'all or nothing' law. Repeated flight was found to lead to adaptation of the sympatho-adrenal system to the flying stressors.

References

Balke, B., Wells, J. G., and Clark, R. T., Jr.: 1957, *J. Aviat. Med.* **28**, 241.
Bloom, G. *et al.*: 1963, *Acta Physiol. Scand.* **58**, 77.
Debijadji, R. *et al.*: 1967, *Physiol. Pharmacol. Acta* **3**, 258.
Demos, G. T., Hale, H. B., and Williams, E. W.: 1969, *Aerospace Med.* **4**, 385.
Euler, U. S. von: 1964, *Clin. Pharm. Therap.* **5**, 398.
Euler, U. S. von and Lundberg, U.: 1954, *J. Appl. Physiol.* **6**, 551.
Euler, U. S. von and Lishajko, F.: 1959, *Acta Physiol. Scand.* **45**, 122.
Euler, U. S. von and Lishajko, F.: 1961, *Acta Physiol. Scand.* **51**, 348.
Frankenhaeuser, M. *et al.*: 1962, *Percept. Mot. Skills* **15**, 63.
Hale, H. B., Ellis, J. P. Jr., and Kratochovil, C. H.: 1959, *J. Appl. Physiol.* **14**, 629.
Hale, H. B.: 1962, Internat. Congr. Endocrinology, Milan, Italy.
Hale, H. B., Duffy, J. C., Ellis, J. P. Jr., and Williams, E. W.: 1965, *Aerospace Med.* **36**, 112.
Klepping, J.: 1963, *Compt. Rend. Soc. Biol.*, pp. 1727–1729.
Kramer, E. E., Hale, H. B., and Ellis, J., P. Jr.: 1966, *Aerospace Med.* **37**, 1095.
Marchbanks, V. H., Jr.: 1960, *Aerospace Med.* **31**, 639.
Marchbanks, V. H., Jr., Hale, H. B., and Ellis, J. P., Jr.: 1963, *Aerospace Med.* **34**, 14.
Ulvedal, F., Smith, W. R., and Welch, B. E.: 1963, *J. Appl. Physiol.* **18**, 1257.

MAN IN HIS THERMAL ENVIRONMENT

TOLERANCE À LA CHALEUR DANS LE CAS DE PANNE DE LA CLIMATISATION SUR AVION DE TRANSPORT SUPERSONIQUE

J. COLIN, C. BOUTELIER, et J. TIMBAL

Laboratoire de Médecine Aérospatiale du Centre d'Essais en Vol, 91 – Brétigny-sur-Orge, France

1. Introduction

En cas de défaillance du système de conditionnement d'air d'un avion de transport supersonique on peut assister à une élévation plus ou moins rapide de la température de l'atmosphère de la cabine. Ainsi se pose la question de la tolérance à la chaleur, car c'est en fonction de cette tolérance que des consignes pourront être données à l'équipage, concernant la poursuite du vol après une panne grave du système de refroidissement.

Lorsque l'on étudie la tolérance à la chaleur il est possible de définir deux zones d'ambiance:

(1) *zone non compensable* – on entend sous ce terme la gamme d'ambiances thermiques dans laquelle l'équilibre thermique de l'organisme ne pourra jamais être atteint, car les limites de la thermorégulation efficace sont dépassées. Ce peut être le cas:

(a) soit d'une ambiance où le degré hygrométrique est trop élevé: la sueur s'évapore mal ou pas du tout.

(b) soit d'une ambiance où la température est trop élevée: la sueur s'évapore bien mais le débit qui serait nécessaire dépasse les possibilités de l'organisme.

Dans cette zone non compensable le temps de tolérance correspond soit au temps que met à se constituer un stockage de chaleur limite, soit à l'apparition de douleurs provoquées par des élévations de températures locales trop importantes.

(2) *zone compensable* – on désigne sous ce terme les ambiances pour lesquelles l'équilibre thermique de l'organisme peut être réalisé. Il est alors évident que le temps de tolérance correspond au temps pendant lequel le débit sudoral nécessaire peut être maintenu. Ce temps limite correspond à divers phénomènes tels que la fatigue des glandes sudorales, la deshydratation, la déchloruration.

Nous allons voir rapidement ces deux cas généraux, en rappelant deux caractéristiques essentielles et heureusement favorables de l'atmosphère de la cabine: (1) la pression, plus basse que celle qui règne au niveau de la mer, diminue les échanges de chaleur par convection et favorise l'évaporation de la sueur, (2) l'hygrométrie très basse à haute altitude, élève le pouvoir évaporatoire de l'atmosphère cabine et favorise ainsi l'évaporation de la sueur: et en rappelant aussi que l'on peut définir deux temps de tolérance: le temps de tolérance correspondant aux limites physiologiques, et le temps de tolérance correspondant à l'apparition d'une détérioration du rendement psychomoteur.

Enfin, pour clore ces généralités rappelons qu'il existe deux méthodes pour connaître le temps pendant lequel un sujet peut endurer une ambiance donnée. L'une,

D. E. Busby (ed.), Recent Advances in Aerospace Medicine, 331–336. All Rights Reserved.
Copyright © 1970 by D. Reidel Publishing Company, Dordrecht - Holland.

empirique, consiste à soumettre des volontaires aux situations prévues et à suivre leurs réactions physiologiques et leur rendement psychomoteur. L'autre, se basant sur des résultats expérimentaux précédemment acquis, qui permet par le calcul de prévoir le temps de tolérance dans des circonstances diverses. Nous nous limiterons ici à cette dernière méthode.

2. Tolérance dans la zone non compensable

Dans cette zone, où, ainsi que nous l'avons vu, l'organisme ne peut réaliser son équilibre thermique, un important stockage de chaleur S apparaît. On peut admettre que lorsque ce stockage de chaleur atteint la valeur de 50 kcal/m^2, il existe un inconfort appréciable et le rendement psychomoteur commence à être détérioré. Lorsqu'il dépasse 80 kcal/m^2 la situation devient dangereuse pour le sujet exposé. Ces valeurs peuvent en réalité varier avec la vitesse d'établissement du stockage (Goldman et al., 1965) mais laissent une marge de sécurité suffisante si l'on en juge d'après les valeurs de stockage observées chez des sujets au travail (Wortz et al., 1967).

Pour connaître le stockage, il est nécessaire d'apprécier la charge thermique à laquelle est soumis l'organisme et la quantité de chaleur qu'il arrive à perdre par évaporation de la sueur. On peut apprécier la charge thermique à laquelle est soumis l'organisme par radiation R et convection C, les échanges par conduction étant négligés, si l'on connaît la température cutanée ou superficielle des vêtements $\bar{T}_s$ la température ambiante T_a et le coefficient combiné d'échange de chaleur h en appliquant la formule:

$$R + C = h\,(T_a - \bar{T}_s).$$

Le coefficient h est la somme des coefficients d'échange de chaleur par radiation h_r et par convection h_c; h_r varie avec la posture du sujet (Guibert et Taylor, 1952), h_c avec l'altitude et la vitesse de l'air (Colin et Houdas, 1967: Timbal et al., 1969; Winslow et al., 1939).

Pour un sujet assis on a:

$$h_r = 3.8$$
$$h_c = (1.9 + 6.4\,v^{0.67})\,(d/d_0)^{0.67}.$$

Pour une pression atmosphérique voisine de celle qui règne au niveau de la mer on obtient:

pour une vitesse d'air nulle $h = 5.75$
pour $v = 0.2$ m/sec $h = 7.85$.

L'altitude cabine restant basse nous simplifierons les calculs ci-après en admettant un coefficient h de 8, donc correspondant à un vent légèrement supérieur à 0.2 m/sec. Pour d'autres altitudes on pourra appliquer les coefficients donnés par Timbal et al. (1969).

Le dernier paramètre inconnu de l'équation donnant la charge thermique est la température cutanée (ou superficielle des vêtements). Il est certain qu'elle est elle-même fonction d'autres variables telles que la température ambiante, l'isolement et la perméabilité des vêtements, l'efficacité de la sudation....

Nous prendrons comme exemple le cas d'un sujet nu pour lequel on peut admettre pour la température cutanée moyenne une valeur de 36 °C. Dans le cas d'un sujet vêtu la température superficielle du vêtement est plus proche de la température ambiante. Il en découle donc que nous surestimons la charge thermique externe dans notre exemple. Certes, il est facile de calculer la charge thermique externe lorsque l'on connaît l'isolement du vêtement porté, mais le calcul dans le cas du sujet nu nous donne sa limite supérieure. Nous arrivons donc à une charge thermique externe de:

$$R + C = 8\,(T_a - 36).$$

En ajoutant à cette charge thermique externe la production métabolique M on obtient la charge thermique totale. Pour un sujet au repos on peut prendre pour M la valeur de 50 kcal/m² hr, ce qui donne:

$$R + C + M = 8\,(T_a - 36) + 50.$$

Une partie de cette charge thermique va être évacuée par la sudation. Pour un sujet moyen non acclimaté le pouvoir maximum de sudation est de l'ordre de 220 g/m² hr, ce qui correspond à 130 kcal/m² hr si elle est totalement évaporée.* Les pertes de chaleur par les voies respiratoires ont été négligées car elles sont faibles par rapport aux pertes de chaleur totales par évaporation que nous avons admis ici.

Le pouvoir évaporatoire de l'atmosphère de la cabine d'un avion de transport supersonique volant à haute altitude dépasse largement cette valeur. On peut l'estimer en effet à plus de 300 kcal/m² hr. Il est cependant douteux que toute la sueur puisse s'évaporer, car une partie importante du corps est en contact avec le siège. Cette partie du corps représentant $\frac{1}{6}$ de la surface corporelle totale on aboutit à une quantité de chaleur perdue par évaporation de 100 kcal/m² hr. Cette quantité de chaleur peut etre limitée par les vêtements, si leur perméabilité est basse. Cependant, sauf dans le cas de port d'une combinaison pressurisée il apparaît probable qu'une évaporation de cet ordre soit possible, compte tenu de l'altitude et de la sécheresse de l'air ambiant.

Nous avons maintenant tous les éléments pour calculer le stockage de chaleur. En négligeant la période transitoire d'établissement de la sudation au cours de laquelle s'établit un certain stockage de chaleur, il est donné par l'équation:

$$S = (R + C + M) - E = 8\,(T_a - 36) + 50 - 100.$$

Le temps de tolérance pour atteindre un stockage de 50 kcal/m² sera alors donné en minutes par l'équation:

$$t_{50} = \frac{3000}{8\,(T_a - 36) + 50 - 100}$$

---

* Pour un sujet très acclimaté le débit atteint 1300 g/hr soit plus de 430 kcal/m² hr perdus par évaporation (lorsque le pouvoir évaporatoire de l'ambiance le permet).

et pour atteindre 80 kcal/m² par l'équation :

$$t_{80} = \frac{4800}{8\,(T_a - 36) + 50 - 100}.$$

Quelques résultats types sont donnés dans le Tableau I qui donne en quelque sorte les limites du temps de tolérance à la chaleur en fonction de la température ambiante.

TABLEAU I

Temps de tolérance à la chaleur avec
$M = 50$ kcal/m² ,hr

$T_a(°C)$	Temps pour atteindre	
	$S = 50$	$S = 80$
50	48	77
60	21	34
70	14	22
80	10	16

TABLEAU II

Temps de tolérance à la chaleur avec
$M = 100$ kcal/m² hr

$T_a(°C)$	Temps pour atteindre	
	$S = 50$	$S = 80$
40	94	150
50	27	43
60	16	25
70	11	18
80	9	14

Un calcul semblable peut être effectué pour des valeurs de production métabolique supérieure à 50 kcal/m² hr. Il suffit de remplacer M par la valeur considérée. Le Tableau II indique les résultats obtenus pour un métabolisme de 100 kcal/m² hr, ce qui correspond à un travail modéré. La diminution du temps de tolérance est manifeste. Comme certains membres de l'équipage peuvent avoir à exécuter un travail de cet ordre, sinon plus intense, on voit toute l'importance de ce facteur. La Figure 1 donne les courbes correspondant aux deux tableaux. Les équations données plus haut permettent de procéder à des calculs semblables pour différentes altitudes et diverses vitesses de vent.

3. Tolérance dans la zone compensable

Sachant, comme nous l'avons vu plus haut, qu'une évaporation de 100 kcal/m² hr est possible, toutes les conditions aboutissant à une charge thermique totale inférieure à

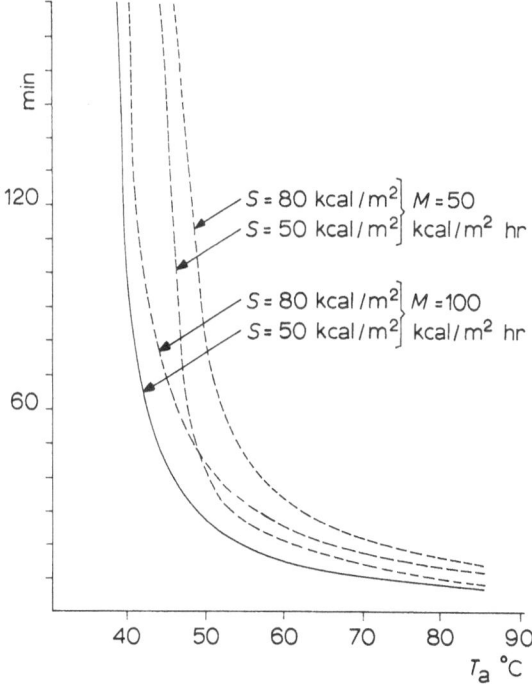

Fig. 1.   Temps de tolérance pour atteindre deux niveaux de stockage de chaleur S, dans le cas de deux niveaux de production de chaleur métabolique M.

ce chiffre pourront être supportées pendant plusieurs heures. Partant de l'équation donnant la charge thermique il est possible de voir que pour un sujet au repos la zone de températures compensables va jusqu'à 42 °C, et pour un sujet ayant une production de chaleur métabolique de 100 kcal/m^2 hr, jusqu'à 36 °C.

4. Conclusions

Dans cette brève étude de la tolérance à la chaleur nous avons vu que pour un sujet au repos, non acclimaté, une panne de climatisation cabine d'un avion supersonique volant à haute altitude ne pose pas de problème aigu tant que la température reste inférieure à 42 °C., le pouvoir évaporatoire de l'atmosphère cabine autorisant l'équilibre thermique. Au-delà de cette température un stockage de chaleur de plus en plus important apparaît. Lorsque ce stockage dépasse 50 kcal/m^2 hr, il existe une atteinte du rendement psychomoteur, c'est pourquoi il nous paraît préférable de ne prendre en considération que le temps de tolérance calculé sur cette base.

Nous avons vu également qu'un travail même modéré abaissait nettement le temps de tolérance. C'est pourquoi il nous paraît souhaitable, pour garder une marge de sécurité suffisante en ce qui concerne l'équipage de ne retenir en définitive que la courbe de temps de tolérance correspondant à une production métabolique de 100 kcal/m^2 hr.

Il est certain que les calculs qui sont exposés ici ne sont valables que dans le cas d'un sujet nu, et sous-estimant vraisemblablement le temps de tolérance de sujets vêtus en raison de la résistance thermique des vêtements qui diminue la charge thermique externe. En effet il ne semble pas qu'avec des vêtements ordinaires la diminution des pertes de chaleur par évaporation puisse annuler ou même dépasser cette action bénéfique. La courbe proposée donne donc une marge de sécurité suffisante.

Il est possible de calculer les temps de tolérance pour diverses altitudes: ils sont d'autant plus longs qu'elles sont élévées (tant que l'on reste à l'abri de l'hypoxie): pour des vitesses de l'air plus faibles: ils sont plus longs également; et enfin pour des hygrométries plus élevées; ils sont plus courts. Mais cette dernière éventualité ne se rencontre qu'en vol à basse altitude.

Enfin pour terminer il faut souligner le caractère théorique de cet exposé. Une étude expérimentale des temps de tolérance en maquette au cours de pannes de climatisation simulée nous paraît souhaitable pour préciser les temps de tolérance à la chaleur dans le cas des avions de transport supersoniques.

Bibliographie

Colin, J. et Houdas, Y.: 1967, *J. Appl. Physiol.* **22**, 31.
Colin, J., Timbal, J., Guieu, J. D., et Boutelier, C.: 1969, *Revue des Corps de Santé des Armées* **10**, 547.
Goldman, R. F., Green, E. B., et Iampietro, P. F.: 1965, *J. Appl. Physiol.* **20**, 271.
Guibert, A. et Taylor, C. L.: 1952, *J. Appl. Physiol.* **5**, 24.
Timbal, J., Colin, J., et Boutelier, C.: 1969, XVIIIe Congrès International de Médecine Aérospatiale, Amsterdam, Pays-Bas.
Winslow, C. E. A., Gagge, A. P., et Merrington, L. P.: 1939, *Amer. J. Physiol.* **127**, 505.
Wortz, E. C., Edwards, D. K., Diaz, A. *et al.*: 1967, *Aerospace Med.* **38**, 181.

INFLUENCE DE L'ALTITUDE
SUR LES ÉCHANGES THERMIQUES DE L'HOMME

J. TIMBAL, J. COLIN et C. BOUTELIER

Laboratoire de Médecine Aérospatiale du Centre d'Essais en Vol, 91 – Brétigny-sur-Orge, France

Les échanges thermiques dans l'air, dépendent de la température radiante, de la température et de la vitesse de déplacement de l'air, de l'hygrométrie et de la pression barometrique. Le rôle de ce dernier facteur est souvent passé sous silence. Les auteurs qui s'intéressent aux problèmes de la thermorégulation donnent des résultats valables à l'altitude de leur laboratoire, en général voisine du niveau de la mer, et ne s'inquiètent pas de la pression barométrique. Ces résultats, suffisent d'ailleurs à résoudre la plupart des problèmes qui se posent dans ce domaine. En aéronautique, il en va tout autrement, et on ne peut negliger ce facteur extrêmement important. Il est toutefois possible à partir des équations régissant les échanges thermiques de prévoir son influence.

Les échanges par radiation sont régis par la loi de Stefan-Boltzmann qui ne fait pas intervenir la pression. Ils sont donc en principe indépendant de ce facteur. Néanmoins, l'air intervient indirectement en formant écran au transfert du rayonnement solaire. Au fur et à mesure que l'on s'élève en altitude, l'écran formé par les nuages disparait. L'action de l'atmosphere proprement dite, diminue également puisque son épaisseur diminue, mais son rôle est moins important que celui des nuages. En effet, l'atmosphère claire n'absorbe que 15% du rayonnement solaire. A 30000 m, le flux solaire est d'environ 1150 kcal/m² hr, pour un angle au zénith de 0 deg. Dans les couches plus élevées, là où évoluent les satellites, le flux de chaleur émis par le soleil n'augmente guère, il est de 1180 kcal/m² hr.

Il faut également tenir compte du rayonnement thermique de la terre. Le flux de ce rayonnement varie avec les conditions météorologiques locales, mais on peut admettre comme chiffre moyen environ 190 kcal/m² hr. Outre ce rayonnement terrestre proprement dit, la terre et son atmosphère réfléchissent environ 36% des radiations thermiques qu'elles reçoivent du soleil. C'est ce que l'on appelle l'"Albedo". Le flux thermique qui lui correspond est d'environ 430 kcal/m² hr.

En ce qui concerne les échanges par convection, le problème est plus complexe et fort mal connu théoriquement. L'approche qui chez l'homme semble la plus valable est essentiellement empirique. Cette étude a été abordée de la façon suivante:

Les sujets étaient couchés nus, sur un lit en treillis métallique placé à l'intérieur d'une chambre climatique, permettant de contrôler indépendamment la température de l'air et sa vitesse, la température radiante et l'hygrométrie. Après un repos préalable de 90 min, à la neutralité thermique pour permettre au sujet d'être en état basal, les conditions d'ambiance sont modifiées très rapidement pour créer une charge thermique importante. L'expérience est ensuite poursuivie pendant 90 min de façon à atteindre un état stable de la sudation et des températures corporelles. Les pertes thermiques par évaporation sont mesurées par une méthode de pesée continue. La température rectale et 10 températures cutanées sont enregistrées en continu à l'aide de thermo-couples Cuivre-Constantan. Les conditions d'ambiance ont été réalisées d'une part, avec une température d'air égale à la température radiante de 30 à 50 °C avec des vents allant de 0.2 à 1.2 m/sec, et d'autre part, en combinant une température d'air constante à 30 °C avec des températures parfois allant de 60 à 70 °C. Au total 69 expériences ont été réalisées de la sorte.

Des considérations théoriques ont conduit à admettre pour les échanges par convection, une équation de la forme:

$$H_c = h_c \left(T_a - T_s \right) \tag{1}$$

avec

$$h_c = \left(a + b \cdot v^n \right) \left(d/d_0 \right)^n. \tag{2}$$

H_c représente la quantité de chaleur échangée par convection, d et d_0 densité de l'air à l'altitude considérée et au niveau de la mer; a, b, n, des constantes; T_a et $\bar{T}_s$ les températures de l'air et cutanée moyenne; v, la vitesse du vent; h_c le coefficient de transfert thermique par convection.

Les résultats expérimentaux obtenus au niveau de la mer, ont permis de déterminer la valeur de ces constantes (Colin et al., 1967). Le coefficient de transfert s'exprime par l'équation suivante, pour un sujet allongé, vent dans le grand axe du corps:

$$h_c = (2.3 + 7.5v^{0.67}) \left(d/d_0 \right)^{0.67}. \tag{3}$$

Lorsque le vent est nul le terme $7.5 \, v^{0.67}$ s'annule, et la constante 2.3 correspond aux échanges par convection naturelle. La plupart des auteurs admettent que l'intervention de la vitesse de l'air obeït à une relation exponentielle de puissance 0.5 (Winslow et al., 1939; Nelson et al., 1947; Bütner, 1934). Par contre Hall (1950) trouve pour n une valeur plus élevée -0.80. Mitchell et al. (1969) donnent 0.60.

Les équations ci-dessus font intervenir l'effet de l'altitude et il est possible à partir des résultats obtenus au niveau de la mer de prévoir la valeur de h_c en altitude. Au niveau de la mer, le terme $\left(d/d_0 \right)^{0.67}$ devient égal à l'unité et l'Equation 3 se simplifie. Avec l'altitude, ce terme diminue, et le coefficient de transfert thermique diminue également. Ainsi, quand la pression barométrique et la densité tendent vers zéro, ce qui est le cas de l'espace, les échanges par convection s'annulent. Figure 1 ci-contre, calculée à partir des pressions barométriques, montre les valeurs du coefficient h_c pour diverses vitesses de vent à des altitudes allant de 0 à 20 000 m et illustre ces remarques.

Les échanges par évaporation dépendent du pouvoir évaporatoire de l'ambiance (PE). Les équations utilisées habituellement pour apprécier ce facteur sont de la forme:

$$PE = k \cdot v^n \left(Pw_s - Pw_a \right). \tag{4}$$

Pw_s et Pw_a représentent les pressions partielles de vapeur d'eau au niveau de la peau et dans l'air.

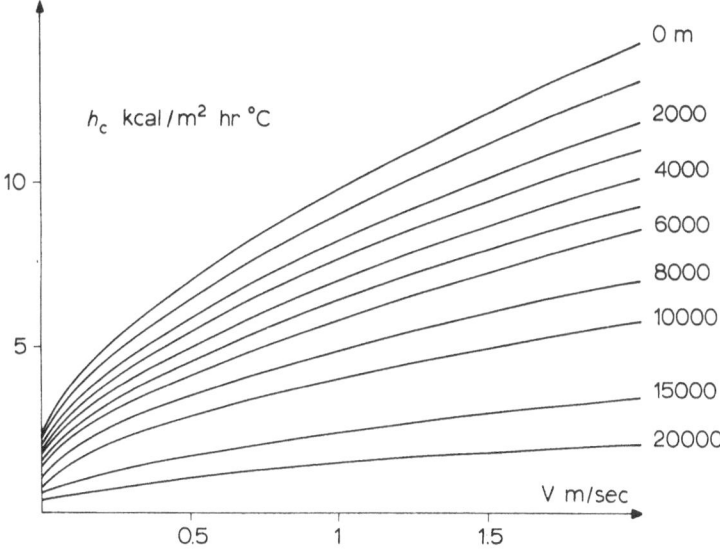

Fig. 1.   Influence de l'altitude sur les échanges thermiques de l'homme.

Le pouvoir évaporatoire de l'ambiance, représente l'évaporation maximale permise par l'ambiance. Si la sudation nécessaire pour assurer l'équilibre thermique du corps humain lui est supérieure, la sueur ruisselle et ne joue pas son rôle. Pratiquement on admet qu'il y a ruissellement dans le cas où le déplacement de l'air est linéaire, lorsque le débit sudoral atteint le $\frac{1}{3}$ du pouvoir évaporatoire maximum.

Woodcock *et al.* (1956) ont admis à partir de raisonnements théoriques que le coefficient d'échange par évaporation devrait être le double du coefficient d'échange par convection. Cette conclusion a été vérifiée expérimentalement sur une peau totalement mouillée par Clifford *et al.* (1959) qui donnent 11.9 pour k et 0.63 pour n, cette dernière valeur étant très voisine de celle que nous avons trouvé dans nos expériences pour la convection. Avec l'altitude Pw_a diminue et le pouvoir évaporatoire de l'ambiance augmente, ce qui facilite l'évaporation de la sudation.

Ainsi l'altitude agit de deux façons différentes sur les échanges thermiques. Elle facilite l'évaporation de la sueur, et diminue les échanges par convection.

Bibliographie

Bütner, K.: 1934, in *Bioklimatologie und Meteorologie, Veröffentlichungen des hanssichen Meteorologischen Institutes*, Abhandlungen BdX, Nr. 5, Berlin.
Clifford, J., Kerslake, D., et Wadell, J. L.: 1959, *J. Physiol.* **147**, 253.
Colin, J. et Houdas, J.: 1967, *J. Appl. Physiol.* **22**, 31.
Hall, Y.: 1950, Memo Rept. MCREXD 696-1058, Wright Patterson AFB, Ohio, U.S.A.
Nelson, N., Eichna, L. W., Horvath, S. M. *et al.*: 1947, *Amer. J. Physiol.* **161**, 626.
Winslow, L. E. A., Gagge, A. P., et Herrington, L. P.: 1939, *Amer. J. Physiol.* **127**, 505.
Woodcock, A. H., Pratt, R. L., et Brekenridge, J. R.: 1956, QRDC-EP-30, U.S. Quartermaster Research and Development Center, Natick, Mass., U.S.A.

MAN IN HIS TEMPORAL ENVIRONMENT

CIRCADIAN PERIODICITY OF REACTION-TIMES

J. C. ASCHOFF, G. GIEDKE and H. PÖPPEL

Dept. Neurology, University of Ulm, 79 Ulm and Max-Planck Institut für Verhältensforschung 8131,
Erling-Andechs, West Germany

1. Introduction

It seems that a competent account of diurnal variations in psychomotor functions, in which men's physical capacity can be expressed, can only be given if factors such as practice or motivation are controlled. If such control does not exist, either daily periodicities are likely to be overlooked or diurnal characteristics, such as amplitude, phase relation, or wave patterns, will be misjudged.

In our epoch of shift-work, frequent transgression of time zones, and space exploration, the autonomous periodicity in human performance which is independent of local time has reached a prominent interest of investigators. One must note that circadian periodicity of physical performance has been studied from various perspectives, whereas psycho-physical criteria are still evading subtle concern. An example of this neglect is the evaluation of reaction times under precise consideration not only of nocturnal sleep or waking effects, but also of practice effects.

Four different experiments were planned wherein it could be shown to what extent influences of task repetition and of diurnal periodicities of reaction times can be statistically evaluated and isolated from each other. Since it had already been shown several times that reaction times have manifold distributions, the distribution-independent Friedmann test has been employed for statistical analysis. Using the Bettendorf apparatus a total of 47000 reaction-times have been recorded.

2. Method

The experimental arrangement and technique of the experiments are shown in Figure 1. Ten subjects participated in experiment A. Over a period of 15 hr, at 1-hr recording intervals, white light and bell sounds at random frequencies were presented to them.

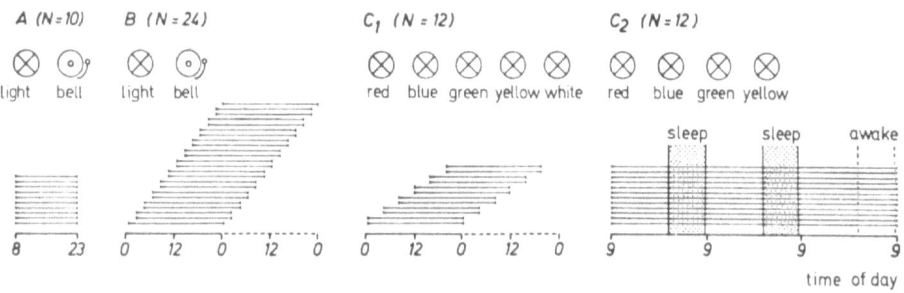

Fig. 1.   Experimental arrangement and technique.

D. E. Busby (ed.), Recent Advances in Aerospace Medicine, 343–347. All Rights Reserved.
Copyright © 1970 by D. Reidel Publishing Company, Dordrecht-Holland.

The effect of practice was neglected. In experiment B the same stimulation program was applied to 24 subjects. Contrary to experiment A, the recordings were made every 2 hr. This time, the effect of practice was eliminated through a sequencing technique; over a period of 24 hr, 2 subjects at a time had to start on the experiment according to the schedule. Thus, at every recording time within the 24 hr identical levels of practice were guaranteed. All subjects were kept awake for 24 hr.

In experiment C_1, during which the subjects again were kept awake, the starting order was maintained. However, the pattern of stimulation was modified so that 4 different color stimuli had to be discriminated. There was no order of succession in the stimuli offered, but the lengths of intervals between stimulus presentation remained constant. This experiment C_1 was meant only to build up a constant level of practice. For the subsequent experiment C_2, extending over 72 hr, the same 12 subjects were engaged. All subjects were allowed to sleep in the first 2 nights and were awakened only for the 5-min test period. All subjects remained awake throughout the third night. Thus it was possible to isolate the tendency of practice, which had nearly reached a constant level, from diurnal periodicities, as well as to assess the influence of nocturnal sleeping or waking on the diurnal periodicity of complex reaction time.

3. Results and Discussion

Figure 2 shows results obtained in experiment A. It appears that reaction times are not equally distributed from 8 a.m. to 11 p.m. The lessening of the reaction time in the

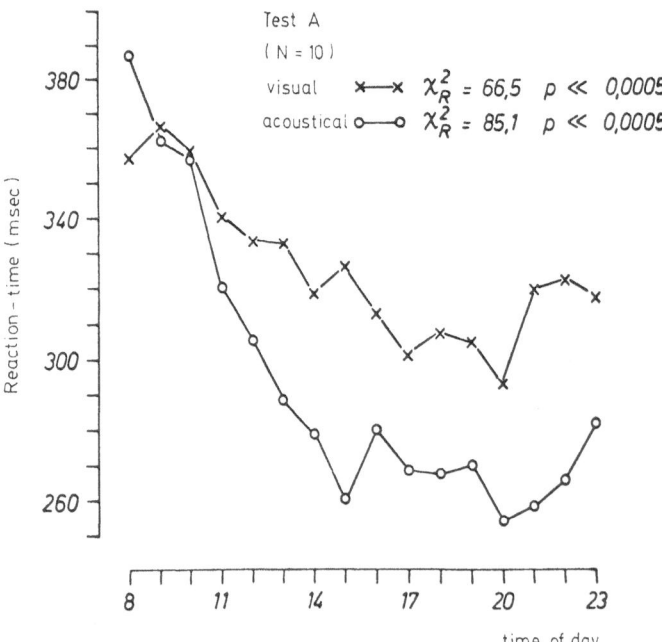

Fig. 2. Reaction times throughout the day.

course of the day strongly indicates the influence of practice. The repeated waxing of the reaction time towards 11 p.m. reflects either the effect of a diurnal periodicity, as observed in other experiments, or the effect of declining motivation.

It was consequently the aim of experiment B to discouple the effects of repetition from diurnal fluctuations through the sequencing technique mentioned above. Figure 3 presents the whole body of results from this experiment. On the left side of this figure, the arithmetic averages are displayed for the optic and acoustic reaction

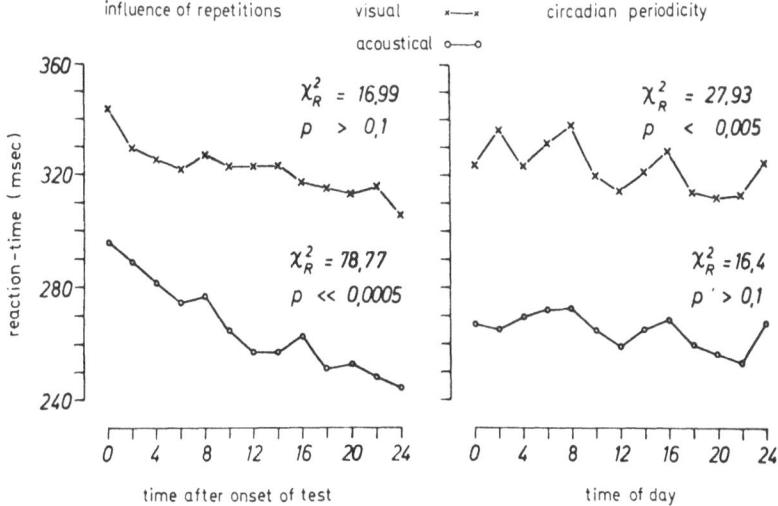

Fig. 3. Reaction times as a function of time of onset of the test and the time of day the test is performed (see text).

times for corresponding experiments as dependent on the starting sequence (influence of practice). On the right side, mean reaction times have been plotted for fixed points of time over the day (diurnal periodicity). As evident in the left graph, optic as well as acoustic reaction times undergo a continual, nearly linear improvement during the experiment; this improvement does not level off towards the end of the test period. For acoustic reaction times, the influence of repetition is more marked than it is in optic reaction times. This might be due in part to the warning property of acoustic signals. On the other hand, long fixation on visual targets produces marked fatigue. The circadian oscillations on the right side of Figure 3 are statistically valid only for optic reaction times (upper curve), which has to be interpreted in the way that functions, where practice plays a minor role, possess larger diurnal amplitudes.

As it had been demonstrated that a constant level of practice would not be reached within 24 hr, and vigilance dampens the amplitude of circadian rhythms, the more complex reaction time to 4 different optic stimuli was determined every 3 hr over 4 days in the final experiments C_1 and C_2. The left side of Figure 4 shows the influence of practice, and the right side the circadian periodicity. The analysis neglects different color stimuli; the whole body of data from one recording event was compounded to

represent one overall optic reaction time. On the average, this has been 240 msec
longer than the simple optic reaction time in experiment A and B.

On the left side of Figure 4, reflecting the effect of repetition, it is recognized that
the wave pattern is not congruent with that of the learning effect observed in experiment B. After an initial decrease, the reaction time increases again towards the end of
the experiment. An explanation might be given by the particular situation of the
experiment, where the subjects knew three further experimental days would follow.
With respect to the circadian rhythm, shortest reaction times appear at 6 p.m., whereas

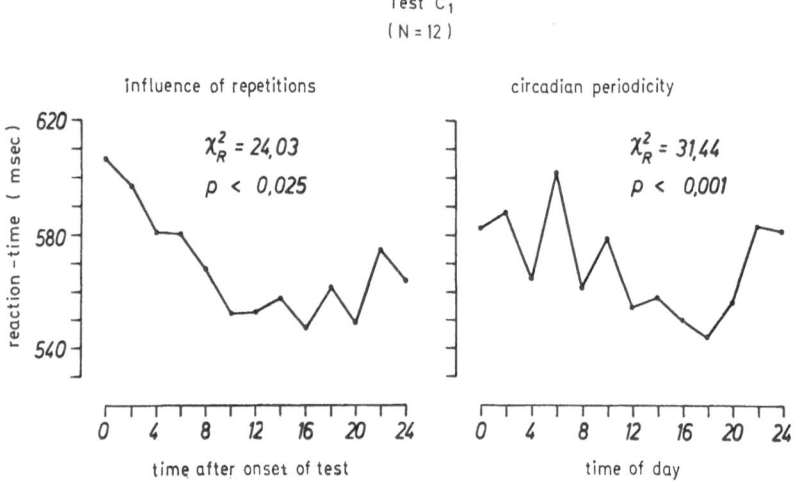

Fig. 4.   Reaction time as a function of time of onset of the test and the time of day the test
is performed (see text).

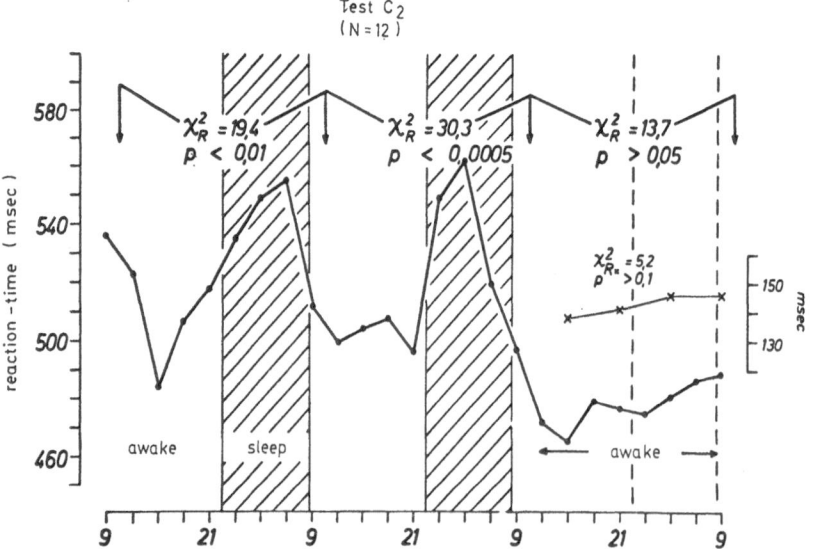

Fig. 5.   Circadian periodicity over a 3-day test period (see text).

during nighttime they grow definitely longer. From the last figure (Figure 5), which represents the circadian periodicity in experiment C_2, it becomes obvious that not even towards the end of this 3-day experiment had an ultimate level of practice been reached. On the contrary, a continual improvement of reaction times, the preceding experiment C_1 included, developed over these 4 days. With sufficient sleep during the first and second night, a clearcut circadian rhythm of reaction-times was demonstrated. During the subsequent final 24 hr during which the subjects were awake again, reaction times remained astoundingly constant, not being prolonged during the nighttime. From this observation, the conclusion may be drawn that by being awake for 24 hr, an individual's performance does not suffer, at least with respect to his reaction time. The depression of the circadian amplitude during the last 24-hr period may arise from an activation of the organism as consequence of the stress to stay awake overnight.

Finally it is noted that where subjects have slept between the short test periods, marked large-amplitude, circadian rhythms in reaction times have become manifest. However, if the subject was awake throughout 24 hr, the diurnal amplitude was considerably shortened, the nocturnal reaction times becoming the same as those recorded in the daytime.

The observed decrement in amplitude during a sleep deprivation period may not be extended to all psychological functions. It could be shown that the amplitude of diurnal rhythms persisted, unaffected as far as acoustic adaptation is concerned, regardless of sleeping or waking during the night. Therefore, it is not possible to generalize from this data that a diurnal periodicity on sleep-waking rhythms exists for all psychomotor functions, not to say of psychological functions. It rather appears that a prolonged waking period causes a dissociation of different functions. Whereas some functions will continue to oscillate with larger amplitudes, the amplitude in some other functions flattens. Possibly this dissociation of different body functions accounts partly for the overall decline of men's performance during nocturnal waking.

4. Summary and Conclusions

In 4 experiments, 47000 reaction times to acoustic and/or different visual stimuli were measured in 24 persons in 2 to 4 hr intervals during normal day/night cycles and during a 24-hr period without sleep. Shortening of reaction time due to learning occurred in the first 24-hr period, and thereafter to a far lesser extent even up to the fourth day. Learning was more significantly increased in response to acoustic than to visual stimuli. A significant circadian periodicity ($p < 0.01$) was observed in experiments with normal day/night cycles; with complex visual stimuli the minimum average reaction-time was 480 msec in the early afternoon, the maximum (560 msec) occurred after midnight. In contrast, when awake continuously for 24 hr, reaction times failed to show any significant diurnal periodicity, and tended to be as short at night as during the day. As far as reaction times are concerned, no immediate danger for task performance seems to arise from a continuous 24-hr awake period.

CIRCADIAN RHYTHM AND PERFORMANCE

M. VAN ZOEREN, L. PANNEKOEK and T. H. H. THIJSSEN

National Aeromedical Center, Soesterberg, The Netherlands

1. Introduction

Fatigue can result from prolonged task performance. It is possible that fatigue is also a function of the time of day the task is performed.

In aviation, both for pilots and for air traffic controllers, it is of paramount importance to quantify fatigue. However, how is fatigue measured? What is it? Is it just a subjective sense of decreased capability or are there measurable psychophysiological and somatic changes which accompany this state and threaten safe piloting and navigation? These changes are the subject of our investigation.

In this study, these investigators were not concerned with the subjective aspect of fatigue but with the measurable psychophysiological effects and their possible correlation with somatic parameters, which closely follow the circadian rhythm. It seemed reasonable to assume that psychophysiological effects would demonstrate themselves in the accuracy, the regularity and the speed with which a task could be performed. A negative correlation will probably obtain between subjective fatigue and task proficiency.

2. Method

In the National Aeromedical Center, much interest has been focused on the so-called 'double task test' as a sensitive indicator of the proficiency of task performance. It was therefore chosen for this study. As the somatic parameter that follows the circadian rhythm, the cortisol concentration of the plasma was chosen. As is well known, this compound follows the diurnal rhythm independently of whether the subject works or relaxes.

The double task test consist of two simultaneous tasks:

(1) The binary choice test. In it high and low pitched tones are presented at varying time-intervals. The left pedal should be pressed in response to a high-pitched tone, whereas a low tone requires right foot activation. Correct and incorrect responses are electronically recorded.

(2) A Bourdon-Wiersma stipple test is the other simultaneously performed task. Errors, omissions and speed with which each single line is scanned are recorded and from it the regularity is computed.

As disturbances of the circadian rhythm are becoming so prevalent in modern aviation, it was felt that a study of fatigue and task performance should not ignore this aspect. In a pilot study it was necessary to refrain from incorporating a time shift in the test program. Thus, in a period of 32 hr (from 16.00 hr on the first day to 24.00 hr on the next day), the double task test was performed by the nine test subjects at

regular 4-hr intervals. Blood samples were taken, at the same intervals for determination of 11-hydroxycorticosteroids (mainly cortisol) and immunoglobulins. The
test subjects were allowed to spend their time as they wished between test periods.

3. Results

The cortisol content of the plasma fluctuated over the test period. This fluctuation
was the same for the 9 subjects, with a coefficient of correlation of 0.50, and was
highly significant ($p < 0.001$). The highest cortisol level was nearly always reached at
08.00 hr (Figure 1).

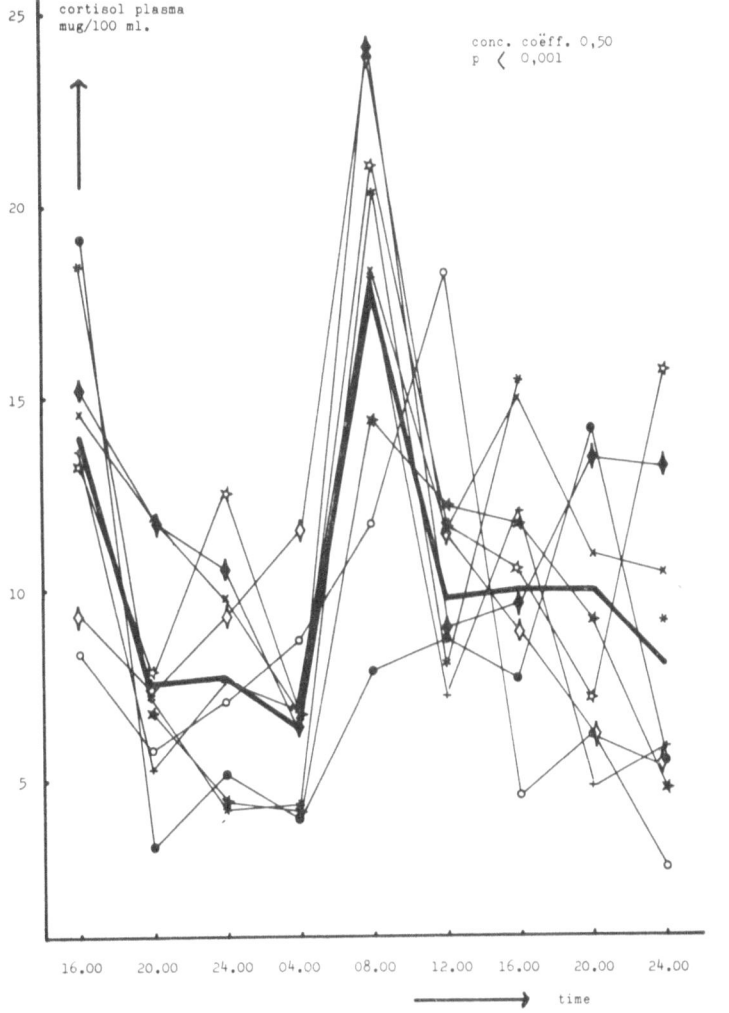

Fig. 1.   The cortisol determinations of each individual test subject, as well as the average of the
9 subjects. The average is represented by a heavy line.

On the binary choice apparatus, the percentage of correct responses showed no fluctuation with time in the 9 test subjects. This would indicate that the test was performed with consistent effort.

The number of omissions in the stipple test decreased with time; this was consistent

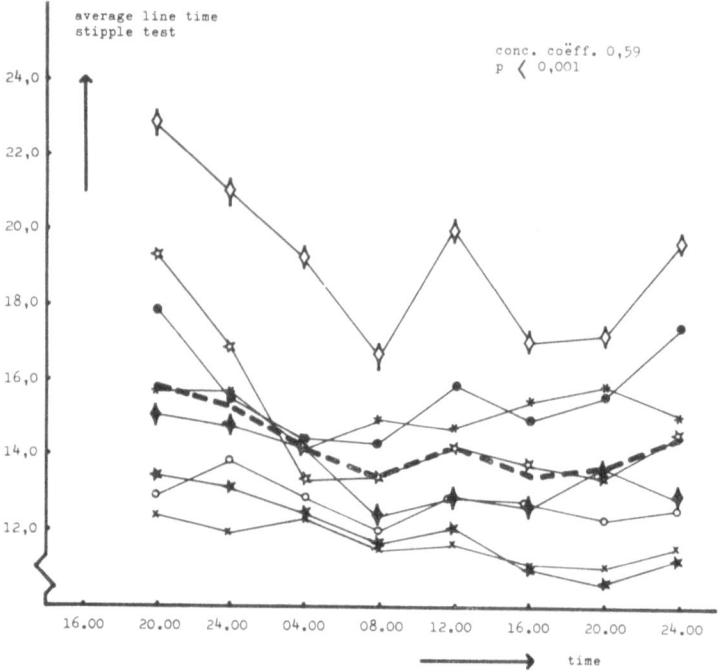

Fig. 2.   The time needed for performing the stipple test, expressed as 'average line time', for each individual and for the group as a whole.

in the 9 test subjects (coefficient of correlation 0.45; $p<0.001$). It is very probable that this is due to a learning effect.

The time needed by the test subjects for the stipple test, expressed as 'average line time', fluctuated with time.

Once again the similarity was highly significant (coefficient of correlation 0.59; $p<0.001$) (Figure 2).

The degree of irregularity with which the stipple test was performed fluctuated with time. Again there was a group consistency (coefficient of correlation 0.37; $0.001 < p<0.01$) (Figure 3).

Finally, it was necessary to determine if a correlation existed between the psychophysiologic and somatic data. This was indeed the case, for cortisol levels and degree of irregularity in performing the stipple test had a negative correlation (product moment correlation coefficient -0.73; $p<0.06$). This correlation was calculated only

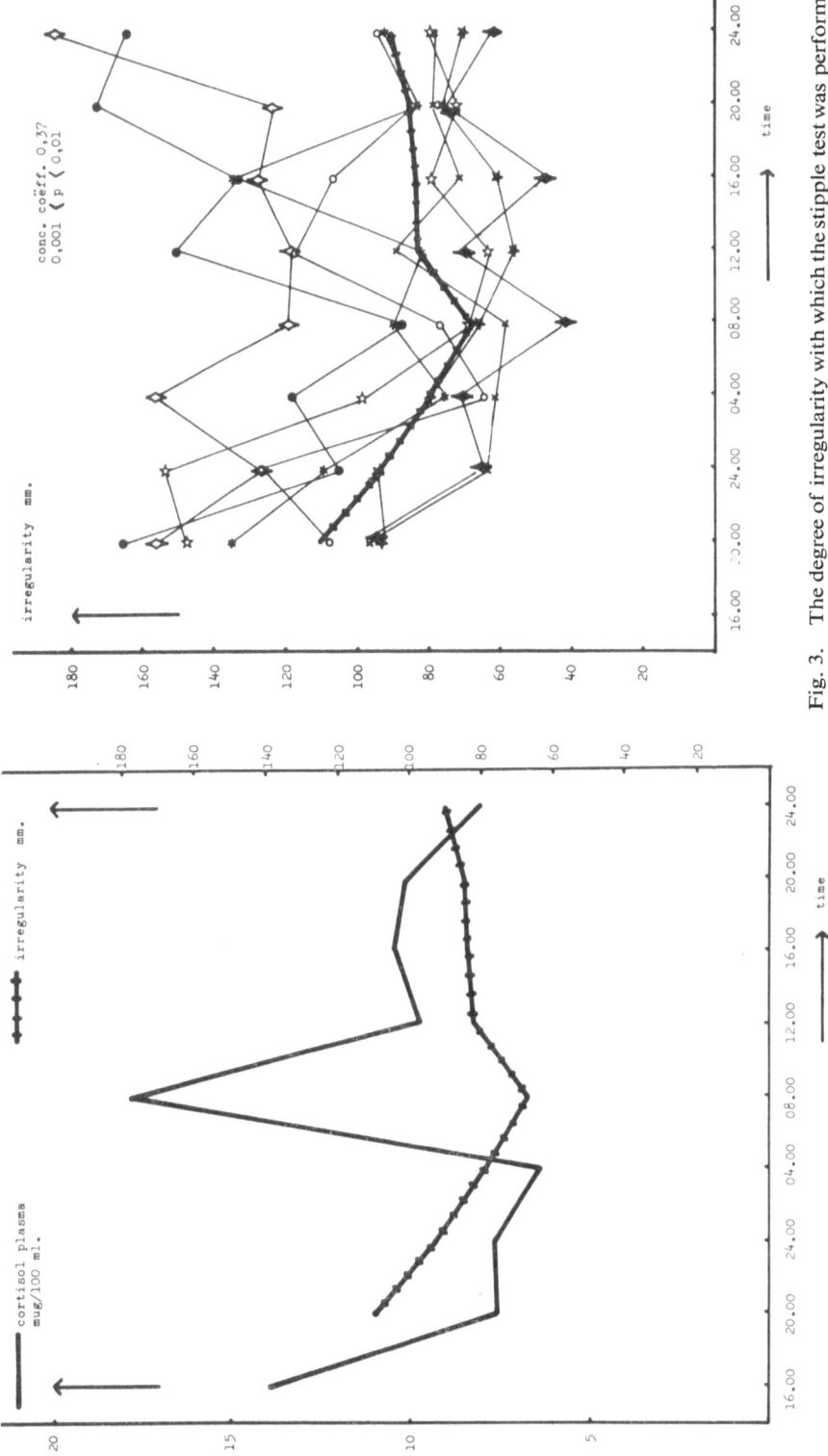

Fig. 3. The degree of irregularity with which the stipple test was performed plotted along the ordinate. It is measured in mm recording tape. The individual values as well as the average of the group are represented.

Fig. 4. Cortisol levels and degree of irregularity in performing the stipple test.

for the last six measurement points. This was done to exclude the learning effect on the stipple test (Figure 4).

It should also be noted that a negative correlation, although of lower significance, also existed between the stipple test time and the cortisol level (product moment correlation coefficient $-0.57; p < 0.10$).

4. Conclusions

In a 32 hr experiment with 9 test subjects, psychophysiologic tests and cortisol determinations were performed at 4-hr intervals. A fluctuation over time was found both in the stipple test and in the cortisol content of the plasma. A negative correlation existed between the degree of irregularity with which the stipple test was performed and the cortisol level in the plasma.

THE URINARY EXCRETION OF HORMONAL METABOLITES

BEFORE, DURING AND AFTER INTERCONTINENTAL FLIGHTS

T. STRENGERS

Clinical Chemistry Department, O.L. Vrouwe Hospital, Amsterdam, The Netherlands, and the
Medical Department, KLM Royal Dutch Airlines, Amsterdam – K. Vaandrager, Head

Gerritzen (1962, 1966), in his studies on the circadian rhythm in kidney function, has stressed the importance of test subjects being investigated under reproducible 'standard' conditions, one of these conditions being the hourly sampling of urine. This condition has made it possible to detect deviations of short duration from the smooth sinusoidal excretion pattern obtained in testsubjects at full rest. This investigator and his associates have found such deviations in the excretion of water, sodium, potassium and 17-ketogenic steroids, thought to be stress-induced, just before and during flights (Gerritzen *et al.*, 1969). From an analysis of this data it was concluded that these findings give strong support to the hypothesis that the pituitary-adrenal cortical system is involved in the maintenance of the homeostatic behaviour of circadian rhythm.

In relation to the main object of these studies, the adaptation of circadian rhythm after time-zone passing flights, the question has been put as to whether or not these effects of stress have any influence on the time of adaptation. In addition to this question, one may also ask if stress experienced during the flight and individual stress susceptibility have a relation to the individual ability to resist the symptoms of time-zone fatigue, these symptoms supposedly being induced by the discongruence of circadian rhythm and local time. The answers to these questions, which are of major importance to air transport operations, need a further evaluation of the role of hormonal activities involved in the maintenance of circadian rhythm in men – in the reactions to stress, as well as in their interrelationship. Therefore, a further differentiation of the steroids excreted in hourly-sampled urines was made in a recent study in which test subjects were flown from Amsterdam to Anchorage and, after a two-week stay, from Anchorage to Tokyo. For this analysis, a recently developed, gas-chromatographic procedure was utilized (Van Kampen and Hoek, 1967; Hoek and Van Kampen, 1968).

In addition to the deviations of short duration in the excretion of 17-ketogenic steroids mentioned above, a very specific abnormality was now found in some test subjects. This abnormality has until now only been found in patients with endocrine disorders. In some test subjects, it lasted for several days, and in others for the whole period of the experiment. It is characterized by a slight elevation in the excretion of etiocholanolone, and an extensive elevation of the total amount of androsterone, androsteendione and dehydroisoandrosterone, these three compounds not being differentiated by the analytical procedure used. There is some evidence that this elevation is a result of increased gonadal activity.

These new findings now give rise to a number of questions. It seems that the somewhat controversial results published in literature on the time of adaptation in part are due to the different conditions under which the experiments were carried out. One main argument, therefore, to study the adaptation time after fast transportation to another time zone under reproducible standard conditions, is the consideration that when studying the influence of a variable, all other possible variables should be eliminated. It appears now that the disturbance of steroid metabolism observed here not only is of rather long duration, but also in some test subjects only arises in the latter periods of the experiment. Therefore, it is possible that the standard conditions themselves have a stressor effect. In view of the great influence of adrenocortical and even of gonadal hormones on all physiological parameters accessible for measurement, this effect could wholly mask the variable being looked for. This consideration is not contradictory to the opinion that adaptation studies should be performed under reproducible conditions, but the experimental design of these conditions seems open for discussion.

An additional problem is related to the postulated influence of stress and stress susceptibility on adaptation time. Such an influence gives a possible explanation of the difference in adaptation time found in test subjects during the former experiment, compared with that of test subjects in the latter experiment. The first subjects were older students. They were very cooperative and interested in the experiment itself. The latter subjects were younger students, who clearly were influenced and occupied with the world-wide unrest at the universities, which also arose in the Netherlands during the period of the experiment. It is concluded that in further experiments cooperation with psychologists is needed. One should mention that the test subject who from the start of the experiment until the very end showed the abnormality of the steroid spectrum was a typical introvert. However, one of the three subjects, who during the whole experiment had a normal urinary steroid spectrum was, even for laymen in psychology, a typical extrovert.

Notwithstanding that the relation between 'time-zone fatigue' and the disturbance of physiological circadian rhythm has been accepted, it cannot be denied that there is a great inter-individual difference in the symptoms experienced after time-zone-passing flights. In addition to the former question, if stress experienced during the flight and individual stress susceptibility influence the time of adaptation, one may also ask as to whether these factors have a relation to the individual ability to resist the aftereffects of the discongruence between circadian rhythm and local time. In this relation, the theory has to be mentioned (Aschoff, 1969) that 'time-zone fatigue' is not the consequence of the discongruence between the circadian rhythm and local time, but of the discongruence in adaptation time of several physiological parameters themselves. Subjects who do not experience such symptoms should be able to adapt their main physiological functions in the same time. Thus this whole problem appears to be a vicious circle. The discongruence of circadian rhythm with local time could decrease physical fitness and stress resistence and increase stress susceptibility. On the other hand, stress experienced and stress susceptibility possibly could retard the adaptation to the local time, respectively promote an internal desynchronization.

In conclusion, attention is called again to the problem which is in discussion – the role of the neurological-hormonal system – in which the steroid hormones are of major importance. The suggestion has been made to suppress the after effect of trans-meridian flights by natural or synthetic steroidal hormones or by compounds which have a direct effect on steroid metabolism. With present day knowledge such medi-cation seems premature and even dangerous. More founded are the recommendations published by the Office of Aviation Medicine of the American Federal Aviation Administration. These recommendations, of which 'rest and sleep' are one of the most physiological features affect the neurological receptors of the system. Indications are that a period of rest before the start of the flight has indeed a direct effect on the time of adaptation, but this preliminary conclusion must be confirmed by the statis-tical evaluation of the results of the last experiment discussed here.

References

Aschoff, J.: 1969, *Aerospace Med.* **40**, 844.
Gerritzen, F.: 1962, *Aerospace Med.* **33**, 697.
Gerritzen, E.: 1966, *Aerospace Med.* **37**, 66.
Gerritzen, E., Strengers, T., and Esser S.: 1969, *Aerospace Med.* **40**, 264.
Hoek, W. and Van Kampen, E. J.: 1968, *C.C.A.* **19**, 371.
Van Kampen, E. J. and Hoek, W.: 1967, *C.C.A.* **16**, 442.

METHODS FOR THE STUDY OF THE BEHAVIOUR
OF HUMAN CIRCADIAN RHYTHMS IN KIDNEY FUNCTION
BEFORE, DURING AND AFTER GLOBAL FLIGHTS

F. GERRITZEN

*Clinical Chemistry Department, O.L. Vrouwe, Hosiptal Amsterdam, The Netherlands,
and the Medical Department, KLM Royal Dutch Airlines, Amsterdam,
K. Vaandrager, Head*

When taking urine volume and the excretion of electrolytes as a parameter of the circadian rhythm, various experimental conditions have to be applied in order to obtain the most reliable and reproducible results. These conditions may be listed as follows:

(1) As diuresis is influenced by water intake, in experiments on rhythmic phenomena in urine volume, the water intake should be kept constant, the most logical method being an hourly supply of equal amounts of water. Apart from this, the most regular excretion pattern is obtained when the water intake is restricted to 30 ml/hr.

(2) Equally important is the constancy of the food intake, as body water may be used for the solution of dry food, thus influencing diuresis, and because water of oxidation may result in an excess of water excretion. Therefore test subjects were given 2 biscuits of known composition every hour.

(3) Collection of urine preferably should be done in intervals of one hour, especially if one wants to know the site of the maximum of the circadian rhythm of the urinary excretion. This is obviously necessary when displacements of the maximum, as an effect of the crossing of time zones, are studied.

(4) Test subjects should maintain the same body position during the entire experiment. This means that they should be kept in lying position.

(5) Though normal persons can empty their bladder completely at hourly intervals, this is not always the case. It is therefore advisable to express urine volume as the reciprocal of creatinine excretion.

If one adheres to these experimental conditions, the average of subjects gives sufficient information to draw conclusions on visual inspection of the graphs. If these conclusions can stand statistical criteria is open for discussion.

Most authors who have worked in this field have used less strict conditions. Part of the present confusion can be explained by this lack of uniformity and reproducibility of the method used when studying urine volume and the excretion of electrolytes as a parameter of the circadian rhythm in the human organism. Moreover, the hourly sampling of the urine has made it possible to detect deviations of the normal excretion pattern. Dr. Strengers, also in this Congress, will deal with the significance of these deviations as to the problem in discussion. It will be pointed out here that part of these deviations probably may be induced by the above mentioned conditions themselves.

*D. E. Busby (ed.), Recent Advances in Aerospace Medicine, 356–358. All Rights Reserved.
Copyright © 1970 by D. Reidel Publishing Company, Dordrecht-Holland.*

In total 6 flights were made:

(1) Amsterdam-New York, *vice versa* – 2 test subjects.
(2) Amsterdam-New York, *vice versa* – 2 test subjects, with immediate return.
(3) London-Johannesburg, *vice versa* – 4 test subjects.
(4) Amsterdam-London   – 5 test subjects.
(5) Amsterdam-Anchorage-Tokyo – 5 test subjects.
(6) Amsterdam-Anchorage-Tokyo – 7 test subjects.

In all flights, the test subjects arrived at their destination with their original maximum of the place of departure. Thus there was a discongruence in flight 1, 2, 5, and 6 between the endogenous rhythm of the test subjects and the local time after the flight. As a matter of fact, no disharmony of this kind was found in flight 3 and 4 (London-Johannesburg, *vice versa*, and Amsterdam-London) where there was no appreciable East-West or West-East displacement.

As it is generally agreed, that this discongruence between the endogenous rhythm of the test persons and the local time might be the cause of symptoms of malaise or fatigue. Therefore, it was attempted in a recent experiment to shorten the period of adaptation.

There are theoretically three methods to suppress the original rhythm:

(1) by preconditioning to the new day-night cycle.
(2) by preconditioning the sleep-wake periods by natural or artificial sleep.
(3) by the application of drugs.

In previous experiments (Gerritzen, 1962, 1966; Gerritzen *et al.*, 1969) an inverse light regimen changed the circadian rhythm in normal subjects. Therefore, before the last flight 4 of the 7 test subjects were exposed to inverse light conditions. However, no difference was found in the adaptation of these four and the three controls. The adaptation of all 7 test subjects proved to be significantly different from the adaptation observed in a former flight. Therefore, this finding is not only not conclusive, but it stresses the importance of the secondary influences on the circadian rhythm, mentioned before and which will be discussed in the paper by Strengers in this Congress.

As to sleep, some authors are of the opinion, that in addition to light, sleep is also a 'Zeitgeber' of the circadian rhythm. However, the author and his collaborators have never seen any influence of sleep, nor on the rhythm itself, nor on the adaptation to a new time zone.

An adequate and effective administration of drugs requires a fundamental knowledge of the mechanisms involved in the maintenance of the rhythm itself, and in its adaptation to other time zones. As long as there are so many gaps in our knowledge, the administration of drugs seems premature.

In conclusion, it may be noted that even though it has been demonstrated that the circadian rhythm persists in continuous light for 48 hr, the question is left open whether or not it would be advisable to guarantee physical and mental fitness of astronauts, to give them a terrestrial light-and-dark cycle, during their stay on the moon for a prolonged period of time.

References

Gerritzen, F.; 1962, *Aerospace Med.* **33**, 697.
Gerritzen, F.: 1966, *Aerospace Med.* **37**, 66.
Gerritzen, F., Strengers, T., and Esser, S.: 1969, *Aerospace Med.* **40**, 264.